ONE REVOLUTION: *Managing the Academic Medical Practice in an Era of Rapid Change*

Contributing Authors:
David J. Bachrach, MBA, FACMPE/FACHE
William R. Beekman, JD
Michael Bowers, MBA, CPA
David Bronson, MD
Ronald Davis, JD, MBA
Rose Ann Frank, MA, FACMPE
Robert B. Jones, MD, PhD
Lindy Kirkpatrick, MBA, MS
Arthur Krohn, MBA, MS, FACMPE
Sara M. Larch, MS, FACMPE
Linda J. Mast, MBA, FACMPE
Anne-Elizabeth McGeary, BSN, MHA
William R. Nicholas, PhD, CMPE
Lee Ann Onder, MBA
Paul Purcell, MBA
Nancy Rhodes, MPH
Judith Roth, MBA
Diana V. Shaw, MPH, MBA
Robert Slaton, EdD, FACMPE
Howard Tepper, MBA, FACMPE
Deborah L. Walker, MBA, FACMPE

Published by:
Medical Group Management Association
104 Inverness Terrace East
Englewood CO 80112
(303) 799-1111

Medical Group Management Association (MGMA) publications are intended to provide current and accurate information and are designed to assist readers in becoming more familiar with the subject matter covered. Such publications are distributed with the understanding the MGMA does not render any legal, accounting or other professional advice that may be construed as specifically applicable to individual situations. No representation or warranties are made concerning the application of legal or other principles discussed by the authors to any specific factual situation, nor is any prediction made concerning how any particular judge, government official or other person will interpret or apply such principles. Special factual situations should be discussed with professional advisors.

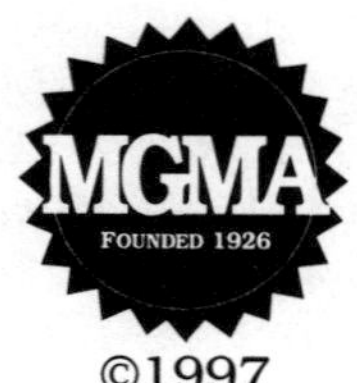

Medical Group Management Association
104 Inverness Terrace East
Englewood CO 80112

ISBN# 1-56829-083-7
Item# 4975

Introduction

Welcome to the world of the academic medical practice and the faculty practice plan. This is not a book that is likely to be picked up by the casual reader looking for an entertaining read on a rainy afternoon. Rather, this is intended to give the administrative and medical practitioner of the art and science of academic medical management and governance a body of knowledge. Within its pages one will discover a unique set of tools that can be used to better practice the craft of academic medical practice management. This text has been assembled by the editors from essays prepared specifically for this purpose by individuals who are actively working in the field; people with first-hand knowledge of the challenges and experience in the tribulations faced each day by the likely reader.

This text begins with three chapters which give the book a degree of comprehensiveness for the readers who have turned to it as their maiden voyage into reading about the world of the academic medical practice. The initial treatise published in 1992, *Managing the Academic Medical Practice: The Two-Headed Eagle*, is a more comprehensive primer, and a proper companion to this text. In the first chapter of this book, we provide readers with a condensed review of the history and development of the academic medical practice as an essential component of the academic medical center. In Chapter Two we look at the essential elements of faculty practice plan governance and update the earlier work with an emphasis on those changes which have occurred during the past five years as these plans have become more thoughtfully and effectively managed. Chapter Three provides the reader with a basic review of medical education and how it has evolved from the 1700s to the present.

This book complements the original text with chapters on the partnership between the physician manager and the practice plan administrator, and looks thoughtfully at the decision-making processes used in academic medical centers as well as the tools of strategic planning and business plan development. Further chapters on measuring productivity and demonstrating value and quality make the discussion on physician compensation all the more relevant in this era of inverse incentives (the less you do, the more you get to keep) found in capitated managed care contracts. Managed care contracting is addressed, as is the market strategy associated with the placement of practice sites at locations convenient to those patients you seek to serve. No longer can we count on patients to travel long distances to enter our health care systems; we must be competitive with the private sector while meeting our academic missions.

As we move from the era of data and information to the knowledge age, we demand that the vast amounts of information be readily accessible, any time/any place, and that it be formatted in a fashion which supports not only patient care and the functions of billing and collection, but also research and teaching. Our academic medical centers and their affiliated teaching hospitals will expend hundreds of millions, if not billions, of dollars in the development and acquisition of software programs, communication networks and necessary hardware for the management and communication of information in the support of physician knowledge. One chapter addresses the challenges of developing and maintaining competitive information systems in this complex environment.

While this has been a period driven by market forces more than regulation, we still find federal policies and state government practices driving what we do, how we do it and how much we are paid for our services for that portion of the population traditionally served by academic medical centers; the poor and the aged. Not the least of our concerns are the Health Care Financing Administration (HCFA) audits of academic physicians. This and other subjects ranging from the basic principles of law and the legislative process, to those structures which uniquely impact health care delivery systems are addressed in a chapter on government regulation. Risk management continues to be an important topic as it represents a major cost element for academic physicians who deal with the most complex illnesses and traumatic injuries while concurrently giving physicians in training the opportunity to learn by example as well as by experience. Thus, this subject has its own chapter.

Finally, the summary chapter looks at the factors driving the entire health care field, with an emphasis on their impact on the academic sector. The reader is provided with a summary of those forces likely to drive change in academic medical groups in the next five years. The author ventures forth with forecasts of how the critical factors which shape and support our academic medical centers will look five years hence. His summary paints a picture of challenges which exceed those of the past ten years as we experience continued market pressures, an apparent mandate to reduce the number of physicians we train, an expectation that we will continue to lead the world in developing diagnostic and therapeutic technologies, and the ambiguity of a nation which wants the best and most accessible health care in the world, but may not be willing to pay for it.

So make yourself comfortable; strap yourself into your seat as we take off on the next leg of our journey, hurtling past the millennium into the next century. Of one thing we can be certain; the future ain't what it used to be!

David J. Bachrach, MBA, FACMPE/FACHE
William R. Nicholas, PhD, CMPE
Editors

August 1997

Foreword

Since its founding in the late 1970s as the University Medical Practice Association, the Academic Practice Assembly has served several important roles in advancing the quality and performance of medical school physician group practices. First, it has served as a forum for those who are engaged in the business of managing these practices. Now with more than 2,000 members, the APA is the second largest of all MGMA Assemblies and accounts for more than 11 percent of all members. Second, from its inception this organization has placed a high value on educating its members through well-designed and professionally delivered annual programs that address fundamental as well as emerging issues facing the academic medical practice. Attendance at these programs has regularly exceeded 700 individuals in recent years. Third, the APA has sponsored or co-sponsored a number of studies of the field of academic group practice administration including annual reports of administrative salaries, academic physician productivity and compensation, and faculty practice benchmarks.

In 1990, a group of APA members, with the support of the MGMA leadership, took on the task of developing a text on academic group practice. Entitled *Managing the Academic Medical Practice: The Two-Headed Eagle*, this 1992 publication represented the first definitive and comprehensive work on the subject. Under the able leadership of William Nicholas, PhD, and with contributions from ten others, this 300-page text covered a range of subjects from the history of academic practice to the rapidly evolving changes in reimbursement. Much of what was presented in that text holds true today and those interested in the field would be well served by including a copy of it among their library of reference books. More than 1800 copies of this text have been purchased by those interested in the field.

One Revolution: Managing the Academic Medical Practice in an Era of Rapid Change takes the study of academic group practice a major step further. It does not restate the basics nor the historical development of these structures, as these were covered well in the first text. Rather, it revisits those topics, such as governance and structure which have evolved substantially over the decade of the

1990s, and introduces important new subjects for consideration by its audience. Under the continued editorial leadership of Bill Nicholas, who was joined by David J. Bachrach as co-editor, this text addresses those factors in the health care environment which are driving changes in the number, size, configuration and governance of our nation's academic medical centers.

The academic medical practice plan has become an essential element in the success of medical schools. Practice income represents virtually 50 percent of all financial resources available to support these institutions which will produce the next generation of our nation's physicians. During a period of stable or declining state and federal support, the faculty practice plan has become the single element which most institutions have been able to utilize to increase available resources. In many cases, these are the most flexible funds allowing deans and chairs the ability to recruit and retain the best faculty; create economic incentives to promote changes in individual and group performance; provide seed money for, if not fund new initiatives in research and education; and often represent the core dollars for construction of medical center-based ambulatory care facilities, offsite care centers, community physician practice acquisitions and even the construction of laboratory research buildings.

Norman A. MacLeod, MSPH
1997-98 Chairperson
MGMA Academic Practice Assembly

Acknowledgments

The editors and authors owe a great deal of thanks to **Alys and Brian Novak**, of Discovery Communications, Inc., and **Mary Wayman Huey**, Denver CO, for their editorial and production assistance. We also appreciate the support of: **Barbara U. Hamilton, MA,** and **Cynthia Kiyotake, MA,** former and current directors of the MGMA Library Resource Center; as well as **Fred Graham, PhD, FACMPE/CAE,** MGMA's former Senior Vice President/Chief Operating Officer, who served as an early supporter of the University Medical Practice Association and the Academic Practice Assembly since their inception and encouraged the preparation of both the present and previous texts.

We are indebted to the leadership of the **Academic Practice Assembl**y for their continuing support of this project with special thanks to its Executive Committee; most notably the current and recent past chairs, **Norman A. MacLeod, W. Robert Wright, Jr.,** and **Stephen A. Valerio.**

And most important, we are indebted to the patience and understanding of our families who have tolerated our assuming yet another responsibility in our already busy lives. For many of us this project has transcended a period of employment transition and family moves, making the fulfillment of this commitment all the more difficult. This is further testament to the turmoil we all face in the field of academic medical practice administration.

David J. Bachrach, MBA, FACMPE/FACHE
William R. Nicholas, PhD, CMPE
Editors

About the contributing authors

Chapter 1

William R. Nicholas, PhD, CMPE, is a professor with a joint appointment in the College of Business and the College of Medicine at the University of Illinois in Chicago. Dr. Nicholas is the Executive Director of the UIC Medical Practice Plan. He earned his MA degree in Administration at Central Michigan University and his PhD in Management and Program Development from Michigan State University. He is a member of the Medical Group Management Association and its Academic Practice Assembly. He is a founding member and past president of the Association of Academic Surgical Administrators. Dr. Nicholas is the immediate past chairperson of the Research Committee for the Center for Research in Ambulatory Health Care Administration. He is a member of the Association of American Medical Colleges Group on Faculty Practice and its Group on Business Affairs. He is also a certified member of the American College of Medical Practice Executives. Dr. Nicholas is a frequent speaker and author on the subject of management in academic practice.

Chapters 2 and 16

David J. Bachrach, MBA, FACMPE/FACHE, is currently Professor of Health Services Management at the University of Texas M.D. Anderson Cancer Center. He served as Executive Vice President for Administration and Finance at M.D. Anderson from January 1989 through October 1996. Mr. Bachrach holds a MBA in Health Services Management and Hospital Administration from the University of Missouri. He is a Fellow in both the American College of Medical Practice Executives and the American College of Healthcare Executives. He has served as an officer of several professional organizations in the health care field, including as the first Chair of the University Medical Practice Administrators (the predecessor of the Academic Practice Assembly) and as a consultant to deans, hospital directors, department chairs, and individual physicians at a number of institutions throughout the country.

Chapter 3

Rose Ann Frank, MA, FACMPE, is the Director of Contract and Government Compliance at Samaritan Health System, Phoenix, AZ, and is a consultant on practice management issues. She earned her MA in Organization Management from the University of Phoenix. Mrs. Frank is a member of the Medical Group Management Association and its Finance Assembly. She is a Fellow in the American College of Medical Practice Executives (ACMPE) and is a member of its Professional Papers' Committee. Mrs. Frank has lectured, published several articles on health care practice management issues, and coauthored *Managed Care Operational Strategies* by St. Anthony's Publishing.

Linda J. Mast, MBA, FACMPE, is Director of Compliance and Reimbursement for the University of Missouri-Columbia, University Physicians. She is a Fellow in the American Association of Medical Practice Executives, and recipient of the President's Award for Research and Education. Linda has been elected to Who's Who of Women Executives and the Pi Lambda Theta honor society for educators, and is a frequently invited speaker at national health care conferences. Publications include: Mast. L. (1997) "Theoretical Framework for Implementing a Managed Care Curriculum for Continuing Medical Education," *American Journal of Managed Care* (3) 1, 68-73; Mast, L. (1997) "Application of the Problem-Based Learning Model for Continuing Professional Education: A Continuing Medical Education Program on Managed Care Issues," *American Journal of Managed Care* (3) 1, 77-82; Mast, L. (1993) "Marketing health care to an aging America," *College Review,* 10(2), 59-77. Linda's education includes: BSN, University of Maryland-Baltimore; MBA, Western New England College; Doctoral Candidate, University of Missouri-Columbia.

Chapter 4

David Bronson, MD, is Chairman of the Division of Regional Medical Practice at the Cleveland Clinic Foundation. He is a graduate of the University of Maine and the University of Vermont College of Medicine. He completed his residency training in Internal Medicine at the University of Wisconsin and the University of Vermont Hospitals. He served on the faculty of the University of Vermont for 15 years where he was Associate Chairman in the Department of Medicine, President of the Medical Staff and Associate Professor of

Medicine. Since 1992, he has held several positions at the Cleveland Clinic including Chairman of the Department of Internal Medicine. He is Clinical Professor of Medicine at the Pennsylvania State University and Associate Professor of Internal Medicine at Ohio State University.

Lee Ann Onder, MBA, is the Administrator for the Departments of General Internal Medicine and Pulmonary & Critical Care Medicine at the Cleveland Clinic Foundation in Cleveland, OH. She has a Bachelor of Arts in Communications and an Executive Master of Business Administration from Cleveland State University. Lee Ann has worked in health care for the past 11 years as an ombudsman at the Cleveland Clinic, Private Patient Coordinator at St. Mary's Hospital in London, England, Quality Assurance Coordinator at Rush-Presbyterian-St. Luke's Medical Center in Chicago, IL, and since then has held administrator positions in four medical departments at the Cleveland Clinic. She is active on most of the clinic's managed care committees and represents both the divisions of medicine and surgery for the managed care operational issues.

Chapter 5

Judith Roth, MBA, is the Associate Director for Administration of the Clinical Cancer Center of the Albert Einstein College of Medicine in New York. While writing this chapter, she was the Administrator of the Department of Anesthesiology of the Columbia Presbyterian Medical Center. Before her 13 years in anesthesiology, Judith held administrative positions in otolaryngology, medicine and psychiatry at Columbia and at Montefiore Medical Center in New York. She was the first editor of the MGMA Anesthesia Assembly newsletter, *Anesthesia Awakenings.* She was appointed the editor of the *APA Matrix,* the newsletter of the Academic Practice Assembly in 1996. She holds an MBA from the New York Institute of Technology and is currently pursuing fellow status in the American College of Medical Practice Executives.

Chapter 6

Michael Bowers, MBA, CPA, is Executive Director of Orthopedic Associates of Dallas, LLP. He received his MBA in organization development and finance and is a certified public accountant. He previously was Administrator of the Surgery Department at the University of Texas Southwestern Medical Center at Dallas. He has published numerous articles, presented at numerous MGMA conferences and educational sessions and worked on the cost accounting task force with CRAHCA.

Robert Slaton, EdD, FACMPE, is the Associate Vice President for Ambulatory Care at the University of Louisville School of Medicine, Louisville, KY. In that capacity he serves as the director of the faculty practice group. Dr. Slaton previously served as Administrator for External Affairs at a large multispecialty group practice. He is also a former Commissioner for Health for the Commonwealth of Kentucky. He holds a faculty appointment in family and community medicine. Dr. Slaton is a frequent speaker on practice management, health care administration, health care reform, and managed care. He earned his degree in Educational Administration at the University of Louisville. He is a Fellow of the American College of Medical Practice Executives. Dr. Slaton has coauthored two books, *From Green Persimmons to Cranky Parrots* and *Caught-in-the-Middle Management.*

Chapter 7

Nancy Rhodes, MPH, is senior administrator, Department of Surgery, University of Pennsylvania Health System. She received her master's of public health in health services administration from Yale University. Ms. Rhodes is a member of the Medical Group Management Association and its Academic Practice Assembly. She also is a member of the Association of Academic Surgical Administrators. She has served as its Education Chair and is currently serving as a Member-at-Large, Eastern Region.

Paul Purcell, MBA, is currently in the Planning and Analysis Group at FHC, Inc., a newly formed Medicaid HMO in Galveston, TX. He is performing business planning and managed care operations analysis in the emerging Medicaid managed care business in Southeast Texas. Previously, he was an analyst with another HMO, PacifiCare of Texas, and a division manager in the Department of Pediatrics at Baylor College of Medicine. He earned a BA from Austin College and an MBA from the University of Houston.

Chapter 8

Ronald Davis, JD, MBA, Attorney at Law, is the Administrative Director of Pediatric Cardiology at the University of Utah and the Administrative Director of Cardiology at Primary Children's Medical Center, a member of the Intermountain Healthcare System, Inc. He is a member of numerous associations, including the Medical Group Management Association and its Academic Practice Assembly and the Healthcare Financial Management Association.

Chapter 9

Sara M. Larch, MS, FACMPE, is the Chief Operating Officer of University Physicians, Inc., the faculty practice plan of the University of Maryland in Baltimore, MD. Ms. Larch has more than 15 years experience in physician practice management in both small and large groups. She is a past national board member of the Medical Group Management Association, past president of the Academic Practice Assembly and the Association of Managers of Gynecology and Obstetrics. She received her MS in Health Sciences Administration from the Medical College of Virginia and is a Fellow in the American College of Medical Practice Executives.

Deborah L. Walker, MBA, FACMPE, is a Principal with BOEHM/WALKER Associates, a management consulting firm specializing in health care and organizational development. Ms. Walker is an accomplished health care executive with more than 18 years experience in academic health care. Prior to entering the field of management consulting, she held management positions in the highly competitive managed care market of Southern California. Ms. Walker earned her MBA degree from UCLA and she is a Fellow of the American College of Medical Practice Executives. She is known for her facilitation skills and ability to institute sustainable administrative improvement in service organizations. In addition to her consulting practice, Ms. Walker is a frequent national speaker on a variety of health care issues including physician incentive compensation and improving productivity and efficiency in medical group practice.

Chapter 10

Lindy Kirkpatrick, MBA, MS, is the Chief Financial Officer for Clinical Affairs for the Indiana University Department of Medicine. She earned her MBA from Old Dominion University and her MS from Virginia Polytechnic Institute and State University. She is a member of the Medical Group Management Association and its Academic Practice Assembly, and the Administrators of Internal Medicine. Mrs. Kirkpatrick is a speaker on physician productivity and practice management.

Robert B. Jones, MD, PhD, is a Professor of Medicine Microbiology and Immunology and Vice Chairman of the Department of Medicine for Clinical Affairs at the Indiana University School of Medicine. Dr. Jones earned his MD and PhD degrees from the University of North Carolina at Chapel Hill with subsequent training in infectious diseases at the University of Washington. He is the former Infectious Diseases Chief at the Indiana University Department of Medicine. He is a member or Fellow in the American College of Physicians, American Medical Association, Infectious Diseases Society of America, Medical Group Management Association and Its Academic Practice Assembly. Dr. Jones is also the Director of the Midwest Sexually Transmitted Diseases Research Center and has been active in restructuring his department's approach to clinical practice.

Chapter 11

Arthur Krohn, MBA, MS, FACMPE, is the Director of Finance and Administration for the University of Virginia Health Services Foundation, a physicians' academic practice plan serving 21 clinical departments consisting of approximately 500 faculty, clinicians and 75 consulting physicians. Mr. Krohn's previous experience includes Vice President of Finance and Administration for Inland Leidy, Inc., a chemical distributor, as well as positions with Exxon Corporation and Price Waterhouse. He received his MBA in accounting from the University of Southern California. Other educational experience includes an MS degree in nuclear engineering from Georgia Tech and a BS degree in chemical engineering from Clarkson University.

Chapter 12

William R. Beekman, JD, is the Acting Chief Operating Officer and Contract Administrator for Michigan State University's MSU HealthTeam, a multispecialty group of more than 200 physicians and other health care providers from the University's colleges of Human (allopathic) Medicine, Osteopathic Medicine and Nursing. In that role, Mr. Beekman drafts, negotiates and monitors for compliance, well over 200 contractual relationships between HealthTeam medical providers and hospitals, health care facilities, clinics, insurance companies, third-party payers, and federal, state and local government agencies. These contracts include both clinical and academic relationships and managed care, fee-for-service and hybrid payment mechanisms. Before coming to Michigan State, Mr. Beekman was an attorney in private practice, specializing in legal issues related to health care and the insurance industry. Mr. Beekman is also an adjunct faculty member at Lansing Community College where he teaches legal research and writing. He received his BA degree from James Madison College at Michigan State University and his JD degree from Wayne State University.

Chapter 13

Howard Tepper, MBA, FACMPE, is the Director of Administration for the Department of Medicine at the University of Medicine and Dentistry of New Jersey, New Jersey Medical School. He holds a BS in accounting and information systems from CUNY Queens College and a MBA from Mount Sinai/Baruch College in health care administration. He is a Diplomate in the American College of Healthcare Executives, a Fellow and Certified Managed Care Professional in the Healthcare Financial Management Association, a Fellow in the American College of Medical Practice Executives, and a member of the Board of Directors of the Administrators in Internal Medicine. He has authored two book chapters on information systems in physician medical practice and is a member of the editorial review board of *Healthcare Financial Management*. Mr. Tepper has taught health care administration and finance courses at the undergraduate, graduate and medical school levels.

Chapter 14

Diana V. Shaw, MPH, MBA, is currently Executive Director of the Department of Obstetrics, Gynecology and Reproductive Biology at Brigham and Women's Hospital, Harvard Medical School, Boston, MA. Ms. Shaw is responsible for all clinical, research and educational activities, including program development, strategic planning, financial management, and human resource management. Prior to her position at Harvard, she was program administrator for the Department of Neurology at the University of Rochester Medical School, Rochester, NY, for nine years. She has been in health care and research administration for more than 15 years, earned a MPH from the University of Rochester and an MBA from St. John Fisher College. Professional activities include memberships in Medical Group Management Association, American College of Healthcare Executives,

Society of Research Administrators, Association of American Medical Colleges Group on Business Affairs, American College of Obstetrics and Gynecology, and American Public Health Association. She is a member of the editorial board of the Journal of the Society of Research Administrators and author of a number of articles. In addition, she has given many presentations, workshops and poster sessions on health care management, ethics and research administration.

Chapter 15

Anne-Elizabeth McGeary, BSN, MHA, is currently the Executive Director of the Integrated Delivery System Partnership between Highmark Blue Cross, Blue Shield and Shadywide Hospital, University of Pittsburgh Medical Center. She has previously held positions as the Executive Administrator for the Department of Obstetrics, Gynecology and Reproductive Sciences, School of Medicine, University of Pittsburgh; as the Assistant Vice President of Ambulatory Care, Allegheny General Hospital; and as the Manager of Risk and Insurance, the Mercy Hospital of Pittsburgh. She obtained her BA from LaRoche College and her MHA from the Graduate School of Public Health, University of Pittsburgh. She is a Diplomate in the American College of Healthcare Executives and a member of MGMA and the Society of Ambulatory Care Professionals.

Table of contents

Table of contents

Table of contents

Chapter 1

The formation of academic medical group practices

by William R. Nicholas, PhD, CMPE

"We had the sky up there, all speckled with stars, and we used to lay on our backs and look up at them and discuss about whether they was made or only just happened."

- From Mark Twain's *The Adventures of Huckleberry Finn*

Just as Huck Finn and Jim drifted down the Mississippi on their raft and wondered about the stars, today people are asking similar questions about the nature of academic medical practices. "Was they made or only just happened?" The answer to this question describes the role, defines the responsibilities and ascribes the authority appropriate to the managers of academic medical practices. If academic practices "just happen," managers should not be expected to lead. Their primary responsibilities would include describing what is occurring, doing things right, speculating on what will next transpire and hoping for the best. In such a circumstance, their role requires little authority. If, on the other hand, academic practices "were made," their managers have an obligation to function as leaders. Executive responsibilities would include interpreting the current state of affairs and deciding on the right thing to do. The resources of the practice would be used to move the enterprise to ever more productive and prominent levels of accomplishment. In this scenario, management authority must exceed the scope of the task. Which is it? Let's go backwards into time to explore this issue.

Medical school as venture

In the 1800s, the typical medical school was a private, for-profit, proprietary venture. Its owners were the attending faculty.[1] It existed as an extension of preexisting medical practices. Abraham Flexner, the famous educator and change agent saw these schools as essentially private ventures, money making in spirit and object. A school that began in October would graduate a class the next spring. Income was simply divided among the lecturers, who reaped a rich harvest besides, through the consultations that the loyalty of their former students threw into their hands. Positions as chairmen or heads of departments were, therefore, valuable pieces of property, their prices varying with what was termed their reflex value. The rivalry between different so-called medical centers was ludicrously bitter. Still more acrid were the local animosities bound to arise in dividing or endeavoring to monopolize the spoils. Sudden and violent feuds thus frequently disrupted the faculties. But a split was rarely fatal: it was more likely to result in one more school."[2] Yet by the 1940s, the typical academic medical practice existed as a minor fiscal extension of its medical school. Just what happened to so radically change the relationship between medical education, academic medical practice and the finances that drive them?

Shortly after the turn of the century, American medical education experienced a radical change. That transformation was triggered, in part, by Dr. Abraham Flexner's comprehensive survey of medical schools. His highly critical findings were published as "Bulletin Number Four" of the Carnegie Foundation for the Advancement of Teaching. Bulletin Number Four altered, for three generations, the relationship between medical schools and their academic medical practices. Now, in the last decade of the 20th century, the academic enterprise is again examining the premise that defines academic medical practice. This reexamination harbors the potential to profoundly change the way in which medical schools relate to their academic medical practices.

The issues currently facing medical schools are reminiscent of the concerns that were raised at the turn of the century. In that era, the stature of American medicine suffered from the unacceptable state of its medical education. A 1901 issue of the *Journal of the American Medical Association*,[3] reported that American medical schools:

- existed far in excess of the public need;
- granted medical degrees to persons with financial ability, however lacking in mental and moral fitness;
- lacked adequate facilities and equipment;
- lacked capital funds;
- had few affiliations with academic centers of scientific and intellectual inquiry;
- were indifferent to curricular reform as their faculty had direct financial stake in the status quo; and
- generally had as instructors men of mediocre or less ability.

While chilling, a similar critique can be made of contemporary medical education:

- The number of graduates, particularly those seeking careers in the specialty fields, appears to exceed the public need;
- The ability to fund one's own education or the willingness to assume significant debt is a key determinant as to which individuals will be granted a medical degree;
- The lack of adequate facilities, equipment and capital funds is a pervasive problem;
- Academic medical centers are behaving more like businesses. This increased emphasis on the financial over the literary marketplace tends to distance the medical faculty from the values and interests of the general academic community. As in 1901, modern medical schools are growing more intellectually estranged from their parent institutions;
- Indifference to curricular reform can still be traced to the faculty's stake in the status quo. Most faculty teach as they were taught. Most faculty accept lower income expectations. In return, they expect an opportunity to earn tenure and with that the freedom of individual action. The protector of intellectual freedom, tenure also allows faculty to exhibit indifference to curricular reform through individual inaction;
- As the traditional sources of funding for research and medical education have plateaued, medical schools have become increasingly reliant on practice-generated revenues. Until quite recently, medical schools offered their faculty secure employment in an environment that valued their contributions to research, education and patient care. Now, the most valued faculty activities are becoming research and patient care. Both of these activities are directly traced to sources of revenue. Should the eclectic appeal of academic careers continue to erode, one might anticipate that more of the brightest and the best would pursue more lucrative careers in the private sectors of medicine and research. Such a trend will leave medical schools with instructors of mediocre or less ability.

Just as when ascending a spiral staircase, one rises relative to its vertical axes; i.e., one will periodically return to the starting point relative its horizontal axes. Over the past nine decades, academic medical centers have advanced on many fronts - only to return to their starting points relative to funding and society's perception of their legitimacy. The relationship between medical education and academic medical practice has again come full turn.

One Revolution: Managing the Academic Medical Practice in an Era of Rapid Change

The Hopkins model

Following the publication of Bulletin Number Four, Abraham Flexner, a graduate of Johns Hopkins in education and the humanities, began to promote a model that the Johns Hopkins School of Medicine had adopted in 1894 for organizing its medical education and patient care services.[4] Flexner argued that bringing medical education and clinical training into universities would bestow a greater legitimacy on medical education. His vision called for an amalgamation of the university's scientific resources with that of its medical school to advance medical research. At Hopkins, unlike the facilities used by most other medical schools, the hospital was owned and managed by the university. This arrangement made the facility exclusively available for the use and the medical administration of the Hopkins faculty.

Flexner felt that the pressure to make money from the delivery of care precluded many medical faculty from pursuing their legitimate role as scientists and intellectuals. He advocated the proposition that residents and students should be taught by a cadre of geographical full-time faculty.[5] Flexner attributed the idea of full-time faculty to Leipzig physiologist Ludwig. Ludwig believed that sooner or later teaching and research in clinical medicine and surgery would have to be organized on the same basis as teaching and research in anatomy and pathology. Both of these disciplines had once been in the hands of practicing physicians, and neither had prospered as they should, until they commanded the full time and strength of the men engaged in their teaching and cultivation.[6] The Hopkins faculty adopted the full-time clinical concept in 1913. At Hopkins it was envisioned that medical practice would exist to provide a laboratory for teaching and research. It would serve to maintain the skills of the attending staff. Medical practice would no longer serve as the engine that drove the finances of the medical school.

At the turn of the century, there was a lot of turmoil in American medical training; 457 medical schools were established in the United States and Canada between 1890 and 1910.[7] Of those schools, 326 closed their doors by 1910. The instability of American medical education was all too evident when on average 3.26 schools went out of business each year. At the time Flexner published his report, 131 medical schools were in operation. During the height of the "Flexnerian Revolution," the rate of medical school closures increased to 4.50 institutions per year. The medical school replacement rate fell to zero. By 1920, the number of American medical schools stood at 85. Between the years 1920 and 1960, the number of medical schools fluctuated very little. In 1961, the total number of American medical schools was 86.[8] One might argue that Flexner's goal of bringing stability and legitimacy to American medical education was accomplished in just one decade. That fact should not be lost on modern medical group managers as revolutionary forces are now reshaping the relationships between their hospitals, their medical schools and their medical practice groups.

Insurance development

During the first half of this century, few employers provided medical insurance benefits to their employees. Much as today, few people felt they could afford to purchase private health insurance. Government programs for the payment of medical services did not exist. In the private sector, patients paid their physicians with cash or they arranged some form of barter. A lack of technical sophistication further contributed to the limited exposure most people had to medical care. Prior to the 1940s, medicine existed in the "pre-antibiotic era." This was a period when the major focus for medical care was either associated with acute trauma, urgent surgery, control of infectious diseases or sanitation.[9] A large portion of society had contact with a doctor or a hospital only when a life was coming into or leaving this world.

The widespread acceptance of prepaid health insurance was a major factor in reshaping the American health system. An early American venture into prepaid insurance took place in Texas in the 1920s in an academic practice setting. Baylor University was experiencing financial difficulties. The top officials of the hospital and the university decided to experiment by enrolling groups of public subscribers for hospital care on a prepayment base. Because the idea fulfilled a need among the teaching staff at the university, in 1929 the Baylor faculty was the first group to sign up as subscribers. The product they created became known as Blue Cross hospitalization coverage.[10]

Early in the 1930s, the American Hospital Association appointed Mr. C. Rufus Rorem as its national consultant on group hospitalization.[11] Rorem developed national standards or "essentials" for Blue Cross plans in 1933. These essentials stressed the quasi-public role of the plans, both as public service agencies organized on a nonprofit basis, and as cooperative local forces designed to avoid competition among hospitals and clashes between hospitals and the medical profession. Approved Blue Cross plans were required to exclude the attending physician's fees. Attending physician fees were to be covered under the Blue Shield plans. They were also required to cover services given by all participating physicians and voluntary hospitals. Voluntary prepayment, as offered by Blue Cross, was endorsed by the board of trustees of the American Hospital Association in 1933. It is interesting to note that none of the initial participants in Blue Cross arrangements wanted the plans to become too successful; that is, to develop an independent power base. Both hospitals and physicians were nervous about the prospect of well-funded, local prepayment associations that might seek powerful organizational alliances with local employers, who even in the 1930s provided the major pool of subscribers.[12]

Modern medical group management

Between 1940 and 1962, science, industry and government championed three unique events which, when combined, laid the foundation for modern medical group management. These events were:

1. The discovery and the use of penicillin, the first commercial antibiotic;
2. The broad acceptance by employers of the concept of purchasing both hospitalization and medical/surgical health insurance for their employees; and
3. The passage of the federal government's Medicare and Medicaid acts.

Penicillin, first of the "miracle drugs," was widely used by the military during World War II. At the end of the war, it became readily available for use by the civilian population. Its impact on physician behavior was enormous. For the first time, doctors could cure rather than simply manage a wide range of infectious diseases. Thanks to penicillin, the general population began to change the way in which they related to the medical establishment. Visits to the doctor for reasons other than acute care became commonplace.

As late as 1940, fewer than one in ten Americans had any hospitalization insurance and fewer than four in a hundred had any surgical or medical protection.[13] During World War II, the federal government placed a freeze on wages. At the same time the worldwide demand for war materials and supplies, insured healthy profits for American industrialists. By 1942, industries were approached by unionized labor with requests to share the wealth. Following complex negotiations, it was agreed that hospitalization and health insurance were benefits that employers could provide their employees in place of increases in their wages. A *Fortune* magazine survey during this period revealed that almost three-fourths of the American public believed that the government should collect enough taxes to provide medical care for all who needed it.[14] By 1965, the federal government enacted Medicare and Medicaid legislation. Medicare insures health care to the elderly. Medicaid insures health care to many of the disadvantaged and the needy. These were two large populations that were left out of the employer-sponsored health insurance programs. Under these programs nonpaying patients, previously classified by academic medical centers as "clinic" or "service" patients, became paying patients entitled to the same treatment as private patients. As the sponsor of these plans, the government became the third-party payer for Medicare and Medicaid patients.

The end of the Second World War saw millions of American veterans, who served in a military that offered full medical coverage, return to civilian life with heightened expectations for access to high quality medical care. Labor-employer health benefit agreements, the baby boom, improved transportation, antibiotics and mass communication changed America's vision for medicine. Policymakers and politicians began to address the belief that America suffered from a distribution problem and a general shortage of doctors. This perception prompted the federal government to take action.

Between 1960 and 1980, the government provided incentives to encourage the development of medical resources with the result that:

- 40 new medical schools opened;
- the number of medical school enrollments doubled; and
- the number of full-time clinical faculty increased from approximately 7,201 to 37,716, and by 1990 that number grew to 59,189.[15]

As the number of medical schools increased, the competition for financial resources became more intense. The result was an attack on all four major sources of funding:

- state appropriations and private endowments;
- tuition and fees;
- research grants and contracts, primarily from the National Institutes of Health; and more recently,
- income from professional services rendered to patients and managed under faculty practice plans.

Of these, the fourth became vital to meet one of Flexner's primary goals. He sought to stabilize medical schools by insuring their fiscal viability.

From the 1950s on, medical schools began to increasingly rely on the patient care revenue-generating potential of their faculty to meet their expenses. The income from professional services has become a very important component in the funding mix that supports medical education. By 1990, on average, 30 percent of medical school revenues resulted from the collection of professional fees.[16]

Faculty practice plans

Practice plans are the management vehicle used to administer academic practice revenue. The Faculty Practice Plan (FPP) is a generic term describing the framework within which clinical practice is conducted by the faculty of a medical school.[17] A practice plan is an organized arrangement for billing, collecting and distributing professional fee income. A practice plan's organizational structure refers to its level of common governance and common management systems. The Association of American Medical Colleges' Liaison Committee on Medical Education recognizes the following categories of practice plan organization:

- Multispecialty groups have a high degree of common governance, one overall governing board, a central administrative and management structure, and pooled income;
- Integrated groups represent a transitional model between federated and multispecialty plans. They may or may not pool income;
- Federated groups share some measure of common governance, a central advisory committee to address issues of common management systems; and
- Departmental groups exist where individual departments are autonomous, no common governance, and there are little or no common management systems.

In 1967, a survey of 84 medical schools reported 22 had operational practice plans.[18] Of the 22 schools with plans, only four had existed as group practices prior to 1945. In 1996, the Association of American Medical Schools reported to its Council of Deans that of 125 medical schools surveyed all but 8 had an organized practice plan. Multispecialty plans accounted for 41 percent of the total. Federated plans were 24 percent. Integrated plans were 15 percent. And, department models were 14 percent of all plans.

The formation of academic medical group practices

While a few faculty practice plans can trace their history back to the late 1920s, the funding of medical education through the fees collected from patient care is an older concept that has found new life in the closing decades of this century. Just as the propriety schools of the 1800s relied on a mix of financial support buttressed by patient fees, today's medical schools are seeking a similar solution to their funding requirements. The successful management of the faculty group practice is every bit as important to the welfare of modern medical schools as state funding, endowments, tuition and fees, and external sources of research support. This emphasis on successful management has led to the development of criteria, objectives and professional support organizations.

In 1968, Clyde T. Hardy, Jr., described nine criteria for faculty practice plans.[19] A quarter of a century later, Hardy's criteria remain relevant and serve as the blueprint for most faculty practice plans. Under Hardy's criteria a faculty practice plan would be or include:

1. All the full-time faculty of the medical school;
2. A subdivision of the medical school, not a part of the teaching hospital and not independent;
3. A separate office for the billing of professional fees;
4. A full-time administrator;
5. A written agreement specifying the uses of the professional earnings;
6. Limits on the time spent on practice;
7. Coordinated clinical practice facilities; and
8. Patients available for teaching and research purposes.

Together with the development of general operating criteria for faculty practice plans, objectives have evolved. These objectives have become increasingly important, as they speak to purposes that surpass making money for the personal benefit of the faculty. Numerous variations exist among medical schools. However, four major thrusts appear in many practice plan governance documents.[20] Practice plans exist to:

- Provide a mechanism for organizing and controlling the practice of medicine that is consistent with the mission of the academic health center;
- Provide a significant source of revenue to support the academic programs of the school of medicine;

- Ensure sufficient numbers of patients for educational and clinical research programs and for meeting the financial needs of the teaching hospital; and
- Provide a vehicle to recruit and retain high-quality faculty members.

As academic medical group practices took shape, nationally recognized organizations began to address the specific concerns of the academic medical group managers. The Medical Group Management Association organized its Academic Practice Assembly (APA). In 1976, the APA held its first annual education conferences. The Association of American Medical Colleges formed a Group on Faculty Practice in 1988. These professional organizations have provided a means for managers to share insights and expand the body of knowledge associated with their field.

It has been suggested that the 1970s were the golden years for American medical education and that the 1980s were the golden age for academic clinical practice. During this period the numbers of medical schools had again stabilized and their clinical practices became more visible, more organized, more successful and more necessary to ensure the salary support for the majority of the faculty.

New challenges

In the decade of the 1990s, academic medical centers and their faculty group practices are beset by new challenges:

- During the 1980s, "cost plus" compensation for hospital care became a thing of the past. Stringent diagnostically related group compensation standards (DRGs) became the method used by third-party payers to determine reimbursements to hospitals. The subsequent reduction in hospital reimbursements has diminished the operating margins of many academic medical centers;
- Managed care, with its risk sharing of the compensation pools and its "gatekeeper" approach to referrals, has altered the way in which primary care providers and specialists interact. Further, as academic provider groups accept the full risk for managing the care of a defined patient panel, the group can find itself negotiating with its own teaching hospital related to the assignment of the component parts of the global reimbursement cap;
- Increased costs of operation, the influence of organized labor, the servicing of wage and benefit packages designed in more affluent times, the cost of technology and facility maintenance and

expansion all challenge the fiscal viability of academic group practices; and

- Academic medical groups are trying to cope with the ramifications of the information age. Electronic information management systems require highly trained and well-paid technical and service staffs. These systems call for sophisticated hardware, software and facilities. Infrastructure development places another draw on the limited capital available to most practice groups.

As the academic medical centers debate how to pay for the administrative and technical services needed to manage a group practice, the faculty see a potential drain on the funds available for provider compensation. The question is often asked, "Who will pay for a new administrative service, the dean, the hospital or the practice?" To be successful in the remainder of this decade, practice managers will have to provide value-added answers for their faculty. At the same time they will have to find a way to balance the traditional administrative prerogatives of the dean and the department heads with the management requirements of group practice.

Some of the issues that will alter the current balance of administrative power and prerogative include:

- The concept of enterprise-wide budgeting and cost accounting;
- Centralization of contracting and risk assignment related to managed care services; and
- Defining, directing, measuring and rewarding clinical productivity.

While addressing these issues, academic group managers must remain sensitive to the fiscal anxiety of their parent institution. University administrators are becoming increasingly aware of the potential for the academic health center to place the fiscal viability of the larger institution in jeopardy. The levels of anxiety are fueled by the national debate over health care costs, the apparent surplus of physicians, and the increased competitiveness in the health care industry. The federal government's aggressive stance on Medicare fraud and the financial penalties that can be imposed have given universities further cause for concern.

Just as at the start of this century, medical schools are striving to redefine their place in American society. Funding, legitimacy and the need for additional physicians are all matters of intense debate. Faced with boundless challenge and endless opportunity, academic medical centers and their faculty practices are brought back to a fundamental question, "Were they made or only just happened?" The answer to this question should become clear as one considers the rest of this text. Already the reader may begin to see that academic medical practice just didn't happen. Academic practices are being made and remade by people of vision and purpose. There is a universal acceptance of the faculty's need to practice, yet the optimal governance and operational relationships of academic practice are still in question. The task of seeking a proper balance between academic and practice governance calls for managers who are visionary and adaptable people, endowed with a high tolerance for ambiguity.

When Dr. Flexner sought to improve and legitimize American medical schools, he built bridges between practice and education. Academic group practices should remember that their legitimacy is tied to the educational and research missions of their medical schools. It is that foundation which provides the stability necessary for academic groups to continually remake themselves and remain viable in the complex and capricious arena of American health care.

References

1. Cunningham, E.R., "A short review of the development of medical education and schools of medicine," Ann. Med. Hist. (N.S.), 7:228, 1935, quoted in James Bordley III, MD, and A. McGeher Harvey, MD, *Two Centuries of American Medicine: 1776-1976* (W.B. Saunders Co., 1976), 13-16.
2. *Abraham Flexner: An Autobiography.* New York: Simon and Schuster, 1960, 77-78.
3. Philbrick, I., 1901, "Medical Colleges and Professional Standards," Journal of the American Medical Association, 36, 1700-1702.
4. Nicholas, William R., ed., *Managing the Academic Medical Practice: the Two-Headed Eagle.* Medical Group Management Association, 1992, 13.
5. Flexner, op cit, 115.
6. Ibid, 112.
7. Nicholas, op cit, 13.
8. AAMC, LCME Annual Questionnaire, Part 2.
9. Lyons, Albert S., MD, and R. Joseph Petrucelli, II, MD, *Medicine: An Illustrated History* (Harry N. Abrams, Inc., New York, 1978), 56.
10. Sloan, Raymond P., *This Hospital Business of Ours* (G.P. Putnam's Sons, 1952), 139.
11. Stevens, Rosemary, *In Sickness and In Wealth* (Basic Books, Inc., 1989), 189-90.
12. Ibid, 191.
13. Knowles, John H., MD, ed, Hospitals, *Doctors and The Public Interest* (The Harvard University Press, 1965), 171.
14. "In the Public Mind," The Fortune Survey, vol. 26, no. 1, July 1942.
15. The Association of American Medical Schools, AAMC Data Book, January 1991.
16. Nicholas, op cit, 34.
17. Ibid.
18. Hardy, C.T., "Group Practice by Medical School Faculty," *Journal of Medical Education*, 1968, 43:907-11.
19. Ibid.
20. Nicholas, op cit, 32.

Chapter 2

Governance of faculty practice plans

by David J. Bachrach, MBA, FACMPE/FACHE

". . . the only legitimate right to govern is an express grant of power from the governed"

- William Henry Harrison, Inaugural Address, March 4, 1841

Governance comprises the exercise of authority, direction and control. A well-articulated governance structure, although periodically re-evaluated to ensure that it is meeting the organization's needs, does not generally change from year to year. However, the era of dramatic change in health care experienced during the first half of the 1990s has resulted in far more substantial change in the governance of faculty practice plans (FPP) than was recorded over the previous 25 years. Such changes, as driven by shifts in the external environment which have lead to reduced patient care revenue to support academic medical centers, will likely drive fundamental changes in the organization not just in its governance. The governance structure must adapt to best meet the needs of the organization in its current and evolving form.

During the 1990s, we have seen emerge a closer relationship between FFPs and their related teaching hospitals; the development of academic medical center-driven integrated delivery systems; community physician practice acquisitions by academic medical centers to build the primary care feeder network; and practice plan-owned health insurance plans and business ventures once thought strictly the purview of the private sector. Such dramatic change in structure has resulted in an even more significant change in the governance of some FFPs; possibly a trend which will affect most practice plans by the end of this century.

The purpose of this chapter is to explore the governance structure of FFPs and to emphasize the importance of effective governance to the plan's success. Supplementing the basis of governance which appeared in an earlier rendition on this topic, this work will reflect the significance of change which is occurring in academic medical centers during this era of rapid evolution in American health care.

The principles of governance

The principles of governance have not been altered by the changes in the environment. The governing body of the FFP serves the plan best by focusing on matters of principle and policy, leaving the execution of business practices, procedures and routine operations decisions to professional and physician management. The governing board must respond to the strategic, programmatic, financial and marketing plans developed by management in concert with members and leaders of the FFP. As is the tradition, the responsibilities of the plan's governing body should include selection, evaluation and compensation of the plan's management personnel, including an increasing number of physician executives committed to management roles within the practice plan.

For those practice plans operating within the traditional university/medical school setting, of which there are still many, the governing body may serve as an advisory group rather than a policy-making body. In such cases, the governance system within the FFP is more akin to an oversight body for management. A true governing board has full legal authority to make a wide range of final decisions concerning the distribution of capital, acquisition of debt, determination of programs, selection of markets and geographic location of delivery sites, building expansion and other matters. FFPs tend to operate within a set of circumscribed parameters dictated by the higher governance structure of the parent institution. This is generally a board of regents or board of trustees whose purview is the entire university.

In some cases, the parent institution's board of trustees is responsible for a number of academic and health-related campuses involving several practice plans, teaching hospitals and medical schools (e.g. the University of Texas, with its four medical schools, three teaching hospitals and six FFPs; and the University of California system, with its five medical schools, FFPs and teaching hospitals). The responsibilities of the FFP's governing body under such circumstances are often well circumscribed and rarely have the breadth of authority found in the governing body of a free-standing plan or private medical group practice. Today the traditional academic medical center structures are under intense review. For example, the University of California System is exploring a divestiture strategy for its teaching hospitals in recognition of the challenges faced by a public institution operating hospitals in today's health care environment.

Such changes will surely impact their faculty practices which are an integral part of their health care delivery systems.

The practice plans which are now operating outside the corporate confines of the parent university must have governing boards which assume full fiduciary responsibility. In institutions that are strictly health-related (e.g., the University of California - San Francisco, the Thomas Jefferson University and the Medical University of South Carolina), the medical school, FFP and the teaching hospital often account for 80 percent or more of the institution with the other health-related schools making up the balance.

Although this chapter refers to the parent body of the traditional FFP as the "medical school," some plans exist within organizations other than medical schools, per se. These organizations include medical school-affiliated teaching hospitals with full-time medical staffs, such as the Henry Ford Health Care Corporation, and a few unique institutions such as the University of Texas M. D. Anderson Cancer Center. This center which, although not a medical school, trains nearly 2,000 physicians, scientists and allied health students at the graduate, postgraduate and undergraduate levels each year and maintains a $120-million per year research institute; funded in part from the margins from patient care.

The increasing pace of change in the 1990s

"The future ain't what it used to be," said the great American past time's philosopher Yogi Berra. While an oxymoron, it reflects the sense many have expressed about what is happening today at academic medical centers as they are buffeted by changes in the field of health care. The range and pace of change is dramatically different today than was experienced by these institutions in the 1980s. Many of the issues FFP governing boards now face are different than in 1990. While a chapter on faculty plan governance penned in the early 1990s by this author spoke to evolutionary change, a review of practice plans since then shows a much more rapid rate of change which more closely approaches "revolutionary"; at least in contrast to what we often think of as the traditional "glacial" pace of change at academic medical centers.

During mid-1996, an inquiry was made of several FFP administrators and consultants who work closely with these plans to determine where and how these changes have occurred.[1] The questions were:

- Recall your FFP governing board's "typical" agenda in 1990, and compare it to your "typical" agenda today. How do they differ?;
- How has the composition of your FFP board changed?;
- How has the role of the medical school dean changed in the governance of the FFP?; and
- How does FFP income, as a percentage of total medical school revenue, compare today to 1990?

Their answers are clear; the focus of FFP agendas has clearly changed. Issues which were important before are still important, but less so in relationship to emerging issues. The board is much more active today and members are committing far more time and effort to the deliberation of organizational, relationship and market issues. The focus is more external than internal. Yesterday's allies are today's competitors, and vice versa as affiliated teaching hospitals are merged into health systems or snapped up by for-profit hospital corporations. Figure 2.1 shows a non-scientific comparison of typical agendas as offered by the survey respondents.

Figure 2.1

Typical faculty practice plan governing board agenda Comparing 1990 to 1996

1990	1996

• Compensation plans
• Malpractice insurance
• Billing and collection systems
• Dealing with HMOs
• Affiliated / university-owned teaching hospital relationships
• Practice revenue growth and productivity
• HCFA / IL372 Compliance
	• Management of clinical activities including efficient utilization of resources; cost management
	• Patient service quality
	• Multidisciplinary care centers
	• Clinical practitioners
	  • Medical center-based
	  • Community-based
	• Clinical information systems
	• Integrated delivery system relationships
	  • Regional PHOs
	• Joint ventures with affiliated hospitals
	• Managed care plans
	  • Ownership / capitalization
	  • Joint ventures with other providers and / or insurers
	  • Risk contract management
	  • Delivery system (community physician practice acquisition) management
	  • Mergers, acquisitions and affiliations
	• Long range strategic planning
	• Near term tactical planning
	• Marketing and advertising
	• Reengineering for cost management and survival
	• HCFA / IL-372 compliance / PATH audits
	• Subsidization of clinical and basic research, the capital needs of the medical school and related fiscal issues

We more frequently find cases of financial integration of the FFP with the primary affiliated teaching hospital, creating a "Clinical Delivery System" with a merged governing board. This has occurred at the University of Vermont and is underway at the University of Michigan. The University of Texas M. D. Anderson Cancer Center has created a single billing and collection process for both efficiency and better patient service, and a merged subcommittee to oversee patient business services. The University of Colorado has created a forum made up of the senior executives of the medical school and hospital. Chaired by the chancellor, this body is committing its time and energy to strategies and tactics to position the medical center for success. They have decided not to spend time sorting out merged governance issues and the consolidation of assets, but rather are focusing their energies on those external factors which are threatening their mutual survival.

Practice plan boards are, with increasing frequency, bringing to their membership affiliated hospital CEOs or chief medical officers; and some have one or more members representing their acquired community practices. The ownership interest in health insurance plans may result in "community representatives" on the more broadly integrated board. With the increasing importance of an effective primary care delivery system to support the often specialty-dominated academic medical center-based FFP, primary care representation on the board is increasing.

We now often find a physician executive, other than the dean or associate dean for clinical affairs (or even medical director/physician-in-chief of the primary affiliated teaching hospital), with a near full-time commitment to practice plan management. This individual is partnered with the practice plan's executive director and together they address complex management issues. The academic preparation of these individuals is often different than it was less than a decade ago; many are dually prepared in medicine and business, health care administration or law. For example, the University of Texas M. D. Anderson Cancer Center recently expanded the role of the individual in this position from 25 to 75 percent time and, in recruiting a new individual to this role, found itself with a candidate pool of 19. Of the six internal candidates, five held both the MD and MBA degree. Of the 13 external candidates, four were MD/MBAs and three were MD/MPA prepared. An internal candidate, with an MD/MBA, was selected.

Medical school deans are still held accountable for the fiscal integration of their medical schools, and FFP income has retained its place as the single leading source of support in most medical schools. Given the broadening scope of practice management and the role of integrated delivery systems, the deans of tomorrow (and many today) may further delegate their traditional academic roles to associates and be selected for their ability to effectively lead and manage these complex medical/business structures. There are examples now where deans have moved into the position of leader of the entire health care delivery system, such as at Fletcher Allen Health Care at the University of Vermont. The regents at the University of Michigan have affirmed their intent to recruit to the new position of executive vice president for medical affairs. This physician will lead the medical center and both the dean of the medical school and the hospital director will report to this position. One thing is assured, we are seeing the pace of change increase markedly in the second half of the 1990s.

Governance structure considerations

Virtually all of the structures described in this chapter are found in both public and private medical schools. During the 1980s, a number of publicly supported medical schools adopted FFP structures that more closely paralleled those previously found only in private medical schools. This trend toward shifting the practice plan into a separate, not-for-profit entity was driven by factors such as:

- statutory limits on physician compensation;
- public disclosure of salaries;
- adherence to untimely and non-competitive state employment practices for non-faculty staff members;
- burdensome and inefficient purchasing practices;
- limited access to outside capital for program expansion and facility construction;
- the need to limit the impact of professional liability claims on the parent institution;
- timeliness in decision-making;
- the desire to protect accumulated assets from sequestration by higher level public-sector authorities;
- changes in Medicare reimbursement procedures under consideration at the federal level which would have adversely affected publicly supported academic medical groups had they been implemented;
- an ability or willingness to assume risk under increasingly common capitated contracts for services; and
- an inordinate amount of time required of the parent institution's board to address complex issues facing their health components.

Among the public institutions that changed their practice plans to private, not-for-profit, separate legal entities were the University of Arizona, the University of Cincinnati, the University of Colorado, the University of Florida, the University of Maryland and the University of West Virginia. More long-standing examples include the University of

Alabama, the University of Virginia, the Medical College of Virginia and the University of Washington. Often concurrent with these changes was a decision to change the university-owned teaching hospital to a parallel, not-for-profit entity.

In recent years the need for capital, coupled with the pursuit of efficient management systems, has led some public and private universities to explore relationships with the for-profit hospital sector. While not all of these explorations produced contracts or sales, several did. The Medical University of South Carolina and Tulane are two examples of universities selling their previously owned teaching hospitals. Such new arrangements will surely impact the related FFP.

Other institutions, such as the University of Michigan, considered the concept. Michigan's Board of Regents, however, elected to increase the flexibility with which the FFP and the university hospital were administered, rather than forfeit control of these substantial economic assets. The consent to greater flexibility may have been more readily achieved at Michigan than would be possible at some other publicly supported institutions because the University of Michigan has operated as a constitutional entity with its own publicly elected officials, independent from direct control by the state's legislature. This structure is now being challenged by the state's governor and this, along with factors related to the size, complexity and risk of operating a $1-billion health care system has resulted in a study of options which may include the movement of this enterprise from the University into a separate but not totally uncontrolled structure as has been the case at some other previously state-owned hospitals which now operate as public authorities.

During the 1990s, the rate and degree of change have been far more dramatic. While occasionally found earlier, the following factors appear with greater frequency today:

- Practice plans have developed a substantial presence beyond the traditional boundaries of their academic medical center campuses through the acquisition of community physician primary care practices or the placement of specialists in community-based clinics with admitting privileges to community, non-teaching hospitals;
- Practice plans have taken an equity interest in managed care health plans, often assuming risk in capitated models. Capital contributions to establish those plans often run to the millions of dollars;

- Relationships with their primary teaching hospital(s) have driven practice plans into integrated clinical delivery systems, sharing risk, resources and often governance; and
- Faculty with clinical-track appointments are receiving greater status within the academic community because of the essential role they play in meeting contractual commitments to clinical service agreements. This permits the more traditionally oriented faculty member time to meet their teaching obligations and engage in clinical and basic laboratory research. Of course, we still find examples of the "triple threat" faculty member who is able to "do it all."

The above notwithstanding, the following factors are important in defining the governance structure of a FFP:

- The structure should be consistent with (even if separate from) that which is used in decision-making related to other policies and resource-allocation mechanisms of the medical school. Because the FFP is such an integral part of the operation and success of the medical school, its activities, priorities and resource-allocation mechanisms must not conflict with those of its parent institution. This is increasingly difficult in the competitive world of managed care and competition for patient market share;
- The board designated to govern the practice plan should include individuals who make policy and resource-allocation decisions for other components of the medical school. Although practice plans may have been originally created to nurture the income needs of the faculty, virtually all plans have evolved as an increasingly important mechanism for financing and managing the medical school. While the "dean's tax" may have previously represented the limit of the practice plan's financial contribution to the academic mission of the school, practice plans are increasingly being looked to as a principal source of funds. In some schools, practice plan income represents the single largest source of the funds that support the institution's activities, and in virtually every case contributes substantially to faculty salary support;
- Responsibility for the capital and operating costs associated with ambulatory care, including physician practice acquisition and capital investment in offsite facilities, often falls within the purview of the FFP. This situation gives the governance board broader responsibility, often including the authorization of debt and the investment of resources;

- Management of the clinical faculty's retirement portfolio may also be a responsibility of the governing board. Academic physicians often trade off near-term earnings for better structured and more robust retirement plans than are found outside the academic community;
- Although the governing body rarely gets involved in setting individual salaries, guidelines for the faculty's annual salary program, especially incentive distributions, are often a function of a subcommittee of the board. With economic credentialing and increased pressure to control the utilization of resources within increasingly rigid guidelines, the governing board is likely to look at this as an essential means of preserving the plan's solvency. Fringe benefits, an important component of the compensation package, are also a topic of consideration by the board; and
- The board may also establish a mechanism for awarding internal grants of FFP funds for such programmatic activities as physician and scientist trainee stipends, and support of clinical and basic research.

Centralized and decentralized FFPs and their impact on governance

Departmental plans are fewer in number as pressure for economies of scale and interdisciplinary care inherent in efficient patient treatment drive institutions toward more centralized structures. They do, however, continue to exist. The mechanisms used to direct a fully decentralized practice plan involve a governance system at the departmental level; assuming that the department is the decentralized unit. This system is usually coupled with some sort of interdepartmental governance structure to facilitate the coordination of the institution's clinical activities. The structure may range from a loose confederation to an integrated system assigned certain well-defined responsibilities and authorities. In a decentralized structure, the governance bodies of the departmental entities sometimes take on rights analogous to those of "states," whereas the overlying governance assumes the responsibilities of a "federal" bureaucracy. The delineation of authority and responsibility between these two layers of governance permits them to operate in relative harmony. There is no easy way to describe governance structures at those institutions with decentralized plans as all are unique unto themselves.

A centralized structure is intended to provide a balanced view of all FFP activities within the school, drawing on the contributions made by each of the operational entities (e.g., the clinical departments). Members of this type of governing board should be expected to "put on their institutional hats" when serving in this capacity, rather than representing parochial departmental interests.

It is hard to imagine how an academic medical center could operate effectively if each clinical department attempted to separately and independently negotiate its own managed care contracts. Institutions such as the University of Minnesota, which had a long-standing tradition of strong departmentalized practice plans with their own governance structures, recognized the need for an umbrella organization in which each of the departmentalized plans participated. In setting up the Minnesota Clinical Associates, P.A. in the early 1980s, it was the institution's intent that the executive director of this entity would negotiate on behalf of all departmental plans with third parties and managed care providers in Minneapolis; a city known to be the seedbed of managed care. Still, this institution was slow to respond to such change and during the early 1990s several of the clinical specialty departments moved outside the confines of the University to community hospitals. During 1996, Minnesota embarked on a radically different plan. It sold a significantly downsized hospital to Fairview Health Systems and the medical school will concentrate on medical education and research. Fairview, which will operate an open staff hospital including the medical school faculty and community physicians, will concentrate on efficient health care delivery at the University Hospital and the other clinical sites. This may be a structure followed by other academic health centers which find that they can no longer carry out their multiple functions in traditional structures.

The University of California - San Francisco developed a similar structure during the 1980s although its practices are no longer separate corporate entities. In the first half of 1997, the regents of the University of California are moving toward the merger of UCSF's Moffitt Hospital with Stanford University Hospital into a separate, not-for-profit corporation which will operate both facilities. While at present it appears that the two FFPs will remain separate, it is likely that there will be a coordination of efforts and the sharing of systems design and development between these two large practice plans as they pursue survival in an increasingly competitive health care environment.

Shifts from decentralized to centralized practice plans will precipitate additional changes and refinements in the governance models. The following section speaks to the governance structure as if all plans are centralized. The models described can be largely applied at the departmental level for the few places which will continue to utilize this structure in the future.

The governing board

Figure 2.2 is a decision matrix that provides a format for: constructing a board; choosing who may serve on the governing board; deciding by what mechanism they are selected; and determining how long they may serve.

Figure 2.2

Faculty practice plan governance committee

Potential Governance Participation	Members						
	Chair	Ex-officio		Selected / Appointed		Elected	
		w/vote	w/o vote	permanent	rotating	length of term(s)	right of succession
Medical school dean							
Associate dean for clinical affairs							
Executive director of faculty practice plan							
Medical schoolís director of administration and finance							
Medical director for managed care and/or administrative director							
Hospital administrator or CFO Hospitalís physician-in-chief or chief of clinical affairs							
Department chair							
Department vice chair for clinical affairs							
Members of the clinical faculty							
Member of the clinical track faculty and/or community physician employed by practice plan							
Members of the basic science/research faculty							
Vice president/chancellor for health affairs							
Vice president for academic affairs/provost and/or vice president/chancellor for business affairs							
Member, board of regents/trustees							

The role of the board's chair is to "set the agenda" for the plan in the greatest sense, but also the agenda for the board meetings, and to advance the decision-making process. The chair controls the agenda and may use this authority in a benevolent or in a totalitarian fashion. Even within our rapidly changing health care environment, most universities still hold the deans of each of their several colleges accountable for the overall performance of that college, including its financial solvency. Therefore, it would be problematic for the dean of the medical school not to either serve as the chair or control the appointment of the chair of the FFP's governing board. Furthermore, if the authority and responsibility delegated to the dean is to be maintained, the dean must be able to directly or indirectly appoint the majority of the board's members.

Although there are examples to the contrary, the most effective governance structures may be those in which the governing board serves as advisory, rather than directive. In such models, the dean looks to the board for the initiation or confirmation of policies relating to the FFPs. As reflected in the quotation beginning this chapter, a dean who wishes to survive generally maintains harmony with the practice plan board. The dean who operates with a board that, either by the incumbent's own determination or the determination of prior leaders, has an authority greater than his or her own, is occasionally placed in the position of having to challenge the authority of the board, or have his or her own authority challenged. For the past 30 years dissent over FFP issues has probably disenfranchised deans from their faculty members more frequently than any other single element of medical school operations. This problem occurred with great frequency in the 1970s when many practice plans were first being formed from cohorts of geographic and strict full-time faculty, and it is still true today. While changes during the 1980s appeared to be more evolutionary than revolutionary, the speed and degree of change in the 1990s, and the ability to sustain faculty salary levels, depend on a financially successful practice plan. This means that deans are expected to lead their institutions through turbulent times or risk votes of "no confidence" from those they lead.

A FFP governance structure in which the dean is not in a position of control is likely at some point to confront the authority of the dean in an unpleasant fashion. Plans which have evolved into separate legal entities usually have governance structures under which the dean, as chair, and a majority of the members, serve *ex officio*.[2] The dean has the prerogative to appoint and remove members, either directly, or *ex officio*, by removing the individual from the appointed medical school position that led to membership on the board. The board of regents and/or university officers indirectly control the plan under this governance structure by controlling the appointment of the dean.

Physicians who go into academic practice usually share certain characteristics. Although most forego considerable personal income to contribute to the academic institution's mission, few are willing to ignore the need for an effectively managed plan if they are to assure continued income and a proper retirement plan. Further, they will want to assure the proper distribution of resources in support of their own and the institution's priorities of patient care, research and teaching. Not every member of the faculty wants to be involved in governance, but many do. Most likely, the chairs of the clinical departments will insist on being involved in the governance system. Possibly because of the size of their departments and their significant dependence on the practice plan for programmatic support, the chairs of medicine and surgery often play key leadership roles on the governance board of the FFP. While others may be elected or appointed, their membership on the board is often *ex officio* and includes the right to vote.

The size of the governing board should be established to meet the following objectives:

- Includes the essential decision-makers and linkage to related organizations;
- Assures a broad representation of the faculty;
- If members serve terms of a defined length, assures sufficient consistency in board philosophy by staggering the terms of service so as to allow turnover without a loss of continuity;
- Assures that the board is large enough for the workload to be distributed among its members;
- Limits board size to assume that the body can effectively function; and
- Uses subcommittees, where appropriate, to support the board. Subcommittees may include off-board members for greater representation and to groom individuals for future board service.

Although selecting board members from several, if not all, departments assures broad representation, it is not helpful to the overall success of the institution if board members consider issues strictly on the basis of what is best for their own departments. Therefore, it is incumbent upon the chair of the board, and the executive director of the practice plan, to spend time orientating new board members with special emphasis on the need for them to give priority to the needs of the institution and not just their own department.

Many boards are composed entirely of department chairs serving *ex officio*, along with medical school leaders such as the dean or associate dean for clinical affairs. In this case, changes in board composition occur only when a chair changes or when one of the medical school leaders is replaced. This may affect the extent to which the faculty feel well represented by the board, because their department chairs are selected by the dean rather than elected by their constituents. On the other hand, boards composed strictly of faculty elected by their constituents - and this conceivably might not include a key department chair - may find themselves in the position of having a membership which does not have a full understanding of the broader and related issues facing the management of the medical school. It is the author's judgment that the ideal governing board membership is composed largely, but not entirely of individuals who concurrently hold complementary leadership positions in the school. The balance of the board's members, within the voting minority, should include members who are elected by or selected from the faculty body and from related organizations important to the plan's success.

The dollar value represented by the practice plan has increased in recent years as medical schools have paid more attention to the business side of managing this important resource. In 1993, the Association of American Medical Schools reported that FFPs represented 32.8 percent of all medical school operating budgets, up from 15.7 percent in 1980, 11.8 percent in 1970 and 2.9 percent in 1960. With annual practice plan revenues approaching $8.3 billion, physician fee income is the largest single source of medical school support, exceeding grants and contracts by several hundred million dollars.

More competitive fee structures, a major increase in the volume of clinical activity performed by medical school faculty and better charge-capture, billing and collection mechanisms have all had an impact on practice plan income. Some FFPs contribute more than 50 percent of the financial resources of the medical school, and the annual collections of several plans exceed $150 million. Next to the operating budget of the teaching hospital and state appropriations, the FFP may be the largest single source of funds for many large universities. The plan's success in these challenging times is likely to be of concern to the university's governing board and officers as the future of its medical school may be tied to this success. As a result, the interest of the university's governing board in the practice plan is expected to increase in the future.

Participation on the FFP board by a member of the board of regents, or by one or more of the university officers may occur with increasing frequency in the future. University officers will certainly expect to receive periodic reports on practice plan activities, measures of plan success and annual independent certified audits of the plan's finances.

Board subcommittees

The full board of the FFP may provide general oversight and may convene only periodically to address broad institutional issues. This arrangement is particularly common if the practice plan has a large board. A smaller board is more likely to be regularly involved in a number of issues, including the oversight and review of the FFP's executive director. Most boards generally operate with a subcommittee structure and elect an executive committee to serve on behalf of the board throughout the year. The following section of this chapter lists several of the subcommittees that may be formed and their functions.

Executive committee

The responsibilities of an executive committee include:

- acting for the board as a whole between meetings of the full board;
- acting within prescribed authority (many actions taken by the executive committee are later confirmed by the full board) to authorize the expenditure of funds above the authorized limits placed on the executive director, but below those requiring action of the full board;
- acting in an advisory capacity to the executive director and medical director of the practice plan and other officers; and
- acting on the recommendations of other subcommittees, as established by the full board.

Members of the executive committee may serve as chairs of the other subcommittees of the board. The executive committee often meets monthly, and sometimes more often, whereas the full board may meet only quarterly.

The chair of the executive committee is often the chair of the full-board. We sometimes find that the chair of the executive committee is an associate dean for clinical affairs who also serves as vice-chairman of the full board, while the chair of the full board is the dean, who retains ultimate control.

Managed care subcommittee

In the chapter on governance penned by this author five years ago in the predecessor to this book, this section received what today would be viewed as a passing comment. Today there is not likely to be a single FFP which is not involved in managed care contracts, and most are looking at managed care payers as the source of 30 percent or more of their income. On the West Coast and in such advanced-stage cities such as Minneapolis, managed care payers account for 65-70 percent or more of practice plan income. This subcommittee is likely to be integrated with or tied to an affiliated hospital's managed care committee and closely linked to the practice plan's strategic planning process. The committee will establish parameters for negotiating contracts and monitor economic performance under capitated agreements where the plan is at risk for the over-utilization of resources.

Strategic planning subcommittee

Strategic planning and tactical implementation are far more essential in today's rapidly changing environment than just five years ago. This committee is involved in:

- planning and expressing the direction the FFP should take as it contemplates growth, resource conservation and its relationship with other parties. This includes strategies for community physician practice acquisitions;
- considering programs or investments that would assure the FFP a viable future; and
- participating in the parent institution's strategic planning process to assure that the FFP is well represented and well informed about the strategic directions being contemplated and that the plans are mutually compatible.

Finance subcommittee

The finance subcommittee addresses a broad range of fiscal and business-management issues including:

- taking responsibility for financial forecasting;
- establishing a fee or pricing strategy;
- establishing the practice plan's collection policy;

- recommending the practice plan's budget;
- recommending the allocation of reserves and special funds;
- developing a plan for the financing of building projects and other large capital expenditures, such as the purchase of major pieces of equipment; and
- being responsible for investment strategies and performance.

Marketing subcommittee

There has been a substantial increase in the resources committed to the marketing of academic medical center health care services during the 1990s. Marketing activities which previously were taboo occur now with regularity. Not only marketing services to employers and payers, but also advertising to the general public is commonplace. This subcommittee will set strategy, policy and propose a budget for these activities and will work with (or be integrated with) its parallel committee at the affiliated teaching hospital(s).

Compensation/fringe benefits subcommittee

The compensation/fringe benefits subcommittee deals with the salaries and benefits of those supported by the practice plan. Although individual salaries are generally set by the department chair and confirmed by the dean, this committee may recommend an overall compensation strategy for the practice plan. Its responsibilities may include:

- comparing the salaries of practice plan members with those of medical staff at other academic institutions to assure a competitive compensation strategy;
- developing and maintaining elements of a competitive fringe-benefit program;
- maintaining a retirement plan, including evaluating and selecting investment managers; and
- in some cases, awarding benefits funded by the practice plan to members of the basic science and research faculty.

The compensation committee, established principally to work with faculty compensation, may also address the compensation of the medical director, the executive director and senior administrative staff. If this committee is not responsible for non-physician/management compensation, a separate committee is warranted for this task. Senior administrative staff often share the same benefits as members of the clinical faculty, assuring the plan's ability to attract and retain well-qualified individuals who will have the maximum incentive to help the practice plan perform in an optimal fashion.

Membership/credentialing subcommittee

The membership and credentials subcommittee is often found in private group practices, but has traditionally had a lesser role in FFP governing boards. This role has been the responsibility of department chairs, the medical school's faculty affairs office and the affiliated hospital's credentialing committee. With the increase in community physician practice acquisitions, this board committee is becoming more important and active.

Academic practice plans have seen increased pressure to enhance and reduce operating expenses. As such, this committee may be involved in faculty "guidance" or discipline (or even dismissal of those not protected by tenure) if the individual faculty member is not in compliance with revenue-generating objectives or expense management limitations. When FFPs assume financial risk under managed care agreements, the plan's solvency is at stake if members are not compliant.

This committee may also make decisions concerning members of the faculty who are retired or semi-retired but who remain involved in practice plan activities or share in practice plan benefits.

Corporate/professional liability subcommittee

Corporate liability and malpractice insurance remain major issues of concern and cost for any group practice. Selection and oversight of an insurance carrier, or the manager of a self-insured plan, is an important role for this subcommittee. The professional liability committee should fully understand risk-management issues and should advise the full board and the membership about mechanisms to control risks. This subcommittee often meets with corporate counsel and retained attorneys to determine the most effective means of mitigating losses and disposing of claims.

Hospital relations subcommittee

The functions of a hospital relations subcommittee may be taken care of by the executive committee or by a group of board members specifically designated to work with one or more teaching hospitals to maintain an open dialogue and an effective working relationship. Issues related to joint ventures, medical-staff coverage and residency training programs may be addressed by this committee as well. Increasing competition and onerous reimbursement rules are factors which make the symbiotic relationship between affiliated teaching hospitals and practice plans all the more important to the success of both parties.

Ambulatory care subcommittee

Many academic group practices are involved in the direct funding and management of ambulatory care facilities. This subcommittee is designed to work with the executive director of the practice plan and the director of ambulatory care in regard to planning and operations of the ambulatory care facility. This subcommittee would also be involved in overseeing the budgeting and managing of operating costs, decision-making about capital expansion and reviewing performance data concerning the use of resources.

Clinical practice subcommittee

The clinical practice subcommittee, which may operate under various titles, is involved in determining which clinical disciplines within the institution's FFPs will be permitted to engage in certain clinical procedures. While the individual's clinical competence must be the overriding factor in determining a physician's performance of specific services, several departmental specialties may offer overlapping services; sometimes with different fee schedules. Some FFPs allow all physician members to provide services within their area of competence, whereas others delineate boundaries and require cross-appointments in more than one department in order for individual faculty members to perform certain procedures. The issue of clinical specialty boundaries is often less volatile if the practice plan is centralized and the income is pooled. However, most practice plans, even those that are highly centralized, distribute resources in part on the basis of individual or departmental clinical productivity. In this situation, faculty members have an incentive to engage in a broader range of activities rather than to have their services circumscribed. This is especially true in highly compensated disciplines such as cosmetic plastic surgery. The violation of clinical boundaries, or the lack of any established boundaries, may be the source of much conflict within a FFP or within any group practice. It is often helpful to establish a committee specifically charged with reviewing new procedures, deciding by whom they will be provided and determining by what mechanism faculty members will be authorized to practice them.

Public affairs subcommittee

A public affairs subcommittee may serve as the mechanism by which the FFP's members relate to organized medicine such as city, county, state and national medical associations. This subcommittee may represent the practice plan in public policy forums relating to health care; including involvement in addressing public health issues such as care of the area's indigent population, contingency planning for natural disasters and the financing of health care at the local, state or national level.

Mechanisms by which board members are selected

As described in Figure 2.2, board members may be selected and appointed, elected or may serve *ex officio* by virtue of their appointment to specific positions in the medical school. Under any of the three circumstances, the individual may serve with or without the right to vote. Boards are often composed of individuals chosen by various mechanisms. For example, some boards are composed of all the clinical department chairs, serving *ex officio* with voting privileges. Other governing boards are composed of a combination of department chairs serving *ex officio*, along with several other (but not all) clinical department chairs appointed by the dean to serve on the board. Boards may have a minority of their voting members chosen by a vote of the entire faculty membership of the practice plan.

Members may be elected by their department, by constituency area (such as the surgical, medical and diagnostic disciplines) or elected from the faculty at large. Governing boards that operate with elected members would be wise to have a well-documented and carefully executed election process. The election process for a large faculty can be time-consuming and every effort must be made to demonstrate that the process is followed with complete propriety and consistency.

Role of the practice plan executive director in governing board activities

The senior administrative officer of a business or academic organization may serve as a full member of the governing board. The governing boards of FFPs often include the plan's executive director as an *ex officio* member; most often without voting privileges. Some state laws prohibit a non-physician from serving as a member of the governing board of a medical group. In cases in which the executive director does not hold a board position, he or she is usually in attendance at all board activities. Executive sessions may exclude him or her, especially when the subject includes their performance evaluation or decisions concerning their compensation.

Among the roles of the practice plan's executive director is supporting the board in its deliberations and activities. Such support comes in the form of agenda development, provision of supporting materials and presentation of all performance data concerning the plan. Most often, the executive director represents the plan in all business negotiations with other parties and may serve as a principal liaison between the plan's administration and that of the university hospital and other teaching hospitals supported by the faculty in the practice plan. The executive director will personally, or through senior staff, support the subcommittees of the board and may serve ex officio on each of these subcommittees. The executive director should be actively involved in the education of the board on matters pertaining to health care legislation and regulation, and should play an active role in the orientation of new faculty joining the plan and of newly appointed board members.

Conclusions

To be effective, the FFP must have a well-defined and highly functional governance structure. The structure must be consistent with that used to operate the medical school, the university and increasingly, the affiliated or owned teaching hospitals with which the practice plan maybe engaged in joint ventures. It should serve as an advisory body to the senior executive of the medical school because this individual is held ultimately responsible for the overall operation and success of the school's constituent units. Membership on the governing board should be broad enough to assure representation of the faculty being served. Members should function with a view of the institution's needs, rather than serving as representatives of parochial interests.

FFP governance structures should be periodically re-examined to assure their efficacy. There should exist a well-understood process for the faculty to interact with the governance structure and it should include built-in mechanisms that will allow it to evolve in response to changes within the institution, within the medical community and within the field of health care. The board should be the focal point for planning and authorizing change in response to what will surely be a dynamic period as we close out the 20th century.

References

1. Participating were James Reuschel, Fletcher Allen Health Care at the University of Vermont; Lilly Marks, the University of Colorado; William Vogt, Vogt Management Consulting, Inc.; and Edward Baloun, Executive Consulting Group.
2. *Ex officio* means, "by virtue of one's office or position"; e.g., the current holder of a department chair.

Medical education: evolution and reform

by Rose Ann Frank, MA, FACMPE, and Linda J. Mast, MBA, FACMPE

The history of medical education in the United States began with colonial women treating the sick at home with herbs while physicians trained under an apprenticeship system. With no method for testing competency and no licensing bodies, William Smith's 1758 *History of New York* accurately described the situation:

"A few physicians among us are eminent for their skill. Quacks abound like locusts in Egypt, and too many have been recommended to a full practice and profitable subsistence; this is to be wondered at, as the profession is under no kind of regulation. Loud as the call is, to our shame be it remembered, we have no law to protect the lives of the King's subjects from the malpractice of pretenders. Any man, at his pleasure, sets up for physician, apothecary, and chirurgeon. No candidates are either examined, licensed, or sworn to fair practice." (Physician, apothecary and chirurgeon refer to the British category of practitioners.) [1]

During the time of Smith's writing only one hospital and one medical school, the College of Philadelphia established in 1756, existed in Pennsylvania.[2] By the Revolution War there were fewer than 400 physicians who received any formal training, of which only about half had college degrees.[3] The remaining practitioners received a signed testimonial from their preceptors certifying their proficiency.

As the trend toward formalized medical education developed, the better trained physicians began lecturing on various medical subjects. In 1847, the American Medical Association (AMA) was founded and established its primary goal to improve medical education. By the beginning of the nineteenth century, more medical practitioners attended universities with the percentage decreasing for apprenticeship-trained physicians. The increasing numbers of new students encouraged the development of a large number of new medical schools.

During this era, all the medical schools did not operate legitimate programs. No forceful requirements were imposed on weaker schools to encourage reform until the AMA was restructured in 1901. A newly created Council on Medical Education began inspecting the schools and concluded that only 51 percent of the schools were acceptable according to AMA standards.[4] To help aid the AMA with the investigation of the medical schools, Abraham Flexner of the Carnegie Foundation was hired to visit and evaluate all 155 medical schools. The Flexner report provided a candid evaluation of the schools, causing some to consolidate or close. By 1920, the number of medical schools was down to 85 and the AMA developed a Liaison Committee on Medical Education (LCME). Its purpose was to develop educational program guidelines, inspect the schools, and be the official accrediting body.[5]

Medical education today

Today medical education includes undergraduate, graduate and continuing medical education. Typically the undergraduate medical school program lasts four years and concentrates on the basic medical sciences with clinical clerkships in internal medicine, obstetrics and gynecology, pediatrics, psychiatry and surgery. Although medical school graduates are awarded a degree, they are not allowed to practice. An additional training period of supervised clinical training through a graduate medical education (GME) program is required, known as the residency. The length of training required varies between one and four years before the physicians are allowed to take a board-licensing examination.

The residency program follows medical school and focuses around clinical practice experiences and rotations through specific specialities aimed at offering "on-the-job" training for the physician. Current graduate education models vary between universities and hospital-based programs. All the models follow strict regulations specifying the required number of clinical hours needed to qualify the programs. It is the universities' and hospitals' responsibility to assure that the requirements are met. Each residency program incorporates specific requirements developed by the specialty's residency review committee. These models and requirements vary by speciality, but all concentrate on providing the resident with training of clinical skills.

The residency curricula are clinically based, leaving minimal time available for any other program content. Practice management, human relations and career courses, for example, are normally not presented. Only recently have a few specialities begun to incorporate these topics into their curriculum. Most models usually require the residents to spend the first training year working as a specialty resource for emergency rooms. The remaining years are then spent expanding the skills acquired in more advance situations such as out-patient hospital or university departments. As the residents acquire more skills, most graduate education models increase their level of medical and legal responsibilities.

The final phase of medical education for the physician is the continuing education period that commences after residency training. It includes continuing education courses needed to keep up to date with medical technology. Annually, mandatory continuing medical education (CME) courses are typically required for physicians to maintain specific credentials.

New developments in medical school curriculum

Impact of health care reform

Health care reform has resulted in an increased focus on managed care and practice management issues for the medical professional. Physicians must now incorporate concepts of practice management and managed care in their practice setting. Economic issues have become inseparably intertwined with clinical practice. In fact, health care reform, and the rapid expansion of managed care, requires changes in the way that reimbursement for medical services and medical outcomes are evaluated.[6] Utilization management, clinical outcomes analysis, and other methods of linking financial accountability to the practice of medicine, demands that medical school programs make adjustments in their curriculum to address the need for new curriculum content as a result of health care reform. Today, practicing physicians must be able to learn and apply managed care strategies in their medical practice to continue to effectively provide services to patients.[7]

Increased emphasis on primary care

The expansion of managed care has brought with it a growing demand for primary care physicians. The concept of managed care includes the use of primary care physicians as gatekeepers who control access to medical services for a designated patient population. It is projected that America will have far more medical specialists than will be required in the near future and not enough primary care physicians. There has been an increased enrollment in primary care programs over the past five years, likely directly related to the impact of health care reform. Primary care in medical education programs has influenced the development of alternative curriculum models. The most prominent change is the growing interest in the adoption of a problem-based learning curriculum (PBL) in many medical schools.

Problem-based learning and dual track

Traditionally, medical education has not been considered to be a leader in innovation. The majority of medical schools still embrace many aspects of the convention curriculum based on Flexner's report in 1910 linking the practice of medicine to its biological foundations. [8] This tradition in medical education curriculum is generally focused on lecture, memorization, labs, and a heavy reliance on the use of multiple-choice questions to measure learning. However, more than 80 percent of medical schools in the United States have now adopted, at least partially, a problem-based learning (PBL) model.[9] This evolving adoption of PBL in medical schools was originally implemented at McMaster University in the late 1960s. PBL has now been adopted by many other medical schools including the University of New Mexico, University of Arizona, Southern Illinois University, University of Missouri and others.[10] Internationally, the PBL curriculum has been implemented in: Beersheba, Israel; Mastricht, Holland; Newcastle, Australia; and medical schools throughout Europe, Russia, Asia, Africa, the Middle East and Latin America. The extent to which PBL models are used in medical education varies from one medical school to another. Many medical school programs offer a dual-track option where students may voluntarily participate in a PBL curriculum, or choose to enroll in a traditional curriculum. In other cases, schools offer a combination of both traditional and PBL courses integrated in one program.

PBL curriculum is an innovation that has global implications for medical education. The PBL model includes five key components:

1. The starting point is a problem;
2. The problem is one that a physician is apt to face;
3. The subject matter is organized around the problem--not a specific discipline;
4. Students assume responsibility for their own learning; and
5. Most learning occurs in small groups.

Clearly, the PBL model provides medical students with opportunities to incorporate cost of care, and medical outcomes issues in the course of their small group learning activities. The collaborative nature of PBL provides opportunity for students to gain experience in the collaborative practice style that is central to managed care. Medical education shows social accountability through a commitment to addressing issues, helping to solve problems, and identifying priorities jointly with society. [11]

Residency programs

The impact of health care reform

Residency programs have been affected by health care reform. The evolution of managed care programs and cost-containment in medicine has caused GME teaching institutions to refocus and expand their markets. It has forced residency programs to develop contractual relationships with insurance companies and compete with community physicians to attract more patients. Residency training programs can no longer solely depend on uninsured or federally assisted programs for patients. State and federal agencies, such as Medicare and Medicaid, have begun developing policies aimed at applying managed care principles to their programs. This situation places GME teaching institutions in an difficult position.

The concept of "managed care" was introduced by the federal government in 1973 as an approach to control utilization, reorganize health care services, and facilitate cost-containment through the usage of group practice.[12] During the 1980s and 1990s, managed care programs further developed as employers and insurance companies viewed them as a method of reducing costs and physicians' reimbursement. The new form of medical insurance requires physicians to provide quality medical care in a cost-containment environment and assume some financial risk for their patients' health care needs. The plans also require patients to seek care from the contracted physicians or incur a substantial financial penalty for services provided outside the network. This situation forced residency programs to participate with managed care insurance panels to retain and attract patients, and become part of competitive insurance plan networks.

Funding of graduate medical education programs

Academic medical institutions are working under increasingly stringent financial constraints. Graduate medical education (GME) is no exception. After graduation from medical school, a residency is completed in an academic medical hospital. An in-depth study of physicians conducted by Renschler & Fuchs[13] revealed that practicing physicians considered that the time spent in their residency had the most value and relevance to their current practice. Residency programs are accredited by the Accreditation Council for Graduate Medical Education (ACGME). The ACGME, among other accrediting agencies, evaluates residency programs based on the types of patients and the volume of patients that residents will have the opportunity to care for. Although residency programs clearly play a critical role in the learning and development of practicing physicians, the funding of these programs is facing challenging times.

Traditionally, GME programs have been heavily subsidized by federal funds funneled to academic medical programs by the Health Care Financing Administration's Medicare program. In recent years, the budget neutrality that Congress mandated for the Medicare program has limited available Medicare funds. Budget cuts have made it difficult for academic medical institutions to continue to maintain their residency programs.

The increased emphasis on primary care has created growing interest in offering residency programs that utilize community practice and other ambulatory care settings more heavily than in the past. Again, these residency programs will increasingly need to expose the residents to experiences with patient care that incorporate practice management and other community-based issues. Providing these learning opportunities for residents becomes difficult in a managed care environment where academic centers must now compete for patients and provide care within cost parameters defined by managed care third-party payers.

Influences of socialization on the medical profession

Houle's model of continuing education for professionals fits well with the educational process for physicians. The model begins with general education followed by specialized training where beginners are isolated and indoctrinated with the necessary knowledge, skills and values of their future profession.[14] The assumption is made that continued education during residency programs results in increased competence leading to improved physician performance, which ultimately improves patients' health. However, research indicates that physicians don't always do what they know should be done.[15] Further, physicians do not always satisfy their own criteria regarding patient care.[16] Educators involved with residency programs are in a key position to structure those programs to facilitate changes in medical practice behaviors and to help physicians develop self-directed learning skills such as self-evaluation.

Residency programs have unique characteristics which may impact adult development. For example, in addition to demanding work schedules, psychological abuse may be experienced.[17] In fact the AAMC (1984) has challenged medical education programs to provide support and guidance to enhance personal development of both medical students and residents. The isolated environment and rigorous demands of residency programs limit the opportunities for individuals to address many development issues that individuals in other professional environments have resolved.

In the multifaceted theory of adult development, Hughes and Graham[18] view the adult development process as one of multiple life roles including relationship with self, relationship with others, relationship with work and relationship with family. This multifaceted viewpoint provides a more useful framework than traditional linear developmental models to consider when developing residency programs. For example, the residency program environment fosters a high value on performance and career achievement. This correlates with an expected highly developed focus among residents on the "relationship with work" role. The demands of a medical career from the perspective of time commitment and educational requirement would most likely be associated with individuals who are either establishing new relationships or striving to balance relationships with career. Thus, a resident physician's life role associated with work relationships would be expected to be more highly developed than roles associated with personal and family relationships. Because of this, residents can be expected to have a strong investment in their perceptions of self-worth based on their clinical performance.

Indoctrination into the profession of medicine involves focused training on choosing the "right action" at the "right time." In the studies of Bennet and Hotvedt,[19] physicians' personal identities with career were intense, and few talked about aspects of their lives that were free of the influences of their practice. This strong link between clinical performance and self-worth may present barriers to consider when changes to residency programs are considered. For example, the inclusion of practice management issues may not receive the desired level of participation from residents because it is not tied to the aspects of their professional performance that they believe to be valuable.

Continuing medical education

Influence of the Accreditation Council for Continuing Medical Education on programming

The Accreditation Council for Continuing Medical Education (ACCME) conducts a voluntary accreditation program for institutions and organizations that provide continuing medical education (CME). Medical schools are among the most prominent providers of CME programs. CME accreditation assures both physicians and the public that the CME activities offered meet accepted standards of education. Continuing medical education plays a critical role in efforts to improve physician competency and performance. However, CME does not automatically ensure continuing competency. Both enthusiasm and doubt have been expressed about the ability of CME to change physicians' behavior and to impact the quality of patient care.[20] Although the need for lifelong learning in medicine appears to be universally accepted, traditional CME programming, with its systematic subject instruction, has met with criticism.[21, 22] The Association of American Medical Colleges Report of the Panel on the General Professional Education of Physician and College Preparation for Medicine (1994) states:

> "Most physicians are keenly aware of the need for continued learning, and they participate in programs for continuing education. Lifelong learning and adaptation for medical practice to new knowledge and new techniques will be even more important in the future."

Although the value of CME is evident, assumptions are made that CME results in increased physician competence which ultimately improves patients' health. However, research by Renschler and Fuchs[23] reveals that physicians consistently report that the lowest contribution to their learning is from formal CME programs. Their study identified that independent learning and informal study groups were most highly valued by physicians in practice. Similar to the traditional medical school curriculum, the traditional CME program model appears to have a perceived lack of value for physicians in practice. In 1991, a first ever "Institute for New

Investigators" was hosted by the American Medical Association and the Canadian Medical Association with the goal of stimulating new research in the area of CME. The focus of the institute was on the role of self-directed learning in changing physician performance.[24] It is through innovative CME programs that practicing physicians will best benefit from hands-on training and real-life situations, which can be applied in the context of their practice setting.[25]

CME is an important component of continuing physician education. The high value our society places on quality medical care is evident since the present expenditure for medical education and health care represent 14 percent of the gross national product.[26] The medical professional must be able to demonstrate physicians are being educated in ways that enable them to: translate their knowledge into performance; recognize their limitations; learn from their mistakes; keep up with technology; and ultimately, provide high quality care at a reasonable cost.[27] The physician today must perform successfully in multidimensional roles, including clinician, patient educator and resource manager.

Increasing emphasis on practice management issues

Physicians' perceptions

Professional medical practice today presents unique obstacles for physicians. Physicians who have not been trained sufficiently in business aspects often find that once they enter practice, much of their time is spent learning basic practice management skills.[28] Society expects physicians to deliver quality medical care and, simultaneously, fully understand the effects that operating a business has on the care. Health care reform, managed care restrictions, and the transition into a medical practice quickly alert the physician that the practice of medicine in the 1990s is also a business – a business that requires practice management skills, knowledge and abilities. This position is confirmed by a 1996 survey of the Society for Physicians in Administration (SPA) of the Medical Group Management Association (MGMA).[29] The results specifically demonstrated physicians' perception of inadequate preparation.[30]

The questionnaire analysis indicated that 71 percent of the physician-respondents felt that residency training programs are not preparing physicians to operate competitively for the 21st century. In addition, 74 percent indicated that they would feel more prepared for practice if management skills were taught during GME and 66 percent said that the inclusion of management skills during GME would make a difference to a physician's initial success. Also, 65 percent of those surveyed concluded that the inclusion of business courses in GME would make a measurable improvement in residents' management skills.

Options for practice management curricula

What are HMOs doing?

Health Maintenance Organizations (HMOs) evolved based on the success of pioneer plans such as Kaiser Pernamente and the Harvard Community Health Plan which offered health care to employers on a fixed (capitated) price basis. The Health Maintenance Organization Act of 1973 required that specific services be provided and that the organizations (initially staff group practices, such as Kaiser) were prepaid for their services. The HMOs' abilities to keep costs down by carefully managing patients' utilization produced new insurance products that place both the physician and hospital at risk. In 1996, there were an estimated 75 million Americans in HMOs and 95 million Americans in other Managed Care Organizations (MCOs), accounting for more than 50 percent of all Americans enrolled in some form of managed care plan.[31, 32]

With the increase in patient volume and the need for employed physicians to understand utilization management and other business principles, some HMOs have developed facets of a practice management curriculum for universities and teaching hospital programs. In fact, the interest in developing educational programs for physicians in the area of practice management has spread to the insurance industry. In 1995, Prudential announced the formation of the Prudential Healthcare Leadership Institute. This insurance company-sponsored program offers managed care training and development programs to physician associates and community health care providers.[33]

Dual MBA/MD degrees

With the growth in managed care plans in the United States has come a new set of demands on the management of medical practice. These demands require that physicians can acquire new information regarding practice management and related issues in the new health care environment created by managed care. Physicians are beginning to incorporate medical practice management information in their educational preparation. Executive MBA programs have been developed to offer professionals an opportunity to learn business theories and applications while maintaining a career. Physicians are enrolling in these programs. The courses help physicians learn basic business skills not taught in residency training programs. For example, some physicians are now seeking programs offering dual degrees such as MD and MBA. In other cases, physicians are participating in weekend and part-time graduate programs in business or health care administration to acquire necessary practice management knowledge while maintaining their medical careers.

Model curriculum

Until recently, undergraduate and graduate medical education consisted almost entirely of emphasizing technical medical skills only. This focus was altered when the Family Practice Residency Review Committee (RRC) mandated 60 hours of practice management education for family practice residency programs. The RRC is responsible for ensuring that residents are provided with a proficient education including fields critical to the program's specialty. The Committee defines the required number of hours and courses of study for the curriculum to ensure adequate standards have been achieved. The Family Practice RRC requirement does not mandate specific courses, but states that practice management education should "emphasize the tools needed to be successful in practice while optimizing patient care."[34]

The need for GME teaching institutions to develop a practice management curriculum brings many challenges and opportunities to the programs. It is during this phase of their education that residents are accumulating additional skills in preparation for entering practice. Courses offered in practice management during the residency years create a heightened awareness of the importance of business management skills. It is during the residency years that physicians begin to direct their careers and, as such, is the most logical time to present the curriculum.[35, 36, 37, 38]

-Practice management curricula used in GME teaching institutions today vary, but generally include basic business disciplines such as finance, accounting, marketing, information systems, human resources, contract negotiations, strategic planning and general management courses.[39, 40, 41, 42, 43, 44] In addition, some specialized medical business courses such as managed care concepts, medical-legal issues, quality outcomes theories, utilization review methods, medical ethics, the economics of starting a practice and personal financial planning may be offered. Such courses provide residents with basic skills and an understanding to help form a core competency for use during the residency years and beyond.

The instructional design methods used to present the information must keep the students' motivation and interest. This applies especially when presenting information that might not be perceived as necessary and relevant by the residents. Resources for practice management presentations can be found both internally and externally. Internally, department directors, administrators and specialists can develop custom programs. Externally, professional resources are drawn from the community.

Methods of presentation may include lectures, local college courses, video distance learning by TV, internal and external rotations, seminars and self-instructional materials. Of all the possible types of presentations, lectures are one of the most economical methods of presentation available to any residency program. Residents may be exposed to this type of environment and programs may present business case management issues using the lecture method.

Similar to lectures, seminars are beneficial to the curriculum. Business seminars are numerous and offer the resident an opportunity to interface with other business professionals. Annually, organizations such as the AMA, Medical Group Management Association (MGMA), Healthcare Financial Management Association (HFMA) and state medical societies present business seminars at various locations throughout the country.

Case studies which use practical, illustrative examples as problem-solving models, are another approach widely applied in many programs.[45] As this method relates to "real world" situations, residents might find the subject matter more enjoyable and retain more information. The case method would help prepare the residents for similar challenges in a management role.

Bringing the "real world" even closer, office rotations or clerkships in private or group practice environments offer unlimited opportunities. Customized rotations arranged through external companies enhance the resident's perspective and provide outstanding educational opportunities. Almost serving as an internship, these programs offer first-hand experience for the residents. Since this method presents the most "hands on" information available, it is especially important that residents who plan on pursuing private practice spend a considerable amount of time in a private practice office.

GME practice management programs are ideally scheduled throughout the residency years with extra emphasis during the last year. Each year the information is pertinent to the resident's interest and commitment level, offering the most flexibility for the program and subject retention. Using both didactic and experiential instruction, the programs offer management material presented through various formats.

Limitations on implementing a practice management curriculum

There are several limitations surrounding the implementing of a practice management curriculum. One of the biggest limitations is the resident's lack of available time. Residents are typically consumed with clinical responsibilities, have hectic schedules, and support emergency rooms and critical care areas. As such, scheduling time for practice management education is limited without extending the program's timeframe or readjusting priorities.

The resident's lack of interest in studying business courses is also a barrier that affects the program. Learning techniques in the forefront of technology appeal to the physician's scientific investigative nature. However, practice management education may not present the same type of challenge nor hold the same level of interest. Unfortunately, it is not until well into their last year of residency that most residents suddenly realize the advantages of learning basic business skills before graduating. In addition, unless the curriculum is a mandatory part of their programs, the residents often do not attend the classes.

Costs are also a limitation when implementing a practice management curriculum. Curriculums with dedicated administrative personnel to arrange lectures and monitor the program are the most effective. Without the benefits of a dedicated program coordinator, the management curriculum becomes a project and does not receive the attention needed to establish a comprehensive program. This is especially critical when developing and implementing a practice management curriculum.

Current management programs

McLennan County Medical Education and Research Foundation provides more than 60 hours of management education for its family practice residency program by merging its practice management curriculum with its business operations.[46] McLennan uses several approaches for the administration of its program. The Foundation incorporates "blocks" of times into the residents' schedules dedicated to practice management. In addition, the importance of practice management education is introduced during the orientation period to new residents. McLennan requires third-year residents' attendance at 25 lectures over a four-month period and provides training throughout the residents' training period and offers practice management electives such as rotations and "on-the-job" training.

McLennan's program was initially developed by the school's associate medical director after his arrival in 1984. It had the support of the top medical officer and was a priority for the facility. As a free-standing entity responsible for its own financial future, the integration of the practice management curriculum assisted in the success of the business operations.[47] It also has assisted in the recruitment process for medical students (future residents). McLennan has found that the residents' knowledge of the comprehensive practice management curriculum is often a major factor in their decision to rank the school high.[48]

The Oregon Health Sciences University (OHSU) created a unique teaching environment intended to assist with successful faculty practice plans and increased ambulatory education for residents. The University created a teaching clinic that integrated medical students, interns, residents and fellows into an academic private practice.[49] The teaching physicians are reimbursed, in part, from some of the clinic's profits, thus encouraging the physicians to maintain an efficient, successfully operating medical practice. The clinic provides monthly rotations for the residents and first-hand exposure to general management areas that would affect the teaching-physicians' compensation formula. "The system may provide physicians in training with experience concerning the operations of a private office, an area of their education that is seldom adequately addressed in their training." [50]

The University of North Carolina KRON Scholars Program is privately financed using locum tenens physicians in private practices to generate income and add in the funding for management training.[51] The program places locum tenens physicians in a five-week management course at the University of North Carolina at Chapel Hill. Both the physicians and the offices benefit from the program. The physicians have an opportunity to receive business training and often receive an additional stipend. The offices fill a vacancy for physicians in a private practice and pay market rates for their services that, in turn, pay for the business training.

Similar to the purpose and principles of a practice management curriculum, the University of Washington developed an annual resident teaching course designed to assist second- and third-year internal medicine residents learn teaching and leadership skills.[52] The program is presented in three sessions and assists residents in gaining more confidence, skills and abilities in assuming a team leader position. The sessions are intended to help the residents become more proficient communicating with the attending staff, managing and teaching medical students and interns, and recognizing problems faced by residents.[53]

The university uses course materials and videotapes of vignettes. The real-life reconstructed scenarios help the students focus on issues in a non-threatening environment. The sessions are interactive and encourage open discussion of the problems presented and help the residents understand that many strategies may be used to handle situations. Experienced third-year students also relate successes and failures of personal experiences and often repeat the sessions to further develop their skills.

Residents' evaluations of the program are "overwhelmingly positive" and attendance has been exceptional at over 90 percent for the first two sessions.[54] Topics are relevant and the program uses faculty facilitators and experienced instructors as necessary. The program is offered in a timely manner in July as internships have concluded and the second year begins.

Summary

The medical education process, including medical school, residency programs, and all forms of continuing medical education, is evolving. Practicing physicians today, and in the future, must have access to effective educational programs that incorporate managed care and other practice management issues into situations that are relevant to their clinical practice settings.[55] Increased emphasis on managing both cost and appropriateness of clinical outcomes will require formalized practice management curricula that work within the context of medical practice. The successful design of medical education programs that incorporate practice management will become increasingly important.

References

1. Packard, F. *History of Medicine in the United States.* New York: Hafner Publishing Co., 1963.
2. Raffel, M. and Raffel, N. The US Health System Origins and Functions. Albany, New York: Delmar Publishers Inc., 1989.
3. Ibid.
4. Ibid.
5. Ibid.
6. Green, J. "A New Physician Educational Paradigm: Facilitating Integration and Change." Presented to the Missouri Medical Association Annual Conference on Continuing Medical Education, September 1995.
7. Rollings, A. "Connecticare sends MDs to Managed Care School." (On-Line), Managed Care Quality. *Internet Journal,* Index 1, Document # 800185, Individual, Inc., 1996.
8. Albanese, M. and Mitchell, S. "Problem Based Learning: A Review of Literature on its Outcomes and Implementation Issues." *Academic Medicine,* 1993.
9. Jones, H., Etzel, S. and Barzansky, B. "Undergraduate Medical Education." *Journal of the American Medical Association.* 1989: 1011-1019.
10. Kauffman, A., *Implementing Problem-Based Medical Education.* New York: Springer, 1985.
11. Boelen, C. "Prospects for Change in Medical Education in the Twenty-first Century." *Academic Medicine.* 1995: S21-S22.
12. Williams, S. and Torrens, P. *Introduction to Health Services.* Albany, New York: Delmar Publishers, Inc, 1993.
13. Renschler, H., and Fuchs, U. "Lifelong Learning of Physicians: Contributions of Different Educational Phases to Practice Performance." *Academic Medicine.* 1993.
14. Houle, C. *Continuing Learning in the Professions.* San Franciso: Jossey-Bass, Inc., 1980.
15. Hojat, M., Gonella, J., Veloski, J. and Erdman, J. "Is the Glass Half Full or Half Empty? A Reexamination of the Associations Between Assessment Measures During Medical School and Clinical Competence After Graduation." *Academic Medicine.* 1993: S69-S76.
16. Johnson, D. *Physicians in Marketing.* San Francisco: Jossey-Bass, Inc., 1983.
17. Collier, J. "People Who Train People." *The Teacher Trainer.* 1991: 16-17.
18. Hughes, J. & Graham, S. "Adult Life Roles: A New Approach to Adult Development." The Journal of Continuing Higher Education. Spring, 1990: 2-8.
19. Bennet, N. and Hotvedt, M. "Stage of Career." *Changing and Learning in the Lives of Physicians.* Edited by Fox, R., Mazmanian, P. & Putnam, R., New York: Praeger. 1989: 71.
20. Rosner, F., Balint, J. and Stein, R. "Remedial Medical Education." *Archives of Internal Medicine.* February, 1994: 274-279.

21. Renschler, H., and Fuchs, U. "Lifelong Learning of Physicians: Contributions of Different Educational Phases to Practice Performance." *Academic Medicine.* 1993.
22. Rosner, F., Balint, J. and Stein, R. "Remedial Medical Education." *Archives of Internal Medicine.* February 1994: 274-279.
23. Op cit, Renschler.
24. Wentz, D., Osteen, A. and Cannon, M. "Continuing Medical Education: Unabated Debate." *Journal of the American Medical Association.* 1992: 1118-1120.
25. Wikenwerder, W. "Prudential Healthcare Leadership Institute." (On-Line), Internet document # 403375, *PR Newswire,* 1995.
26. Gonella, J., Hojat, M. Erdman, J. and Veloski, J. "What Have We Learned, and Where Do We Go From Here?" *Academic Medicine.* 1993: S79-S87.
27. Ibid.
28. Ridky, J., and Bennett, T. "Training Surgery Residents in Group Practice Management." *Medical Group Management Journal.* September/ October,1991: 38-39.
29. Frank, R. "The Physician Manager, Practice Management Education in the 21st Century." *Medical Group Management Journal.* (44)4. July/August, 1997.
30. Ibid.
31. American Association of Health Plans, 1996 annual report.
32. American Association of Retired Persons, November, 1996, "What Is Managed Care?"
33. Op cit, Wikenwerder.
34. American Medical Association, *1995-1996 Directory of Graduate Medical Education Programs Accredited by the Accreditation Council for Graduate Medical Education.* Chicago, Illinois: American Medical Association, 1995: 50.
35. Cordes, D., Rea, D., Rea, J., and Vuturo, A. "Introducing Management Skills and Issues in Preventive Medicine Residency Programs: A Survey." *Journal Of Occupational Medicine.* September 1991: 977-979.
36. Ridky, J., and Bennett, T. "Training Surgery Residents in Group Practice Management," *Medical Group Management Journal.* September/October, 1991: 38-39.
37. Frank, R. "Practice Management Education - Are Residency Programs Properly Preparing Physicians for the 21st Century?" *College Review.* Fall, 1993: 23 - 46.
38. Op cit, Frank, "The Physician Manager."
39. Ramsey, C., and Durrett, J. *Practice Management for Family Practice Residents.* Kansas City, Missouri: American Academy of Family Physicians. 1992.
40. Ortho Laboratories. *The Ortho Institute of Physician Practice Development Workbook.* Ortho Institute of Physician Practice Development.
41. Sullivan, K. and Luallin, M. *The Medical Marketer's Guide.* Denver, Colorado: Medical Group Management Association. 1989.

42. Macdonald, M., Meyer, K., and Essig, B. *Health Care Law: A Practical Guide.* New York, NY: Matthew Bender & Company. 1991.
43. Frank, R. "Practice Management Education - Are Residency Programs Properly Preparing Physicians for the 21st. Century?" *College Review.* Fall, 1993: 23 - 46.
44. Op cit, Frank, "The Physician Manager."
45. Cordes, D., Rea, D., Rea, J., and Vuturo, A. "Introducing Management Skills and Issues in Preventive Medicine Residency Programs: A Survey." *Journal Of Occupational Medicine.* September 1991: 977-979.
46. Pattersen, A. "A Successful Practice Management Curriculum." *MGM Journal.* September/October, 1995: 28-33.
47. Ibid.
48. Ibid.
49. O'Hollaren, M., Romm, C., Cooney, T., Bardana, E., Walker, J. and Martin, C. "A Model for Faculty Practice Teaching Clinics Developed at the Oregon Health Sciences University." *Academic Medicine.* January 1992: 51-53.
50. O'Hollaren, M., Romm, C., Cooney, T., Bardana, E., Walker, J., Martin, C. "A Model for Faculty Practice Teaching Clinics Developed at the Oregon Health Sciences University." *Academic Medicine.* January 1992: 51-53.
51. Shulkin, D., Kronhaus, A. and Nash, D. "A Privately Financed Fellowship Model for Management Training of Physicians," *Academic Medicine.* 1992: 266-270.
52. Wipf, J., Pinsky, L. and Burke, W. "Turning Interns into Senior Residents: Preparing Residents for Their Teaching and Leadership Roles." *Academic Medicine.* July 1995: 591-596.
53. Ibid.
54. Ibid.
55. Mast, Linda. "Theoretical Framework for Implementing a Managed Care Curriculum for Continuing Medical Education." *American Journal of Managed Care,* Vol. 3, No. 1, January 1997: 68-74.

Chapter 4

The academic physician manager and practice administrator team

by David L. Bronson, MD, and Lee Ann Onder, MBA

In 1992-1993, $2.4 billion dollars of medical school revenue was derived from clinical practice of the medical faculty,[1] representing 32.8 percent of all medical school income. Clinical science departments at most institutions are increasingly dependent on physician practice revenue. In 1995, 57 percent of the income of academic clinical science departments was derived from clinical practice, compared to 52.9 percent in 1992.[2] This dependence on clinically derived revenue is threatened by declining reimbursements, and increasing expectations for participation in managed care contracts. In addition, it comes at a time when funding from research dollars is more competitive, further challenging the fiscal health of medical school faculties. Not only are clinical science departments dependent on practice income, but the majority of clinical departments now derive at least some income from at-risk managed care.

At the same time, university and medical school support for clinical science departments has dropped. The 1995 Academic Practice Management Survey from the MGMA reports that university and medical school support dropped from 14.7 percent of revenue in 1992 to 8.9 percent in 1995.[2] The increasing reliance of clinical science departments on income derived from practice and the growth of at-risk managed care demand effective management of the academic clinical enterprise. The attention of clinical department leadership to this important activity cannot be overemphasized. Failure to manage these resources impairs the ability of clinical departments to meet their missions, demoralizes faculty, and decreases the competitiveness of the academic medical center in the new practice environment. New strategies for departmental leadership now emphasize the importance of faculty clinical effort in supporting the mission of the institution and the fiscal health of the departments.

In this chapter, we will describe the role of the academic practice physician manager and his or her relationship to the department chair and the faculty. We will then specifically define a well-balanced, functional physician/administrator team and the roles and responsibilities of each component.

Academic department structures and leadership roles

The organizational structures of academic clinical science departments vary widely based on multiple factors, including institutional norms, departmental history, number of faculty, and departmental mission. The chairperson leads the department, commonly with various "vice" or "associate" chairs, often for clinical affairs, education and research, followed by section or division heads. A vice-chair of clinical affairs frequently serves as the physician manager over all or most clinical activities. In smaller departments, the department chairperson usually takes on these responsibilities. Various forums for decision-making are used, including large and small executive committees, but the specific structure is less vital than seeing that informed decisions are made efficiently and implemented effectively. The precise form of the department structure is less important than the clarity of mission and the willingness of the chairperson to be flexible in accomplishing the goals.

Chairperson

The chairperson has a number of responsibilities in an academic medical practice. These include the overall performance of the department, the department budget, managing the department's mission, recruitment, promotion and tenure of faculty physicians, continued development of the research programs, managing the department's relationship to the dean and hospital, and defining clear expectations of what is required in the clinical arenas.

The department chairperson usually enters the position with a record of established academic success, frequently in leading and managing successful research programs. He or she will often have support from research grants, be well known in a clinical discipline, and usually have excellent teaching skills. Unfortunately, most new chairpersons have less strength or experience in academic practice management and may have even less interest. The challenge for the chairperson is in balancing the overall mission of the department and seeing that clinical activities get the same attention to detail that research enterprises demand.

The academic physician manager and practice administrator team

Academic physician practice manager

There are several organizational approaches that can be taken to manage the clinical activities of the department, but the role of a physician in a clinical leadership position is central to achieving success in nearly all models. The department chairpersons can choose to manage the clinical efforts themselves, and this approach is usually successful in smaller clinical departments such as otolaryngology or physical medicine and rehabilitation. The core clinical departments, such as medicine and surgery, are multimillion-dollar clinical and research enterprises, especially at larger medical schools. The size and scope of activities usually require the chairperson to delegate leadership of various programs to other faculty in the department. The position of academic physician practice manager is often designated as a vice-chair for clinical affairs, or similar title, to emphasize the critical importance of this activity to the department's success, and to display the close working relationship this individual has with the department chair. Although, in many larger departments, section or division heads have had full responsibility to manage the clinical activities of their sections, this fragmentation often leads to unbalanced clinical efforts across the department and disparate approaches to managing clinical practices areas. This is increasingly so as managed care contracts require enhanced coordination of clinical efforts across the department's and academic medical center's product lines. The most common approach is a combination of delegation to a designated physician practice manager (vice-chair) and then to section heads in a matrix approach.

The selection of the physician practice manager is a critical decision for the chairperson. The selected individual must be both clinically respected and have appreciation of and experience with meeting the academic missions of the department. The tendency to assign this important task to new junior faculty or less successful academicians will position clinical programs as secondary or tertiary in importance to the faculty. At the same time, the physician practice manager must have a good working relationship with the Chair and other physician leaders in the department. The attributes of an effective physician manager are shown in Figure 4.1.

Figure 4.1

Attributes of the Physician Manager

Clinically respected
Academically oriented
Leadership skills
Excellent communication skills
Integrity
Openness
Good team player
Solid business instincts
Commitment to excellence and success in practice
Confidentiality

The chairperson should grant the physician practice manager the authority and support to accomplish a defined set of responsibilities, based on that individual's skills and experience. There is no set formula for defining the responsibilities of the physician manager and each department must consider the attributes of the department and individual. However, failure to clearly define responsibilities and authority will undermine the role of the physician manager and potentially lead to an ineffective leader and unsuccessful practice effort. A particular challenge for the physician manager is to manage other faculty with national academic and research reputations and limited interest in clinical practice. Boundary areas of authority become difficult to define and matrix relationships are challenging to manage. The ability to effectively manage these matrices varies by institution based on such factors as its history, the size of its sections, clinical geography, but is most importantly based on the skills of the physician manager.

The physician practice manager needs to participate with the chairperson in the development of the annual budget for the clinical sections and plan for faculty resource allocation. It becomes increasingly imperative that the chairperson and the physician manager develop great familiarity with the financial aspects of clinical practice. Budgeting may not have been a high priority in the earlier stage of these physicians' careers, but they must now step forward to the challenge. They should be reminded that clinical revenue is important because it represents more than 50 percent of the department's income and serves as a major resource of internal department research support. An academic practice is at risk of increasing Medicare fraud and abuse scrutiny, breaking teaching physician guidelines and decreasing direct and indirect Medical education support from Medicare. Budgeting faculty efforts essentially means managing the allocation of physician professional activity. The practice budget and clinical time spent by each faculty must be coordinated to meet both the needs of the practice, and the missions of the department. A successful clinical practice cannot allow physician clinical activity to be the least important activity of the faculty and the reward systems must value excellent clinical effort as well as traditional academic effort.

The chairperson should set clear expectations with the practice manager for clinical faculty practice commitment, including the percentage effort in clinical activity and goals for revenue. MGMA practice data serves as a useful benchmarking source for staff productivity and a valuable tool for the chairperson and practice manager.

Compensation for the faculty of an academic medical practice often comes from both the medical school and clinical practice, frequently in two paychecks. Productivity formulas may be created and incentives established usually with input from the faculty. As managed care, particularly capitation, expands resource utilization is also evaluated as a measure of performance.

In the changing academic environment, medical school clinical department faculty are often pursuing one of two major tracts for advancement–a traditional tenure track, and the increasingly important "clinical" or "clinician educator" track. The physician practice manager must participate in promotion and tenure decisions by reporting practice effectiveness and quality as well as productivity. Research and education effectiveness may be easier to measure by considering the number of papers, external grant support–particularly from the NIH–and education scores, for each faculty member. It is much more difficult to measure the effectiveness and quality of clinical practice. This is usually done through an assessment of referring physician satisfaction, patient satisfaction and benchmarking against other similar practices. The productivity of clinical faculty is easier to measure, but does not give the full picture of the contribution of the faculty member's clinical effort.

The physician practice manager's responsibilities typically include development of the clinical practice budget to meet departmental needs (e.g., meet budget, break even, contribution margin goals), oversight or collaborative oversight with administrative manager, daily operations of clinical areas, management of coverage for hospital rotations, vacations, meetings, development of business plans for practice expansion, and development and implementation of practice guidelines. The physician practice manager must participate in decisions to use faculty practice resources for education and research. He/she should help bring economic reality to discussions and decisions about faculty clinical efforts. The physician practice manager may be involved in negotiations or in implementing physician practice changes in response to a managed care/capitation practice environment.

The least effective way for a physician manager to manage academic practice is to serve as a clinical advisor to the administrator with no functional authority or control.

Administrator

The role of the administrator in the academic clinical practice is a central theme of this book and well described in other chapters. The most effective administrators will bring a set of attributes to the position that will complement the strengths of the physician manager. A suggested set of attributes are shown in Figure 4.2.

Figure 4.2

Attributes of the Practice Administrator

Solid financial management skills
Excellent communication skills
Conflict resolution skills
Process improvement skills
Enthusiasm
Confidentiality
Innovative thinker
Leadership skills
Honesty
Good team player
Positive attitude

The importance of the combination of business/financial skills and the desire to be innovative are amongst the most important attributes of the administrator. The rapidly changing practice environment requires leadership that will look for as yet undiscovered solutions to the problems that will present themselves in the near future and balance those solutions with a solid understanding of the realities of the business of medicine. Managing the impact of HCFA's medical teaching physician rules is an excellent current example of the types of issues that must be approached with creative and defensible solutions.

The academic practice manager or administrator serves as partner to the chairperson and/or the physician manager. The administrator's primary role is to manage the clinical practice and its daily operations. He or she usually has little involvement in the research or education efforts of the faculty. The experienced academic practice manager has developed practice management skills through years of work in similar practices and comes with a strong educational background. Many administrators come into these positions with master's in business administration or similar graduate degrees as the practice management field becomes increasingly competitive. A clinical background is not essential, but many practices find this type of experience helpful.

The administrator works in concert with the physician manager in managing the daily operations of the clinical practice. This includes development of the annual budgets and management of the associated expenses and revenue. They must keep current on the reimbursement trends specific to their specialty. The administrator should also become involved in the negotiations for managed care contracts. Reporting of activity and costs by physicians is also increasing important for the capitated contracts. The administrator plays a primary role in collecting and reporting this information.

Management of the non-physician staff is usually primarily handled by the administrator through direct reporting relationships. It is his or her duty to handle the hiring, firing and promotion of these individuals. There may or may not be a separate clinical manager over the nursing and technical staff, depending on the administrator's background and competence.

Daily operations matters such as facility maintenance, purchasing, accounts receivables, etc., may also be directly overseen by the academic practice manager depending on the size and scope of the practice and whether or not the practice is part of a larger group or institution. The academic practice manager also assists in management of the physicians' schedules and patient access into the clinic. The manager frequently also has involvement in patient satisfaction issues, particularly the handling of complaints.

The physician manager-administrator team

A physician-administrator team is becoming increasingly important for achieving the goals of the department and academic medical center. The need for an effective team approach has never been more critical. The increasing complexity of the business of medicine demands the strengths of an effective administrator. These new challenges include the increasing emphasis on utilization and cost management, Medicare teaching rules, and the highly competitive practice environment. The physician manager is the best person to translate the mission to the administrative staff, and also to translate the realities of the new business of medicine to the clinical faculty. The relative strengths of the physician manager were shown in Figure 4.1 (i.e., clinically respected, academically oriented, good communication skills, good business instinct, honesty, integrity, good team player). The most important strengths of the physician manager are his or her credibility as a effective clinician and credibility in understanding the academic mission of the department. A leader without respect for the academic mission of the department will suffer from a credibility gap similar to a non-clinician leading the practice effort. The physician leader must also be a guardian of quality, while functioning as an agent of change. This balance requires a clear understanding of both the nature of quality in practice and the future directions of medical practice.

The administrator has traditionally been focused on operational issues and the implementation of policy. Personnel issues often require much of his or her time. In the current environment, this separation of effort by the physician manager and administrator into policy and implementation is less effective in moving the faculty practice forward. The physician manager and administrator must work jointly to establish priorities, establish policy, and seek implementation of effort. As insurers and government agencies require clear evidence of effectiveness and improvement in clinical efforts, the physician manager-administrator team must agree upon measures of outcomes and definitions of success. Although the administrator may be more focused on implementation of efforts, the team must both plan and take responsibility for the program. A suggested set of responsibilities for both the physician manager and the administrator are shown in Figure 4.3.

Communication is the most vital component of an effective physician manager-administrator team and must constantly be nurtured. Confidentiality, trust and mutual support are critical. Regular meetings should be held between the physician manager and the academic practice manager to serve as a forum for brainstorming issues and as a safe place to discuss confidential issues that will not leave the room or the relationship.

Access for patients into the practice is critical. New patients are the life blood of the clinical practice enterprise. These patients require greater use of department clinical resources and serve as an important source of clinical revenue for both the teaching hospital and faculty practice. Access for all patients, particularly new patients, needs to be a focus for academic practices. Under managed care, academic clinical practices are now responsible for handling the health of a population. They are also competing against non-academic practices that understand this very well and do it efficiently. It is no longer an avocation for the faculty to go to the clinic a few days per week. The academic medical practice now needs to mimic the private practice environment in efficiency to remain economically viable and support the mission of the academic medical center. An effective physician practice manager-administrator team will help ensure that success.

Figure 4.3

Joint Responsibilities for Physician Manager and Administrator

Creation and management of budgets
Evaluation of financial performance
Periodic financial reporting
Compensation administration
Resource utilization and management
Quality reporting
Implementation of practice guidelines.

References

1. Jones, R.F. and Sanderson, S.C. "Clinical revenue used to support the academic mission of medical schools, 1992-93." *Academic Medicine.* 1996; 71:299-307.
2. *Academic Practice Faculty Compensation and Production Survey: 1996 Report Based on 1995 Data.* Medical Group Management Association: Englewood, Colorado; July 1996.

Chapter 5

Decision-making in the academic medical center

by Judith Roth, MBA

This chapter will look at decision-making in the academic medical center (AMC) and describe examples of the way things are commonly done at the departmental, interdepartmental, institutional and interinstitutional levels. Exploration of the reasons for the style of decision-making existing; i.e., the differences between physicians and administrators as managers, will provide insight into why we are the way we are. The closing section will discuss various management and decision-making techniques that have been tried in some AMCs and are recommended by experts in the field.

Academic medical centers are institutions which combine professional schools with teaching hospitals and have simultaneous commitments to teaching, research and clinical care.[1] Such institutions have been described as among the most complex organizations existing[2] today and as a result, decision-making, especially decision-making which affects the whole organization, is a time-consuming and labor-intensive procedure at best. Decisions are often avoided and the status quo continues. While this inability to make timely decisions has undoubtedly caused frustration and led to missed opportunities, it has been accepted as the modus operandi in most AMCs. Whether AMCs can continue in this mode is a question of some concern.

Any review of the health care literature will tell you that whatever year(s) it is, you are in the most perilous time for health care and change must be instituted if one is to survive. While DRGs, Medicare fee freezes, closing of rural hospitals and even the proposed Clinton health plan(s) certainly created stirs in the past and made the need to act more pressing, AMCs weathered the storms and most continued doing business as usual.[3] However, the period of the mid-to-late

---

Written in fulfillment of the requirements for advancement to Fellowship Status in the American College of Medical Practice Executives, 104 Inverness Terrace East, Englewood, CO 80112-5306; 303-397-7869

1990s is turning into a momentous era in health care, bringing with it greater pressure for change than we have ever experienced. AMCs are confronting tremendous growth in the acceptance of managed care and risk contracting by insurers, employers and consumers. Medicare audits of teaching physician practices may cost the institutions multimillions of dollars and loss of public trust. Reductions in reimbursement for graduate medical education threaten the viability of medical schools. Mega-mergers between centers will result in staff reductions and constraints on freedom of action at all levels. With these decisions facing academic health centers, which decisions they make and how quickly they make them will likely determine their success and possibly their survival.

Most faculty and administrative staff would say that "complex" does not begin to describe the organizational structure at most AMCs. Unlike a business with a hierarchical structure, a financial definition of success, and a single person or small group of people authorized to say yes or no, the dynamic areas in academic medical centers, such as in biomedical research,[4] involve individual clinicians or investigators or small groups, not whole systems. The faculty very much see themselves as individual professionals and are jealous of their independence. One of their historic rights has been to partake in deliberations and to play a role in a participative democracy in making decisions which affect their daily activities.[5] Add to this the existence of practice plans with their own agendas and needs (which are often so independent that they are unflatteringly called by their own faculty "fiefdoms") and you begin to get the flavor of the problem.[6] Put it simply, decisions which may be in the best long-term financial interest of the medical center may not be in the best short-term interest of some faculty members.[7]

Within these institutions there are different levels at which decision-making takes place. While none is straightforward, it is important to identify which playing field you are on to better assess your options and pitfalls. The scope of decision-making can be broken down into different areas: intradepartmental decision-making, interdepartmental decision-making, institutional decision-making (i.e., between the department and the university or hospital) and interinstitutional decision-making (i.e., between the department, the university and the hospital or between AMCs). Each is now described.

Intradepartmental decision-making

At the departmental level, there are two players who are empowered to make decisions which affect the lives of the individuals within the department. These individuals are the department chair and the department administrator (alternatively called the administrator, the executive director, the chief executive officer). The job of each of these individuals is complementary and while the chair bears the ultimate responsibility and authority for all intradepartmental decisions, the chair and the administrator share a mutual goal to successfully carry out the mission of the department. Traditionally, the chair is focused on clinical, teaching and research aims. The administrator focuses on assuring that these aims can be accomplished--by providing that the financial resources and the administrative structure are capable of supporting and achieving the department's goals.

When it comes to facing the outside world, whether it be faculty, staff, other departments or institutions, the chair and the administrator must appear as one. The decision of the chair must be supported and put forward by the administrator regardless of whether or not the administrator's views agree with those of the chair. This is no different in academia than it is in the business world. What is different is that often, the chair, who is trained to be a leader in medicine, is making business decisions for which he or she has little or no experience. A chair's very training as a physician teaches him or her to act independently, want immediate results and be data driven in approach. An administrator, on the other hand, while certainly trained to work with and rely on data, negotiates and builds consensus, measures effectiveness over time and uses intuition frequently. [8] The different way that physicians and administrators at all levels of the institution, look at the world affects all decisions in AMCs and is very much what drives or fails to drive the decision-making process in our academic medical centers today.

Figure 5.1 shows some of the areas where chairs and administrators can exercise decision-making authority fairly independently of the external environment. This is not an exhaustive list, but it is typical for most departments. The areas are routine and may involve large sums of money and many people, but they do not involve highly complex negotiations or any outside individual inputs and sign-offs.

Interdepartmental decision-making

Examples of interdepartmental decision-making include program development, space utilization, shared resources, billing services, etc. While the institution may have a role in all of these areas, the issues are usually departmentally driven and the departments are directly involved in the outcomes. From the countless examples of the need to make decisions on an interdepartmental basis, here are several which will resonate with the reader of this chapter.

Example: The need to market the breast cancer services of the AMC has been decided by the Department of Surgery and the Division of Medical Oncology. They have put up seed money and engaged a noted advertising agency to prepare a campaign with brochures, radio advertising, etc. They believe that the patients to be brought in via this campaign will benefit several departments and they have broken this down by percentage (Surgery - 35 percent, Anesthesia - 35 percent, Oncology - 15 percent, Radiation Oncology - 10 percent, Pathology - 5 percent) and are approaching these departments to put up a share of the cost of the campaign based on this breakdown. Since these services were not involved in the initial decision to go forward on this project, their willingness to do so now will be highly questionable. As there is no comprehensive institutional marketing program in place, the ancillary services, in particular, have no way of knowing that the Neurosurgery or Orthopedic Departments are not waiting in the wings with other campaigns which might cost less to market and bring in more patient revenue than a breast cancer program. Here is a perfect example of the "individual fiefdom" syndrome at work where department independence hinders decision-making on an interdepartmental level. A multidisciplinary team approach described later in this chapter could have been well used in this process.

Example: A simpler incident is the matter of professional courtesy on reducing or eliminating payment for services for specific groups of patients. A uniform policy on courtesy would present a more user-friendly view to patients and be easier for billing staffs to administer. Yet in many institutions one department may give courtesy to all physicians in the institution, their spouses and children. Another may do this and extend courtesy to all physicians in general. Some may extend courtesy to staff nurses and union members. The variation is endless and usually physician-specific. Personal experience has shown that trying to craft a joint policy in this area runs into difficulty because of the individual wishes of faculty members. Often the ancillary departments, such as anesthesiology and radiology will have group policies. However, when you have hundreds of physicians with a broad variety of views, and independent styles, decisions of this type are hard to achieve. In this instance, the arrival of managed care will have the positive effect of reducing the need to think about professional courtesy for many groups of patients.

Managed care presents another challenge for interdepartmental decision-making--in the area of global or package pricing. Trying to bring five or six departments together to discuss and agree upon discounting of charges is an exercise which requires extreme patience and trust in your fellow administrators and their recordkeeping. As this is an issue which has such direct impact on everyone's revenue, it gets everyone's attention. This confrontation with the "business world" and the need to determine if you can actually make a profit on a package, has prompted AMCs to learn to make more rapid decisions based on plain old dollars and cents or risk losing business or ending up with business on which they will lose money on each case. Difficulties encountered in this process have led to the need for outside consultants to come in and negotiate between the departments. Consultants not only add a sense of impartiality to the proceedings but also bring data to support their recommendations based on their experience.

Another good example of the AMC at work on the interdepartmental level which involves faculty is the selection of a new chair. This very process can be a defining moment in how time is wasted and how the process itself is fraught with delay. Here are some common steps:

- A search committee is appointed. It usually contains no member of the department for which the search is being initiated and no administrator of any type. The committee's size will vary but usually is not less than 10 people. In a medical center with a university affiliation as opposed to just a medical school affiliation, the committee will often contain people from the university campus who have no idea of how a medical department is run or what is needed to run it;
- Letters are sent out to departments all over the country asking for candidates. The people responding to such a mailing may have little idea as to whether the person they are suggesting has the remotest interest in the job being offered. Everyone who is suggested is sent a letter asking them if they are interested and, if so, to submit their curriculum vitae;
- At the same time, the grapevine is in full gear and people are being suggested to the committee and are being asked if they would like to submit their vitae;

- Simultaneously, members of the search committee begin to interview members of the department to find out their views on what the department needs in a chair, what they think was wrong with the last chair, what they think is right and wrong with the department, etc.;
- The dean's office, with the help of the departmental administrator, prepares a financial analysis of the department, which will be given to candidates (usually on their second visit). This will often be shared with the committee so that it is knowledgeable about the department's finances;
- Candidates are invited for interviews. On a first interview the candidate will generally meet with the committee and key members of the department and the school/hospital. An informal feedback process is used by the committee to learn what was thought of the candidate by the interviewers. The candidate may or may not meet the administrator;
- Candidates who make it to the second cut definitely meet the administrator and other members of the department and the school/hospital up to and including the dean and the president;
- If the department is fortunate, the chair of the search committee is doing a good job of keeping the process on track and of informing the department of the search's progress;
- While there may or may not be formal reference checking taking place, there is certainly an active rumor mill, which cannot only damage a candidate's chance at this job but may damage his or her reputation outside of the search. As reported by George Longshore in his paper on "Managing the Search Committee, "[9] "One member of a search committee seeking a chief of medicine for a large, university-affiliated hospital torpedoed a nearly closed search by calling a candidate's former colleague. Although the candidate had already agreed to return from an overseas pharmaceutical job to fill the post, this colleague painted such a negative portrait that committee members panicked. Unfortunately, news of the underground reference check got back to the candidate who withdrew his name from consideration. In the end, the committee discovered that the colleague's opinion was unfounded, but it was too late. A top candidate had been lost." Such is the danger of a loosely managed search;
- Once a candidate is selected by the committee, his/her name is put forward to the dean/president. Then negotiations begin on "the package" which the candidate is going to obtain for himself/herself and the department. A smart candidate at this point will have gathered information from the department members as to their needs/wants;

- Negotiations of this type can drag on for months with letters going back and forth between the candidate, the university and the hospital. I know of one instance where the search committee set out to find the absolutely most prestigious person they could find to head a major department. Naturally, this most prestigious person had a very large shopping list, one which was well beyond the means of the institution to satisfy. After this candidate was nominated and negotiations begun, it quickly became evident that this candidate's requirements could not be met by the school and the committee had to go back to the drawing board. This highlights the problem wherein a search committee is not given guidance by the institution as to what its financial limits are. In fact, committee members are frequently told that this part of the decision-making is none of their business. In contrast is Longshore's story where the committee was not told not to talk money and after months of wrangling offered a candidate for a chair of neurosurgery twice the market value of the position![10]
- Once agreement on the contract is made and the offer duly accepted, it is very unlikely that any chair will move to any institution in any other month than July. So, even if an offer is made and accepted in September, it is rare that the new chair will physically arrive on campus until nine months later. What will ensue is frequent or infrequent visits, telephone calls and faxes and general frustration on all sides. One can only wonder what captains of industry think of this genteel artifact of the academic medical center.

Administrators will realize that there are several steps missing in this structure, the first of which is agreement on a detailed job description. What is needed for the department at this point in its development? Is the department financially strong but weak in research? Are there many junior members who need a seasoned leader to help them grow? Should a candidate have been a vice-chair of a large department or served as a division chief? Or is the title of professor the only qualification needed? In the AMC, all seem to agree that a chair must be a clinician, a teacher and usually a researcher as well. This too often suffices as the "job description." It is far from adequate in offering guidance to a disparate group of people given the important task of finding a leader who will hold the position of chair–usually without review–for at least two years.

Search committees will find that members do not come to all meetings, and that all do not meet the candidate or are present for important discussions. Also committee members come to the task with varying skills in interviewing. It would be advantageous to have someone from the human resources department train committee members in interview techniques so that they can elicit informative answers from the candidate. The use of questions beginning with "who," "what," "when," "why" or "how" make a candidate think before responding. While a search committee rightly feels that part of its job is to sell the institution's merits, some members may spend too much time talking about their own accomplishments and forget their main mission of selecting the candidate on his or her merits. Another decision-making tool which is often not used is to determine the decision-making process of the committee; e.g., will voting be used and if so by secret or open ballots, etc.

Each of these techniques can enhance the process. Not using any of them hampers and lengthens the decision-making process (or at least an effective decision-making process) incalculably.

Although it might be considered blasphemous, medical centers might do well to engage the services of a search firm at least to identify potential and interested candidates. The money saved in person hours spent on this part of the activity would easily offset the cost of the search company's fee.

Institutional decision-making: balancing department needs

There are many loci of power within AMCs. As stated earlier, departments, particularly clinical departments, are akin to individual fiefdoms. Each has its own source of funds from clinical earnings which provides great independence of action. The latest *Academic Practice Management Survey*[11] reports that practice earnings as a percent of all departmental revenue have grown from 52.9 percent in 1992 to 57 percent in 1995. Conversely, funds received by departments from the university/school has dropped from 14.7 to 8.9 percent while affiliated hospital support has gone up to 12.4 from 11.2 percent in 1992. This shift in funding gives the department a greater sense of independence and power and plays a central role in influencing university and/or hospital decisions which affect the department.

If a dean or president is faced with two requests for utilization of the same space and one department has the money to go forward on its own and the other department is relying on the school/hospital to foot the bill, how is the decision to be made? One might think that cases like this are decided on the merits of the request or simply "on the money," but that would be naive. Side issues will enter into the decision-making such as available swing space for one or the other requesters, previous space awards, commitments to third and fourth parties which may be impacted by one or the other of these relocations, etc. Meetings will be held - drawings may even be made of how the space will be utilized and alternative sites discussed. Cost/benefit analysis of who will use the space to generate income may or may not be done, and if done, may not be important to the outcome. In the AMC, academic office space often bears equal weight with income-producing clinic space. Eventually, the dean will be pushed into a decision by any one or a combination of these factors. But the time spent in discussion, raised and dashed hopes, and the department's continued feeling that a decision will never be made--and this is just business as usual–contributes to the lethargy that has traditionally gripped the AMC.

If an eminent researcher brings in grant funds and with them a large injection of indirect money to the institution, how does the dean balance the needs of this individual against the needs of an established individual who has failed to gain an award in the last three grant cycles and seems to be nearing the end of his or her research line? This problem in decision-making raises the whole arcane, but hide-bound issue of tenure and continuation of support regardless of productivity and success. In instances like this, the chair may come to the dean for assistance. This request for assistance may take many forms. Can you find space for this individual in another lab? Can you provide central university funds for this non-producing citizen? Can you help to arrange a buy-out? Granted this is not an easy decision to make, but the respect for tenure and the self-interest of many who have attained it, tie a dean's and a chair's hands and prolongs decision-making and often makes it more costly than it would have been if the decision was made quickly.

Interinstitutional decision-making

Mergers, acquisitions, downsizing, elimination of medical schools, closing of beds. Less than ten, even five years ago, some of these words were not in the vocabulary of university and hospital officials. Today one can hardly open a newspaper without reading of the merger of another major academic hospital system. How are these types of decisions made? It is well known in New York that the now failed merger of Mt. Sinai Hospital and New York University Medical Center was eased along because of close ties between members of the boards of trustees of the two institutions. The merger of Columbia Presbyterian

Medical Center and the New York Hospital (making it the largest medical center in the New York metropolitan area - a claim that Mt. Sinai/NYU held for approximately six weeks!) followed closely on the heels of the Mt. Sinai/NYU merger. This latter move was driven quickly by market forces after a clear, hard look at the remaining partners left at the dance in the highly over-hospitalized New York market.

Although personal relationships undoubtedly play a large role at this level of decision-making, all stops are pulled out as far as the use of consultants, due diligence on financial statements, and long-range planning strategies. Stakeholders, such as physicians and administrators, may be kept informed at monthly meetings, but have little if any input into these discussions. The boards of trustees are, if not the driving forces, intimately involved in the negotiations. Indeed, Lawrence Tisch, the Chairman of the Board of Mt. Sinai, had a letter of intent to pursue a merger between the two institutions, the existence of which was largely unknown to all but a handful of people.[12] When one reflects on the scope of these decisions, the speed with which they are taking place is breathtaking. Time will tell if this style is followed as the new institutions begin to look at merging departments and services. Parenthetically, the Mt. Sinai/NYU merger fell apart when the physicians and chairs and even deans found that their styles and expectations for the merged institution were so at odds that not even pressure from their boards could hold them together.

On a less global but still interinstitutional scale, consider the issue of fund raising. Usually the hospital, the medical school and the university will have fund-raising or development departments. Each will have a mission and a goal. Very often each will also be approaching the same donor for funds. If there has been no high level strategy set between the institutions as to who will ask who for what, you end up with annoyed donors and less than successful campaigns. This is an area where coordination of effort between the institutions should take place.

In the clinical arena, one can find that the hospital may unilaterally make decisions which impact the university. For example, the hospital may decide that an executive director for the operating rooms needs to be recruited and hired to improve the efficiency of the operating rooms. This person will clearly affect the day-to-day lives of all the physicians in that area and may have an impact on the income generated to the practice plan. However, despite the fact that the physicians are probably employees of the university, it is unlikely that the dean will have any role in deciding whether this position should be created, what his/her role will be vis a vis the school, etc.

These interinstitutional dilemmas have an impact on the overall effectiveness of the organization. A study by D'Aunno et al[13] showed interesting results on effectiveness of the institution in regard to how decisions were made. They looked at university hospitals and their academic health centers, both private and state, and measured performance factors such as patient satisfaction, financial performance, research funds, education index, etc., to see how the decision-making style affected performance. They found that if decisions were made at the lower levels in the organization and if these decisions reflected the consensus of the key stakeholders, particularly the medical school and the university/hospital, then the institution was more successful with these performance factors. D'Aunno cited previous work on this interesting topic by Choi, Allison and Munson and Scott and Shortell (see references). He further found that having the more knowledgeable stakeholders involved led to greater speed in decision-making. For those AMCs which have state and university officials looking over their shoulders, it was confirmed that a decrease in involvement by these parties in AMC management and policy decisions leads to better AMC performance.

Decision-making styles: why we are the way we are

As put very straightforwardly by Dr. Gerald S. Levey, Dean of the School of Medicine at UCLA, "The development of educational and clinical partnerships on an individual departmental basis, without concern for the institution and its goals, is no longer tenable in this practice environment. Departments must coordinate educational and clinical efforts to serve the academic health center's overall interests. Chairs of all departments must take the lead in aligning their parochial departmental goals with goals in the best interests of the institution."[14]

This statement of a problem so common in the AMCs is repeated by many people in many ways. Certainly, we all know that the more homogeneous the people in a group, the easier it should be for them to make decisions. People from the same background, with similar education, same age cohort, same religious orientation, etc., should be able to reach conclusions with relative ease. Yet we all know from experience that this is not always, if ever, true. While a group of friends may fairly easily be able to decide on what restaurant and movie they want to go to, when it comes to whether or not after-school programs should be supported by taxpayer dollars for the "convenience" of dual-parent working families, it is amazing how much friction a homogenous group can generate when trying to answer a more difficult question..

As we move into the workplace, we begin to encounter different people and different styles of decision-making. In large corporations, one will find marketing people and R & D people, accountants and engineers, people with advanced degrees and those with a high school education. Foremost in the minds of corporate executives is the need to keep the company profitable and to produce their good or service and satisfy their shareholders. They must find ways to manage their people so that they are all pulling in the same direction regardless of their place in the organization; their goal is what is best for the business. This single mindedness on achieving a unified goal is not a tradition of AMC behavior.

The orientation of physicians run counter to this concept. In single practice settings "a major decision tends to be made on the basis of what best serves the doctor(s). Since each physician's style is based on independent action, steeped in the need for professional quality, he or she thinks first how a course of action suits personal preferences. Then that personal judgment dictates how the practice should act. In a group practice, the mix of personal preferences may cancel out any decision at all. The best business decision often conflicts with some partners' views of what is personally desirable."[15]

It is important to know the traits which drive the faculty who represent such a major force in a group practice or a clinical department. Physicians do not shed their training when they become a member of a prestigious university's clinical department. Physicians are trained to be individualistic and most often deal one-on-one with a patient. They have difficulty dealing with confrontations in a group environment. Some physicians will have a "business" orientation and will be interested in the business aspects of the department; others, particularly those in academics, will want nothing to do with such matters. [16] When physicians do enter the management world, according to Ruelas and Leatt[17] they often hold on to their professional stature when attempting to make management decisions. Their lack of management savoir faire may cause a lack of credibility in their ability as leaders (in the clinical arena). In the clinical/patient care setting, physicians hold a level of authority based upon clinical expertise and will tend to confront management functions from their traditional clinical roles. When confronted with opposition in management decision-making, they are likely to become authoritarian and resistant in nature.

Training in taking care of human lives also tends to make other decisions seem less important. If a physician is appointed to head a committee to decide on the voice mail system for the department and also to a committee to decide which new anesthetic should be introduced to counteract nausea, it is easy to know which is going to attract his or her primary attention. The latter decision-making can be based on facts - what do the studies show, how much will it cost, etc. The former decision means looking at competing products, balancing the needs and desires of all individuals in the department, being involved with training questions. These are not the strengths of physicians who want to act independently, are trained to want immediate results, seek rapid feedback, and are scientific and data driven in their approach.[18]

Administrators, as stated by Royer, are most comfortable negotiating on consensus, work with larger groups of individuals and are trained to be dependent on networking and team efforts.[19] They are comfortable looking at their effectiveness over time, and they frequently utilize intuitive skills sets. Physicians tend to dominate in professional relationships; managers must delegate and cooperate.[20]

Decision-making techniques at work

With these disparate styles, and yet the need to bring the parts together to make decisions which are critical to the institution as a whole, what are some of the approaches which might be tried?

First, recognize that groups generally are superior to individuals in making decisions when an issue is relatively complex, since members of a group can generate more creative solutions than one individual working alone. On the other hand, an individual's decision is apt to be more effective when value judgments must be made and individual initiative is required to implement the decision in a timely manner.[21] At AMCs both physicians and administrators are involved in groups which make decisions all the time. One has only to reflect for a moment to come up with the Infection Control Committee, the Quality Assurance Committee, the Practice Plan Management Committee. These committees are groups of people, physicians, nurses, managers, who work as a group to make decisions to achieve both short- and long-term goals.

Any experienced administrator has sat on and chaired committees which were more or less effective in their ability to move quickly and make good decisions. Simple techniques, such as the use of an agenda, and setting time limits for the length of the meeting are often overlooked. Vasilios J. Kalogredis, writing in the *American Medical News*, comments that as cited earlier in this chapter, there is a fundamental conflict between the individualistic mindset of the physician and the need for a common purpose of the group which, if not managed, can lead to anarchy.[22] Experienced administrators also know how frustrating it is to have spent hours as part of a group which supposedly has decision-making authority only to find that when the decision is presented, it never gets implemented. In any decision-making exercise, it is vital to know who your stakeholders are, who can stand in the way of the decision becoming reality, and making sure that these people are involved and committed to at least trying the solutions that will be the outcome of the problem you are analyzing.

An interesting approach is being used at the University of California, San Francisco Medical Center's Center for Clinical Effectiveness. In attempting reengineering projects, the rule is that the idea and the leadership must come from a "clinician champion." This individual must be a force in the area to be reengineered and must be able to bring other clinicians along to follow his/her lead. No meeting can be held without the "clinician champion" present. This puts the leadership and responsibility for outcome clearly in the hands of one person who must bring a high degree of commitment to the project to even suggest its initiation. This is a unique model and one that bears watching for duplication at other centers.

It is true in AMCs, as in any other organization, that subjective views are an inevitable part of the decision-making process. Studies have shown that people's subjective or intuitive judgments tend to be biased and inaccurate.[23] Some of these biases include making predictions on only the available data, ignoring the basic laws of probability by estimating the likelihood of an event by the degree to which it is similar to other events, becoming entrapped by a previously chosen course of action, being unwilling to ignore sunk costs, etc.[24]

There are many techniques which are used to help groups make better decisions. Some are used informally by experienced practitioners. Some require special assistance such as consultants being hired to help groups work through tough decisions using these techniques.

Decision analysis is one of the tools that can be used to devise answers to problems of large import for an institution. As it is a time-consuming process, those who engage in it, whether with consultants or with in-house experts, should be prepared to act on the decision alternatives generated.

According to Ketchen and Thomas of Pennsylvania State University, the first step is framing the issue or defining the problem.[25] They stress that all stakeholders must help to define the problem or you can end up finding the right solution to the wrong problem. The next step is coming up with alternative courses of action. In this step, they use techniques to generate alternatives which are utilized in many other programs such as brainstorming, interviews, etc. The last step, and the most important, is to weigh the advantages and disadvantages of the various alternatives generated by using a weighted linear average. The aim of decision analysis is not necessarily to make a decision, but to help people involved to be creative, look at various probabilities, and realize that there is no one answer to a problem.

The idea of weighting advantages is used in many different decision-making techniques. This author has long used a device learned about in an earlier career in organization development. The Kepner-Tregoe grid is excellent for helping you to decide if gut feelings have any validity.[26] The technique works as follows. Say you are trying to decide where to spend your summer vacation. You have several ideas ranging from spending time at the beach, to fishing and boating in the mountains, to traveling to Paris and Provence, to visiting Washington, D.C. and historic Virginian homes. There are many criteria you want to meet for you to enjoy your vacation. These include spending no more than $3,000, enjoying the summer weather, getting exercise, seeing things you've never seen before, learning about new places, and relaxing. Satisfying some of these criteria is more important than others so you arrange them in weighted order from 6 to 1 across the top of your grid. You list the places to go on the left side of the grid.

Then you go through each place and put in the top half of a divided box, how this choice satisfies the criteria. For example, seeing Paris would rank a 10 for learning about new places (assuming you've never been to Paris before), but would probably get a 2 for relaxing, perhaps a 5 for exercise (assuming you're walking around the city) and a 1 for costing less than $3,000. The lake vacation would score high for exercise and cost and low for learning new things, etc. Once you have scored each box, you multiply the result by the weight you have given it, add across and you have found the answer to your question and made your decision! Hopefully, the answer will bear out what you really do want to do and you won't throw out the paper in disgust. This technique can be used in simple decisions in the workplace, is not time consuming and is a good guide to help give you direction.

We are all familiar with the hierarchical decision-making model which tends to be very department focused. This style can work well within a department, but can wreak havoc if its results stray beyond the borders of the unit. For example, the anesthesia department of an AMC wanted to redesign its record to include the charge voucher as an integral part of the record and eliminate the need for a separate document. To make this design change work, it was decided that the last page of the record (a three-part carbonless form which had become a throw-away), would be converted to the charge document thereby providing totally accurate data and reducing physician writing time in the operating room. The work in progress was shown to many people within the department and to the medical records committee of the hospital. The change was approved and the order was placed. After the new records were introduced, a frantic call was received from the obstetrics department. Where was the third copy of the anesthesia record which was put into the baby's chart? Obstetrics always gave the third copy to pediatrics and the second copy went into the mother's chart. Obviously one of the stakeholders had been overlooked - neither the OB anesthesiologist nor the OB department had been consulted on this matter which was seen as a totally departmental issue (except for medical records) and the decision was made without all of the needed input. The solution, although not thoroughly satisfying, was to retain the old three-part record for the obstetrics division with the OB anesthesiologist still filling out a separate billing voucher.

As described by Fargason and Haddock from the University of Alabama at Birmingham,[27] the use of cross-functional teams can reduce this type of error and result in higher quality, more long-lasting decisions. Multidisciplinary team decision-making will bring together more people and thereby more ideas, and hopefully better understanding of the problem and greater acceptance of the solution even if it is one which is not favored by all players. These types of approaches are indeed one of the cornerstones of the total quality improvement process.

Other techniques with which most readers are familiar include: brainstorming, which is not a decision making tool as much as it is a means to come up with alternative ideas in a non-threatening forum; and the nominal group technique where individuals who have thought about a question or problem privately write down their ideas, then take turns going around the room and presenting them. The listeners ask questions to gain clarification and when all ideas have been presented, they are ranked and voted on by secret ballot. The Delphi technique uses an iterative approach to getting to the best idea by voting and re-voting on ideas until the remaining choice becomes the evident winner.

The leadership exercised in any group or committee embarking on finding a decision to a knotty problem is critical. The best kind of leader will use informal authority to gain group support and to have his or her leadership and choice accepted without criticism.[28] There are times when managers or chief executives should not make a decision. This is particularly true when you are being pressured by those below and you feel you don't have all the information you need to move ahead. A leader must always think about the priorities of the institution and not give in to others who are looking at things from a narrower perspective. In situations like this, managers might have some tentative decisions made but keep their flexibility until the deadline. This will certainly give your subordinates a feeling that you can make decisions but that you are also after the best decision.[29]

In summary, we all know that decision-making is not an easy task in a large organization. There are conflicting needs, constrained resources, many points of view and often too many options to choose from. There are techniques that can be used to assist us in these efforts which are often overlooked. Sometimes, however, as in the megamergers, the will to decide is enough to generate movement. As we approach the 21st century, perhaps we can be optimistic that the pressure and the lessons of the 1990s will help the AMCs as they confront difficult decision-making in meeting the challenges ahead.

Figure 5.1

Intra-departmental decision-making roles of department administrator and chair

	ADMINISTRATOR	CHAIR
Personnel Recruitment and Retention	Within budget constraints, decides on size of staff and evaluates, promotes, terminates all administrative and clerical staff necessary to carry out dept. mission. Deals with unions where applicable.	Within budget constraints, decides on size of staff and recruits, selects, evaluates, promotes, terminates all physician and research faculty.
Space Utilization	Decides office space allocation for administrators and clerical staff in dept. designated space.	Decides office and lab space allocation for faculty in dept., designated space.
Salary Administration	Decides administrative, clerical and research staff salaries in accordance with medical center guidelines.	Decides salary, productivity, bonus plan for clinical faculty in accordance with medical center guidelines.
Purchasing	Decides and approves all day-to-day purchases; delegates approval authority as neecessary. Adheres to medical center guidelines foradditional signature authority.	Decides on and sets broad guidelines for purchasing needs of the dept.
Planning	Plans for administrative needs. Assists chair in long-range planning.	Works on long-range plans for direction of department. Decides on programs for research, residency recruitment.
Research	Provides staff to assist researchers; manage grants; knowledgeable on how to apply, implement NIH funds.	Decides on research agenda by selection of faculty; allocation of dollars; seeks grants.
Non-Clinical Time	Lets chair know cost of non-clinical time.	Awards non-clinical time to faculty based on established criteria; i.e., research, administrative duties.

References

1. Blumental, D. and Meyer, G.S., "Academic Health Centers in a Changing Environment," *Health Affairs*, 15(2), 200-215, 1996.
2. Rogers, M.C., "The Present and Future Impact of Market Forces on Academic Health Care Centers," presented at the APA meeting, April 28, 1996.
3. Blumenthal, D. and Meyer, G.S., "The future of the academic medical center under health care reform," *New England Journal of Medicine*, 1993:329:220:1-2.
4. DeBakey, M.D., "Medical centers of excellence and health reform, Science 1993:262:523-5.
5. Rogers, M., "Cultural and organizational implications of academic managed-care networks," *New England Journal of Medicine*, 1994:331:1374-1377.
6. Fox, P.D., and Wasserman, J., "Academic medical centers and managed care: uneasy partners," *Health Affairs* (Millwood) 1993:12(I):85-93.
7. Rogers, M., op cit.
8. Royer, T., APA *Matrix*, Summer 1996, 8-10.
9. Longshore, George, F., "Managing the Search Committee," *Healthcare Executive*, 29-31, May/June 1989.
10. Ibid.
11. *Academic Practice Management Survey:* 1996 Report Based on 1995 Data, Medical Group Management Association, Englewood, CO.
12. Finkelsteinm, K.E., "In money-saving move, Mt. Sinai and NYU plan hospital merger," *The New York Observer*, June 12, 1996, 1,21.
13. D'Aunno, T., Hoojibert, R., and F.C. Munson, "Decision-making, goal consensus, and effectiveness in university hospitals," *Hospital & Health Sciences Administration*, 36(4):505-523, 1991.
14. Levey, G.S., "Academic health centers: facing the new reality of a changing health care system., *American Journal of Medicine*. 1995:99:227-230.
15. Beck, L.C., "Your benchmark for decision-making: What's best for the company?" *The Physician's Advisory*, 93*4):8.
16. Latham, W., Jr., "Can your group make decisions?" *MGM Journal*, 89:36(4):23-24,26.
17. Ruelas, E. and Leatt, P., "The roles of physician executives in hospitals: A framework for management education," *Journal of Health Administration Education*, Spring 85:151-169.
18. Royer, T., "creating the culture for team building with physicians and administration," *APA Matrix*, 1996:(2):3, 8-10.
19. Ibid.
20. Friedman, E., "Physicians-Administrators Decision-Making," *Medical World News*, June 1986, 34-8, 40-3.
21. "Group decision making, approaches to problem solving," *Small Business Report*, 1988:13(7):30-33.

22. Kalogredis, V.J., "Groups need central authority to make decisions," *AMA News*, 1988, Mar.11, 31(10):17.
23. Chow, C.W. and K.M. Haddad, "Improving subjective decision making in health care administration," *Hospital and Health Services Administration*, Summer 91,36(2):191-210.
24. Ibid.
25. Ketchen, D.J. and J.B. Thomas, "Breaking down complex problems: the use of decision analysis," *Health Progress*, 1990,71(7):64-65,67.
26. Kepner, C.H., and B.B. Tregoe, "The rational manager: A systematic approach to problem solving and decision making," Kepner/Tregoe, Inc., Princeton, NJ, 2nd Edition, 1976.
27. Fargason, C.A. and C.C. Haddock, "Cross-functional, integrative team decision making: essential for effective QU in health care," *QRB*, 1992m18(5):157-163.
28. Alie, R.D., "Ethical issues in health care institutions," *Radiology Management*, 1991,20(20):1,8-9.

Chapter 6

Strategic planning

by Robert Slaton, EdD, FACMPE, and Michael Bowers, MBA, CPA

It seems that every academic medical center (AMC) is either developing, implementing or talking about a strategic plan. Why is this? Survival! Financial reality is driving this rush to develop strategic plans.

Why strategic planning is a hot topic

Rapid and profound change

Change is sweeping over the field of health care, and academic health care is no exception. Environmental forces are causing change in finance, operations, and relationships within academic medical centers. Coping with these changes requires action. Yesterday's lucrative payment process is gone. In its place are new payment mechanisms that demand more service at lower reimbursement rates, while at the same time requiring that quality be documented as never before.

Historically the patient base of the AMC was conceded; now it is competed for - sometimes ruthlessly. It used to be that patients with good insurance and/or money could go wherever they wanted without any controls. In many cases they sought out the AMC because of the perception of high quality. Today, at the direction of their carriers, many of these patients are diverted to specific providers outside the AMC.

On the other end of the social spectrum, many of the centers' patients (Medicaid recipients and the indigent) were not considered desirable by other providers. In managed care plans, Medicaid becomes an attractive payer for outside organizations. Academic medical centers must now compete to keep these patients. The indigent is the only population now conceded to them.

But health care is different!

Those of us in health care who have smugly stated for years that health care is different are getting a wake-up call. In the June 1996 issue of "Integrated Health Care Report," John L. Miller stated that "In today's supercharged competitive market such industries as retailing, computer technology, defense and health care all share the same challenge - to provide a better product at less cost....After decades of inefficiency, the health care industry is facing the same pressures that other industries have had to address over the last 10 years."

In banking before deregulation, it was hard not to make money. The federal government, in its regulation of banking, required banks to charge two percent more in interest than was paid out for the use of money. In health care it was much the same. It wasn't just the government, but all payers who virtually assured a *profit.*

Providers were paid on a *fee-for-services* basis for whatever they did. The providers set the fees. The payers paid on a usual-and-customary basis. Providers raised their fees annually, and payers kept paying more each year. It was the rare provider who got fees so high as to attract concern from the payers. When occasionally criticism was heard from the business community, a carrier, the government or a consumer group, the system responded with "health care is extremely complicated, and you just don't understand. . . . "

"In the good old days," only very inefficient banking or health care organizations had financial problems. But the world is changing. The lessons of banking are now being applied to health care.

Quick–do something

Health care is faced with rapid change. There is no choice but to do *something.* One of the somethings that everyone is *doing* is *strategic planning.* Strategic planning is becoming as much a part of the language of AMCs as "curriculum revision" or "focusing on primary care."

An academic departmental business manager was told once by a management consultant that another major client, a sheet metal fabricator, was having similar problems–but that organization is handling them better. A rude awakening for the administration. Administrators in AMCs, university hospitals and faculty practice groups are suddenly supposed to know all about strategic planning. It's not quite socially acceptable to ask *"what is strategic planning"*? It's as if this fairly new endeavor has fallen from the sky and we must find an expert to do it for us.

What is strategic planning?

Just what is different about strategic planning from any other planning? Our answer is, less than many people want us to think.

The term comes from the military term strategy which is defined as a detailed plan for reaching a goal or an advantage. So strategic planning is *goal-oriented planning.* But isn't all planning goal oriented? Yes, at some point, but as will be discussed, too often doing the plan becomes the goal. In today's environment, strategic planning does not mean moving toward a clear goal, but instead strategic planning is a way to identify and capitalize on emerging opportunities. More about this later.

Long-term planning

As one reviews the literature it is obvious that most writers have viewed strategic planning as being long term. Mazanes identifies the strategic planning process as focusing on establishing an organization's long-term direction. However, it is now being noted that "long term" isn't as long as it used to be. Health care is changing so rapidly that planning must be flexible, and must focus on shorter periods than in the past.

Jackson et al, states that "change is happening so quickly in our industry that to predict the future any farther than 18 months (at least to predict it accurately) is nearly impossible." Following an out-of-date strategic plan, as if it were *holy writ*, is a sure prescription for disaster. As the environment changes, the plan must change.

Shea agrees and notes that strategic planning has historically implied long term (which she says, "many people define as five, ten or even twenty years"). She adds that multi-year planning is no longer meaningful. Mazanes sees strategic plans as covering three to five years, but notes that plans must be reviewed on an ongoing basis.

The relationship to business planning

We recognize that experts do not agree on the relationship between strategic planning and business planning, or even that there is a difference. What some call a business plan, others call a strategic plan, and vice versa. Beck states that people use long-range planning, business planning and strategic planning interchangeably.

Is strategic planning the same as business planning? The answer, to us, is NO.

Strategic planning should be completed first and is usually conducted at the highest level of the organization. In an academic practice, this is the medical center (or health sciences center) which may be comprised of the schools of medicine, nursing, dentistry and allied health as well as one or more university hospitals.

Business planning is conducted after the strategic planning is completed. It relies heavily on the departments of the institution and will include strategic programs and other initiatives intended to accomplish the strategic objectives of the organization. Finally, program planning is carried out at the operational level within the departmental sub-units (see Figure 6.1).

Figure 6.1

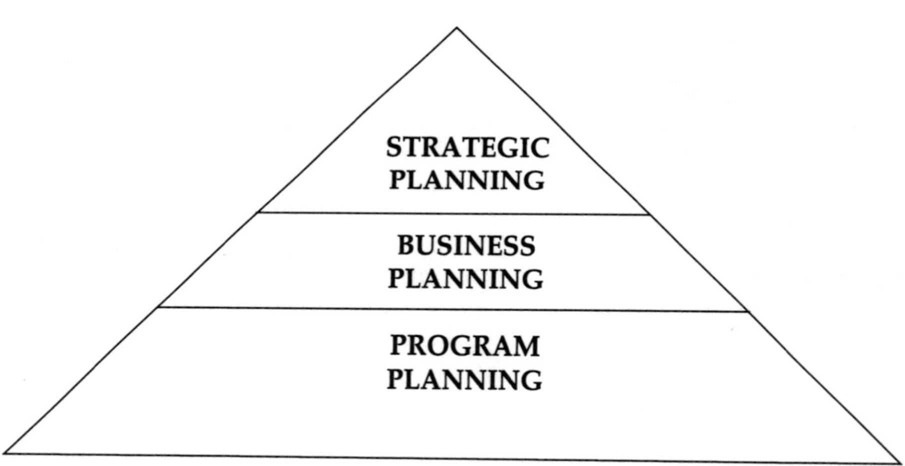

Strategic planning - At the institutional level, the primary strategic task is to develop a strategy for diverse activities by providing a balance set of "legs" for the medical center - a balance between education, research and patient care. The institution will be primarily focused on identifying resource flows to and from the various schools and departments and on providing a strategy for improving the quality of performing activities and delivering services. A key issue in the strategic planning process is the assessment of risk which will significantly impact the eventual allocation of resources among departments, programs and activities.

Business planning - At the departmental, or business unit level, the primary strategic task is to determine how resources will be obtained and utilized to achieve the strategic goals of the institution while carrying out the mission of the organization. Development of strategic programs and implementation is the primary focus at the departmental level.

Program planning - Following this planning structure, program planning occurs at the sub-departmental level and is primarily focused on operations.

Strategic planning finds the academic medical center

Once upon a time, not so long ago (although it seems like a lifetime), those of us in academic medicine did not talk about strategic plans or strategic planning. However, during the 1980s, strategic planning in AMCs spread across the country like a virus.

It was, to say the least, an odd fit because of the uniquely different evolution of the university and of the practice of medicine. The strange mix of lucrative cash flow, tenure and academic freedom created a complicated world of interrelated, overlapping and competing *fiefdoms* all presided over by princes with varying power – usually related to money.

Limitations

Strategic planning, as we shall show later, requires a high degree of candor on the part of the participants to be successful – candor about capability, financial reserves, goals, motivations, etc. As we know, candor has not always been in style in AMCs. Instead, frequently, contentiousness has existed when anyone attempted to get various fiefdoms to work together. Tremendous battles have raged over the differing motivations and competing interests.

This is compounded by the way that university planning has evolved over time, by the typical physician disdain for planning, and by experience with government-mandated health planning.

University planning - Universities evolved over the centuries as isolated, usually slow moving, thoughtful entities where detailed processes for doing any and everything (usually VERY detailed processes) were viewed as sacred. Planning in these institutions developed in a complicated bureaucratic, ritualistic way. This planning process produced periodic tomes of little relevance to day-to-day operations. Plans took a long time to develop and were difficult to change.

Physician planning - Conversely, physician practice evolved as *mom-and-pop* operations in which the owner was on site constantly and oversaw every detail of the operation. No one else needed to think. To the extent that planning existed, it was *seat of the pants* by the owner. These independent strong-willed physicians who entered academic practice were forced into a seemingly endless, and to them, irrelevant process. The typical reaction of the physician was to not participate or to be disrespectful of the process.

Health planning - Planning became a dirty word to hospitals and medical professionals as a result of their experience with government-directed *health planning* in the 1970s. That planning was seen as being directed at limiting expenditures. Academic medical centers were constantly dealing with the question "Do we need a Certificate of Need"?

Academic medical center planning

As a result, planning responsibility was abdicated by academic physicians to either the university or to the teaching hospital(s). Planning in AMCs had little buy-in from the medical school faculty, but was viewed as something that administration had to do at set intervals.

Plans developed in this context sat on shelves somewhere and were only looked at when the university asked for an update. At that point someone in administration was asked to review the plan and draft a response for the dean. Once the update was completed, the whole thing was forgotten until the next request came, at which time the process was repeated.

Strategic challenges to the tripartite missions

The tripartite missions of the AMC consisting of education, research and patient care create special challenges that private practices do not face. This situation is the cause of many debates among clinical and research faculty and, without a skillful leader, can render the faculty unable to communicate with each other and unwilling to pursue goals that are contained in the strategic plan. One challenge having a major impact is the transition of most major population centers to managed care with specific effects on each component of the mission.

Education - Managed care has constrained faculty patient care collections, a critical source of funding for the AMC. In many instances, it has reduced the patient base below the level required for adequate teaching about patient care. The demands of this new environment for lower cost and utilization controls creates new challenges in the teaching environment. What has become obvious in many markets is the realization by AMCs that their academic reputation is not valued in the delivery of routine patient care.

Research - Managed care, and the competition it has spawned among health care providers has introduced, and in fact mandated, patient-friendly service requirements which serve to constrain an emphasis on research. Significantly, no longer can research costs be shifted onto private payers. This results in increasing demands for federal and private research funding at a time of economic shifting and downsizing by most governmental agencies and private businesses.

Patient care - Managed care and the mandate for patient-oriented delivery of care, has resulted in a greater demand for services to be delivered in the communities where patients live, not at the inner-city location of so many AMCs. In addition, larger groups of patients are being channeled away from faculty physicians and hospitals by managed care plans due to the high-cost image of academic practice. Finally, AMCs are losing patients to more organized physician groups and hospital systems. Bureaucracy and the lack of effective governance in academic practice is a major disadvantage cited by managed care executives.

Examples of academic plan strategies

As a result of the changing health care environment, academic practices across the country are examining their strategies for achieving their missions. While the strategic planning process will be discussed in detail later in this chapter, we want to focus briefly on how environmental changes should trigger a review of goals, the possible setting of new goals and finally the development or revision of operating plans. As Figure 6.2 illustrates, this creates a ripple effect - like throwing a pebble in a pond. Action in the middle necessitates change in all directions.

Figure 6.2

Analytical Steps
- Developing Strategies -

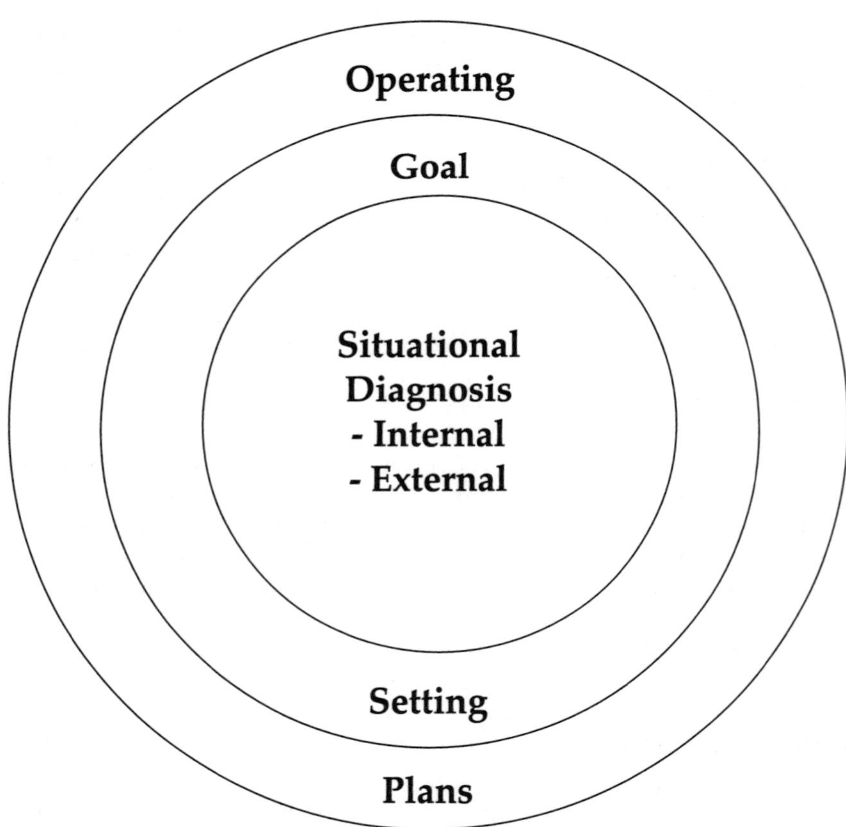

Described below are some examples of the types of strategic goals being pursued as a result of the environmental change to wellness-focused, value-managed health care.

- One West Coast AMC is aiming to provide joint managed care contracting for all clinical departments and hospitals. It plans to facilitate joint marketing of hospitals and clinical services and to build an efficient primary care and ambulatory care system;

- A Midwestern AMC is creating a multi-hospital health care system and expanding the primary care physician base. It also is developing a proprietary health plan;

- Another Midwestern AMC has a goal to develop new practice sites for training and patient care and to secure its speciality referral base;

- A Northeastern AMC is focusing solely on establishing a strong primary care base covering its regional communities to provide this essential component for managed care purposes, to enhance the ability to channel patients within the network, and to utilize these sites for student and resident education; and

- A mid-Atlantic AMC is focusing geographically on the very local, local, regional and statewide markets. These specific strategies exist for the various markets:

  Very local - re-recruiting specialist who left for community hospitals;
  Local - matching market price for secondary referrals;
  Regional - creating a delivery system to access large numbers of patients; and
  Statewide - expanding the centers of excellence speciality contracts.

The real world

Suddenly in the 1990s AMCs found themselves in need of plans - relevant plans; plans to gain or keep market share, plans to obtain covered lives, plans to bury the competition, in effect plans for survival. Neither the university nor the medical school faculty group, in most cases, had the expertise to develop such plans. They also each lacked credibility, one with the other. Suddenly health care consulting became a major growth industry as organizations in need started looking for help.

The strategic planning process

To us, the steps in the strategic planning process are: organizing, developing a mission statement, conducting a situational analysis, setting goals, developing business plans, developing a financial plan and writing the document (see Figure 6.3). There is nothing sacred about these steps and other writers/consultants offer slight variations. However, in nearly all cases the steps are essentially the same.

Figure 6.3

The Strategic Planning Process

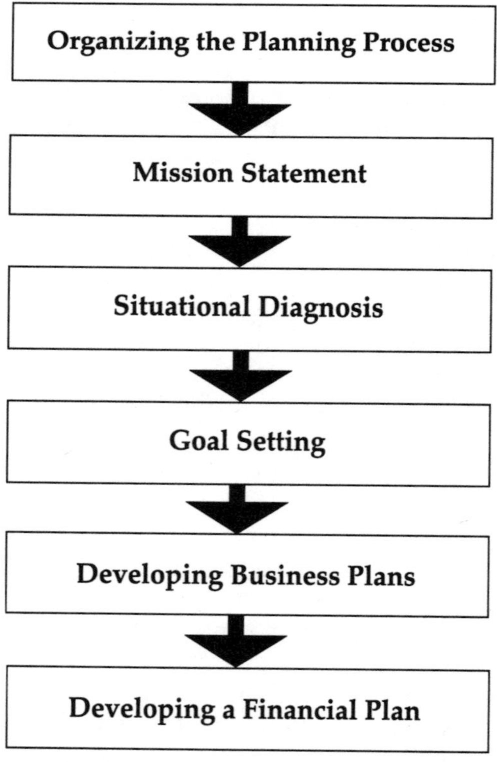

Organizing the planning process

The first step in organizing the process is to get help. Structural conflict makes it necessary to get an outside facilitator. Trying to do a strategic plan for your own organization is like physicians trying to treat themselves or their families. You cannot be as objective as is necessary and you will not have the credibility needed. On the other hand, you do not need to spend ten zillion dollars on the effort and you certainly do not want to abdicate to a consultant.

In the past, with buckets of money spilling all over AMCs, price was not an issue. There was a certain amount of prestige in saying which big name firm you had engaged and how much you had spent on your strategic plan. Today more and more of us in health care are learning frugality - welcome to the American business world that everyone else in business (except defense contractors) has understood for a long time. By the way, one consultant once said that a strategic plan can cost whatever you have to spend. Some questions to ask when considering a consultant are:

> How do you find the right consultant/facilitator? Use your network, call your peers, ask MGMA. In many cases it is worth the cost and time to develop a request for proposal (RFP) and go through a structured selection process. It may even be worth getting a consultant (who will not bid on the job) to draft the RFP. Notice that we said *draft*, not write. Everything written by a consultant should be a draft. Finalization should always rest with the contracting organization;
>
> Commitment - It is important to remember that no consultant/facilitator can help an organization in which leadership does not agree that there is a need to change. No one can save an organization from itself, unless it is committed to being saved; and
>
> Stay involved - Selecting a consultant/facilitator is just the first step in the process. Don't abdicate; doing a strategic plan is not something that an "expert" can do properly in a vacuum. Institutions which turn the process over to outside consultants and let them do whatever they want usually live to regret their decision. The ideal approach is to see yourself as the prime contractor who will select sub-contractors as needed and monitor their work closely.

Who is 'we'?

It is useful to look at planning as figuring out how we get from here to there. This approach introduces one new element to the traditional process - it introduces "we." While it's always implicit in other definitions, it's important to place major emphasis on who is involved.

In developing a strategic plan the first thing to clarify is *who are you?* By this we mean, what is the administrator's role, responsibility, authority, etc? Review exactly where you fit in what organization. This analysis must include an honest assessment of what others view your role to be.

The next question is *who else needs to be involved?* Plans cannot be very valuable if developed in a vacuum. Everything is interrelated.

Departmental administrators, faculty practice managers or administrators, health science center administrators, and university administrators are all involved today with each other, and with outside organizations, to an unprecedented extent. The pressures on health care are creating the need to get bigger, to merge, acquire, sell, buy, to create systems. If we are not able to redefine we, planning will be unrealistic.

Historically there has been great mistrust within academic medicine. Competing interests and conflicting values existed all over the landscape. The department hid things (usually having to do with money) from the dean and (vice versa). The school hid things from central administration (and vice versa), and the chairs hid things from faculty (and vice versa). No one trusted anyone else. Frequently heard lines include, *what are they up to, don't let the fox in the henhouse, or simply I don't trust them.*

We believe that this fear must be overcome, and relationships of trust must be established that are much broader than we are used to. Otherwise plans developed will have little relevancy and little chance of success. If you are not willing to let others be part of we, don't bother to plan; in fact, don't bother to read any further in this chapter. Skip to the next one.

<u>The mission (or vision/mission statement)</u> - Where is *"there"?* Clearly a mission statement is critical. However some experts start with a vision statement which means a statement of where you want your organization to be at some future point in time. Vision statements are *we are* statements. They are statements from the future looking back. They force you to say *what you want to be.* Some examples:

"We are the premier academic medical center within ____ miles";

"We are the center of excellence for _____"; and

"We are the most efficient academic medical center in the entire region."

The mission statement then becomes a *we will* statement. They are looking forward statements. They answer the question *what do we want to do*? Examples:

"We will become an integrated delivery system";

"We will develop a primary care network";

"We will bury the competition" (who by the way, has a consultant working on plans to bury you);

"We will survive" (What does "*survival*" mean - that you have a job, that your institution exists in five years, or that the teaching, research and service mission is still being met?);

"We will make this the best managed medical center in America"; and

"We will obtain X number of covered lives."

Without a vision statement the mission statement becomes a combination of the two. In either case, the purpose is to clearly articulate where you want to be at some future point.

An example of not knowing where there is: A health care system spends $1.3 million on a strategic plan and sets out methodically to follow it. Within one year the market changes, but the plan does not. While following the old plan step-by-step, the organization gets further from reality. It is trying to go to a *there* that is no longer relevant.

The situational diagnosis - where is here?

Do we really understand where we are? Are we in touch with reality? (Was it Lily Tomlin who said that "reality is just society's collective hunch?") Do we have the data to support our perception of reality? How do you determine where here is? The foundation of any strategic planning process is to understand the current external environment and its potential impact on the AMC and on the academic practice plan. This process is referred to as situational diagnosis.

All diagnosis, assessment, or analysis must be based on data, not on opinion. The components of a situation analysis can differ depending upon the target market and the specific practice plan. However, the following components are usually necessary to provide a comprehensive look at the environment and the practice plan's position in it:

> Demographics - The demographic profile of the practice plan's service areas contains important information about the population in terms of age, sex and socioeconomic data. A comparison should be made to the plan's existing patient profile to determine if it reflects the general population profile and, if not, why;
>
> Providers - A comprehensive listing should be compiled of all physicians by speciality, age and service area (location) to understand who and where the providers are. These data may provide insight into threats or opportunities later in the *strategic planning* process. In addition, attention should be focused on provider consolidations and affiliations (both physician and hospital) which may affect the ability to achieve the geographic coverage necessary for managed care purposes. Finally, obtain any information made publicly available regarding the financial conditions of hospitals and medical groups. A review of the financial statements may reveal debt to equity positions, debt service requirements, and excess funds available; and
>
> Health care purchasers - This group consists of managed care plans and large self-insured employers who purchase service directly from providers. Market share data is available from the state department of insurance and can be calculated for self-insured employers by obtaining employment data from local business journals. Opportunities and threats can be determined with an understanding of these data.

An example of not knowing where here is: A hospital decides it needs a primary care base and decides to buy practices. It does this without really understanding the mentality of the referring physician community and offends hundreds of referring physicians, who form an alternative group and refer elsewhere.

A bad trip

Without properly defining *here* and *there*, it is highly unlikely that any trip will be worthwhile, or that any planning will be successful. It's as if you have been kidnapped, blindfolded, transported around, placed in a car and told to go home. If you don't know where you are, any decision about which way to drive is a guess. You may or may not be moving closer to your goal. If there was not agreement about *here* in the President's efforts to reform health care, there was certainly a lack of agreement on *there*. The goals of health care reform were not clear to major constituencies or to the public. Was the intent for every American to have health insurance, or was it for everyone to have health care?

Tradition

While data is essential, so is dialogue. It is essential that key decision-makers participate and communicate. An organization in which leaders do not tell the unvarnished truth to each other is an institution in serious trouble. All cards need to be on the table face up. No matter how much strategic planning is desired, there are two attributes of academic medicine that get in the way of the kind of planning needed today - the traditions of independence and structural conflict. These can be described in this way:

> Independence. An interesting image of the academic medical center is to visualize 20 or so very expensive high powered cars barreling toward a cliff with each driver oblivious to the cliff or to the other cars. The successful strategic plan requires that they all stop their cars and get on a bus together and take a different road. Unfortunately many of the drivers are in denial. To plan strategically we must first get their attention, then help them get past denial. If they persist in denial, all the strategic planners in the world cannot save them;
>
> Structural conflict. Because of the independence of various entities, structural conflict frequently exists within AMCs. Too often, what is perceived as good for one entity (in the short run), may not be good for another. To overcome this conflict, the participants must understand that they are about to *go over a cliff and splatter on the rocks below* if they do not work together in unprecedented ways and dramatically change their behavior.

Such built-in structural conflict can only be resolved with help from the outside.

Goal setting

Goals are statements of major things to be done to achieve the articulated mission/vision. Goals cannot be precise. At best, in today's environment, a strategic plan offers a way to respond to opportunities and to make intelligent guesses as to what opportunities will look like next month or next year. Goals are the way we get from here to there. Each major goal becomes an area for a business plan. Sample goal examples for the mission - *We want X number of covered lives*:

1. To enroll at least 20 percent of the employees of ABC Company;
2. To capture X percent of a Medicaid managed care patients by XX/XX/XX; or
3. To participate in a Medicare risk product.

Opportunity or problem?

A large manufacturing firm approached an academic practice with a request to do pre-employment physicals. The manufacturer offered an opportunity, but not one recognized by the practice group. The manufacturer wanted a physician on-site to perform physicals and decide on the spot whether an applicant could go to work. The practice wanted a few candidates per day to come to the office between the hours of 8 and 11 a.m. or 1 and 3 p.m, except on Tuesday morning or Thursday afternoon.

Guess what, the manufacturer contracted with a physician group in the community and the academic physician group continued to look for ways to survive. The new opportunity was too different from their perception of how things should be done for them to even consider responding. They could not grasp the idea of leaving their large building, driving across town and doing what the customer wanted. As of today they are still looking for customers.

Developing business plans

Each goal in a strategic plan should result in a set of objectives each of which should become the subject of a business plan. These objectives become the items on which effort is focused on a daily basis. Example of objectives for the first goal above:

1. To establish evening/weekend hours to increase our accessibility; and/or
2. To establish a marketing program designed to reach our target population (you are marketing to get covered lives).

As with the vision and/or mission, goals and objectives should be developed in a structured process with a facilitator.

Developing financial plans

If the budget doesn't follow the plan, the plan won't be implemented. Plans are nice, but usually meaningless unless appropriate funding underlies the plan. Likewise, if the numbers don't work, the plan won't be successful. There is no point in developing a strategic plan that you can't afford.

Get your own house in order - A strategic plan without buy-in and support is going nowhere. So take these steps:

1. Be sure the budget follows the plan;
2. Go where the money is, go where the patients are. As traditional sources of patients and revenue continue to shrink, look for new ones - jails, state departments of corrections, worker's compensation, managed care, etc.;
3. Make a commitment to long-term to change. A strategic plan must reflect a commitment to significant change in the organization;
4. Look for a win/win. Plans call for change. Changes is painful. Try to minimize the number of losers, and try to find ways to help those who lose; and
5. If the deal looks too good to be true, it probably is.

Techniques

SWOT/SWOP - We are all familiar with the SWOT analysis - strengths, weaknesses, opportunities, threats. Many consultants use it just that way, while others do only strengths and weakness (folding threats and opportunities into one of them). Another calls it SWOP (strengths, weaknesses, opportunities and problems). Whatever it is called, the technique is a useful way to analyze the situation.

Nominal group process. One of the simplest techniques for doing planning is nominal group process. The participants sit around a table. The facilitator goes around asking each person to state one item, issue, etc., on the topic at hand. Each person can list only one on each turn. The process continues until everyone has listed everything they can think of. The facilitator then starts grouping items and condensing the list. The group then votes on the ranking. Invariably, someone will not vote for an item that they listed. They will have seen that other things are far more important. This is a simple and almost foolproof system for identifying and prioritizing key issues IF you have the right facilitator.

Small groups. Another simple but effective technique for a larger organization is to have a facilitator meet with everyone in small groups and hear their concerns, ideas, etc. After a complete cycle, the facilitator combines in a short report all the items listed and goes back through another round of meetings. In the second round, the groups react to the report. In these sessions nominal group process is always used to prevent anyone from dominating the outcome or of anyone not participating. It is important to be inclusive not exclusive.

What to do to make your plan successful

Be flexible

Relevant planning must be seen as the art of the possible, not a road map to a certain destination. You cannot control the outcome; it's a moving target. Don't follow it too closely. Don't substitute activity for accomplishment.

Don't copy

Just because everybody is doing it doesn't mean it's right for you. After all, the old joke is that once you've seen one medical school (or one teaching hospital), you've seen one medical school (or one teaching hospital). Why should someone else's solution work for you? It's possible that a lot of people could be following one "cookie cutter" plan down the wrong path.

Listen

Talking less and listening more facilitates dialogue. You don't have to say everything that you know and feel. If you take a deep breath and listen, someone else may say what you wanted to say. Try not to feel the need to say it yourself or repeat what they said. The worst offender is the person who waits for the other person to stop talking then says essentially the same thing they just said. It seems they have no realization that the other person has already said the same thing.

Communicate

It must be clear to the reader that we think relationships are the most important aspect of the planning. Doing anything is relatively easy, once relationships are worked out. If there is a relationship between two or more parties and if they maintain dialogue, they can plan together. If there is not a relationship or if dialogue stops, then meaningful planning is not possible.

Give feedback

An important way to enhance communication is by giving frequent feedback. This enables listeners to be sure that what they thought they heard is what the speakers thought they said. It is important to hold regular and frequent participatory review meetings because things are changing so rapidly.

The paradigm has shifted

At the broadest level, health care delivery and financing is undergoing a fundamental shift away from managing episodes of illness toward managing the health of a defined population on a proactive basis. The strategic implication is now well known among health care executives and is often referred to as a paradigm shift.

The *historical paradigm* consisted of treating illness after onset as an episode of care. Optimum performance was focused on the individual physician provider and clinical efficacy was measured at the time of intervention. Hospitals were at the center of the delivery system. Utilization, necessity and other health care decisions were at the sole discretion of the physician.

One Revolution: Managing the Academic Medical Practice in an Era of Rapid Change

Under the *new paradigm* of managing health, the focus is on the health status of specific populations. Optimum performance is measured on the entire health care delivery system, with primary care physicians at the center of the system. Clinical efficacy is driven by prevention and minimally interventionist methods, in addition to clinical efficiency at the time of the intervention. Utilization and medical necessity are based upon shared physician group values, protocols and shared incentives.

Strategic planning that recognizes this paradigm shift enables your organization to identify and capitalize on opportunities that are nothing like you have ever seen before. Looking for yesterday's opportunities or adhering to a plan designed for yesterday dooms you to fail. Academic medicine is not moving on a fixed path to a clear goal in a stable environment.

There isn't ONE strategy. Look at what others have done, assess your own situation, and modify your activities to do what makes sense. AMCs that do not change are in grave danger of becoming marginalized instead of being major players. Tremendous power and major egos are at stake. The vice president, the dean, the chairs, division directors, departmental administrators, faculty and staff must meet the challenge of playing in a new game or becoming irrelevant fringe players.

References

Books

Annison, Michael H., *Managing the whirlwind,* Englewood, CO: Medical Group Management Association, 1993.

Jackson, Clyde, et al, *Caught-in-the-middle management: taking care of yourself and your organization.* Englewood, CO: Medical Group Management Association, 1996.

Lorange, Peter, *Corporate planning and executive viewpoint.* Englewood Cliffs, NJ: Prentiss-Hall, Inc. (1980)

Senge, Peter M., *The fifth discipline: the art and practice of the learning organization.* New York: Currency Doubleday. (1994)

Slaton, Robert, et. al, *From green persimmons to cranky parrots; practice management axioms to live by.* Englewood, CO: Medical Group Management Association, (1993)

Journal Articles and Professional Papers

"Strategic planning is critical." *American Medical News* 35(18):13,15, May 11, 1992.

Miller, John L., "How virtuous is "virtual" integration?" *Integrated Health Care Report,* June 1996.

"Developing your practices' business plan." *The Management Consultant's Advisory,* July 1984.

"Strategic planning." *Journal of AHIMA* 64(1): January 1993.

Bouchard, Eric A., "Management tools." *Radiology Management* 16(3): 10-12, Summer 1994.

Moldof, Edwin P., "Do it yourself strategic planning provides map to the future." *Health Care Financial Management* 48(2):27-31, February 1994.

Shea, William F., "Market planning - competitive advantage." *Group Practice Managed Health Care News* 10(10):28,35, October 1994.

Rich, Stanley R. And Gumpert, David E., "How to write a business plan. "*Harvard Business Review* 63(3): 156-158, 160, 166, May-June 1985.

Jackson. Clyde W.," Strategic planning: how to envision your company's future."

Clark, Brendly and Boissoneau, Robert, "Strategic planning and the health care supervisor." *The Health Care Supervisor* 14(2):1-10, December 1995.

"Planning your year for profitability." *Cronomikes Report* 13(8):4-5, March 1994.

"From involvement to results: 10 secrets of successful market-based strategic planning." *Health Care Strategic Management,* April 1994.

Yarington, C. Thomas, "Implementation tough in strategic planning." *MGM Update* 33(2): 15, February 1994.

Beard, Philip L., "How to capture market share while your competition sleeps." ProSTAT Resources Group.

Chapter 7

The business plan for the academic clinical department

by Nancy M. Rhodes, MPH, and Paul M. Purcell, MBA

A business plan clearly defines what an academic clinical department intends to accomplish, how and when this will take place, and who will be held accountable. While a strategic plan defines the goals and mission of the department, the business plan addresses implementation of the strategic plan and production of short-term results. It defines the day-to-day operations that the faculty, administrative staff and clinical staff must perform to achieve the department's goals. Business plans may address programs at the division, subdivision, or physician level, or initiatives across divisions or departments. Ideally, perhaps, all aspects of an academic clinical department's work would be organized under carefully constructed and regularly updated business plans. In practice, however, most departments' business plans are developed as part of proposals to secure funding or other resources. Figure 7.1, therefore, presents the elements of a typical business plan as they might appear in a formal proposal or application for funding.

It is assumed that the reader will be able to develop the straightforward aspects of a business plan simply from the outline. This chapter will focus on business plan issues specific to the academic health care industry, particularly those which make developing and implementing business plans more complex. Topics will include general obstacles as well as the integration of the business plan with various institutional components.

Figure 7.1

Elements of a Business Plan

1. Executive Summary

2. Background

   Purpose of this particular initiative
   Historical perspective/relevant past experience

3. Product/Services to be offered

   General trends and characteristics of such an initiative
   Uniqueness of this initiative

4. Marketing, Target Customers, Competition

5. Proposed Management Structure

   Rationale and integration with existing structures
   Authority for making decisions
   Competencies required
   Specific skills of individuals required for the initiative

6. Marketing Strategies

   Short- and long-term strategies
      Market penetration
      Growth
      Distribution
   Marketing staff
   Marketing materials

7. Operations -- how customers will access and use

   Programmatic and financial goals
      Services to be provided directly; those to be obtained through vendors
      Key statistics to be monitored
   Implementation plan
   Projection of program growth

Figure 7.1

Elements of a Business Plan (Continued)

Facilities
Staff
Equipment
Supplies
Major leases/contracts
Evaluation of customer satisfaction
Research and development
Distribution of profit

8. Financial Pro Forma for five years or until financial goals have been met

Past relevant financial performance
Assumptions regarding future expenses and revenues
Funding of start-up costs and deficits, if any
Distribution of profits

General obstacles

The longevity factor

Academic clinical departments as well as their parent institutions typically have a long tradition of providing educational and clinical services. The first medical school, and thus the first academic clinical department, were established in 1765 at the University of Pennsylvania.[1] This longevity fosters the perspective that academic clinical departments are essential and will always be needed to maintain the overall vitality of the parent institution. However, this myopic perspective fails to shield a department from the internal and external changes that threaten its identity, prosperity and even its existence.[2] Furthermore, it clouds the development and implementation of meaningful business plans.

Academic clinical departments are also often marked by an air of superiority in which they view themselves as the pacesetters – those who set the standards which others must attain. This view may be partially justified by their cutting-edge research and their innovative clinical techniques. However, except for the small number of truly rare or especially complex cases, the advantages of an academic clinical department over a competent, non-academic clinical department may not be apparent or persuasive to patients, insurors, or employers who are purchasing health insurance benefits.

Community hospitals: friends or foes?

A business plan for a new program has to be developed within the context of the physical and cultural environment in which it will operate. Increasingly, academic medical centers (AMCs) are viewed as the setting of choice for only unusual or extremely serious conditions.[3] In many markets, community hospitals are viewed as more friendly and responsive to the needs of patients, family members and physicians.[4] Few patients have the ability to distinguish between the education and background of different providers. Most, however, understand easy physical access to the health care facility, parking, the availability of appointments within a reasonable time period, short waiting times on the day of their visits, clean facilities and good food. AMCs often do not compete favorably in these areas. In addition, community hospitals near AMCs are frequently staffed by graduates of the medical center's training programs. Consequently, patients do not have to choose between excellent physicians, patient-oriented services and amenities. Business plans, therefore, must state their assumptions about the impact of these factors on their initiatives.

Community hospitals serve as important training sites for academic clinical departments. They are critical to a department's ability to provide strong educational programs characterized by training in ambulatory settings, a wide variety of cases, high volume, a high level of disease severity, and a high level of surgical complexity. Many community hospitals have new or recently renovated ambulatory facilities which offer opportunities for training residents in outpatient medical and surgical services in this increasingly popular and cost-effective milieu. Their extensive patient base is also becoming more important for clinical research initiatives, including the development and use of critical pathways for the entire process of treating a disease and the collection of data related to long-term patient outcomes.

However, what may further the educational objectives of a department may at the same time undermine its ability to compete effectively. The presence of residents at community hospitals makes it attractive for private practitioners to practice at the hospital because of the availability of the residents for on-call responsibilities and for assistance with rounds. These hospitals frequently market themselves as affiliated with the AMC and thus the AMC's reputation as an exclusive facility is lost. In addition, community hospitals may be affiliated with more than one academic institution. The relationships between the AMC and the community hospitals may change abruptly based on changes in the ownership of the hospitals. A business plan needs to take into consideration these positive and negative factors. Relationships with affiliated community hospitals should be viewed as tenuous. Decisions to share information related to new initiatives should be done with the knowledge that the community hospital may at a point in the not distant future become a key competitor.

Technological advances

Technological advances pose another obstacle to the development of sound business plans for an academic clinical department. These advances can erode the academic clinical department's unique identity and role. A business plan's projections that patients in a given geographic area will participate in a new technologically-advanced initiative are frequently based on the assumption that the program is unique and will remain unique and that patients are restricted geographically in their access to health care. Technological advances have meant, however, that community hospitals can safely perform relatively complex procedures such as coronary artery bypass surgery with good outcomes. The time during which a procedure formerly under the purview of the academic clinical department is transported to community hospitals can be as short as the time until the resident who trained in this technique completes his or her residency and is recruited by the community hospital.

Technological advances also mean that procedures formerly under the domain of one department are now performed by another department. For example, interventional radiology and invasive cardiology have provided alternatives to surgical interventions. Patients with varicoceles can undergo an interventional radiology procedure rather than urological surgery. Patients with a blockage in their hearts can undergo ablation procedures rather than cardiac surgery. Currently surgical departments' revenues are only minimally affected by these changes, but an additional erosion of surgical revenue should be expected. Business plans must acknowledge the effect of technological advances in other specialties on the department's proposed initiative.

Technological advances have also meant that telemedicine opportunities are rapidly expanding. This will serve to increase the competition among AMCs because geographic boundaries will not serve as the barriers that they did previously. An example of the effective implementation of telemedicine is the Mayo Clinic's development of satellite operations in Jacksonville, FL, in 1986 and in Scottsdale, AZ, in 1987.[5] Remote consultations are conducted on a daily basis in real time via satellites between the two remote locations and the parent institution in Rochester, MN. Numerous medical centers have also developed various bulletins or news items for the public which are available via the Internet. The business plan's assumptions about which patients will utilize the new program must take these technological advances into account.

Revenue projections – how accurately can the past predict the future?

The development of a sound business plan for an academic clinical department is predicated upon accurate projections of departmental or programmatic revenue. Clinical department administrators are responsible for developing business plans which accurately predict their departments' or programs' expected revenues and are accountable to their department chairs and the medical centers' senior managers for meeting these projections. As will be discussed later, clinical department administrators may also be expected to include projections of hospital revenue in their business plans.

The sources of revenue that must be considered are listed in Figure 7.2. Although revenue from professional services is difficult to predict, accurate projections are critical to the development of meaningful business plans. The matter of identifying appropriate sources of revenue for the business plan is complicated by the fact that lower payments by insurors have decreased the clinical revenue base of academic clinical departments at the same time other sources of funding are decreasing even more rapidly. During the period 1984-1994, revenue for professional services as a component of total revenues increased from 30 percent to more than 46 percent.[4] Consequently, a department's ability to subsidize teaching and research activities as well as new program development is also at risk. A typical institutional requirement is that the business plan show a new program operating at a breakeven point or at a profit in three to five years. The dollars to subsidize the start-up losses, however, are shrinking.

Insurors are no longer willing to pay an additional 20-30 percent for services provided at an AMC.[6] Usual and customary fees are no longer the predominant method of determining payments. When "the best" physician is providing the care, there is typically no longer a higher payment. Payments, instead, are based on fee schedules or relative value units (e.g., Medicare's Resource-Based Relative Value System).

At the time of this writing, an extensive review of the literature (including *MGM Journal*, *Academic Medicine* and *Healthcare Financial Management*), as well as contacts with the major vendors of physician billing software and several professional societies, revealed no known models for accurately predicting physicians' clinical revenue. Numerous articles have been written on the topic of compensating physicians, but these articles focus on the role of benefits as part of the compensation package,[7] the appropriate remuneration for administrative services, research and teaching, [6, 8, 9, 11] the development of incentives based on the severity of illness[12] and measuring physician productivity.[10] These articles do not address the determination of clinical revenue.

Figure 7.2

Potential sources of revenue [8, 9, 10]

- Clinical revenue derived from professional fee billing
- Clinical revenue derived from allocations of global (hospital and physician) or capitation contracts
- Hospital support for administrative services, supervision and teaching – these monies are commonly referred to as effort reporting dollars
- Hospital support for new programs which will favorably influence hospital revenue
- Medical school support for teaching activities
- Contracts for physicians' services
- Veterans Administration Medical Center support for clinical, research and teaching activities
- Research support
- Continuing medical education courses
- Departmental rebates on indirect costs recovered by the institution
- Interest from special accounts such as endowment funds or clinical reserve funds

The revenue from professional fee billing is dependent upon price, charge mix, volume and payer mix. Actual clinical revenue is not known until the charges are paid. Accurate predictions of the timing of payments and amount of payments are difficult. According to the grading criteria in "Score Your Practice™," average performance in accounts receivable management results in 30-40 percent of a department's payments being delayed greater than 90 days.[13] Some payments are delayed as long as nine-twelve months due to coordination of benefit issues between two or more insurors.

The industry standard used by most clinical department administrators to develop the financial projections for their business plans is to analyze historical revenue data at a macro-level; i.e., charge mix, payer mix, percent of accounts receivable greater than 90 days, percent of charges written off to bad debt, and days in accounts receivable for the previous six-twelve month period at the divisional or departmental level. However, there are numerous limitations to the use of historical revenue data in developing financial projections. One limitation is that with the advent of managed care, clinical departments have experienced significant, but not prospectively quantifiable, shifts in their payer mix within a three-six month period. As patients shift from indemnity plans to managed care plans, the clinical department collects less money for the same volume and type of services because of the lower payments by the managed care companies.

A second limitation is that historical trends may not accurately reflect the level of collections possible if the billing office is not performing its tasks well. (When developing a business plan, the credibility of a billing office's efforts should be evaluated by using various criteria such as the adjusted collection percentage, cash collected, and days revenue in accounts receivables. Tools such as "Score Your Practice™" may also be useful[13].) A third limitation is that although department revenue projections for annual budgets based on historical revenue data may be within 0.5-1.0 percent of actual department revenue,[14] there is typically significant variation between projected revenue and actual revenue at the divisional and individual physician levels. Most business plans for new program development are at a division, subdivision or physician level.

A fourth limitation is that historical data do not reflect the changing reimbursement methodology of managed care companies. Initially, many managed care companies paid for services at 60-75 percent of charges. With the renewal of their contracts, these managed care companies have generally changed to payments based on their own fee schedules or on a percent of the Medicare fee schedule. These managed care fee schedules are substantially lower than the previous percent of charges. The Medicare fee schedule may be used to set reimbursement across departments; e.g., 120 percent of the Medicare fee schedule for all physician charges submitted by the medical center in the aggregate, or to set reimbursement per CPT code; e.g., 120 percent of the Medicare fee schedule/CPT code. The methodology used must be understood as well as any institutional reconciliations which transfer funds collected by one physician or department to another entity.

A fifth limitation to the use of historical data is the lack of an external standard or database against which the data may be compared. Consequently, what may appear to be a trend, could be an aberration due to the limited volume of data being analyzed. A sixth limitation of historical data is the lack of comparability between charge and payer data. This is due to the lag in payments as calculated by the days in accounts receivable ratio and the inability of professional fee billing systems to assign any charges to the secondary insurors.

In summary, historical data are limited in their usefulness because they are not sensitive to shifts in charge and payer mix. They assume the billing office is routinely collecting all appropriate revenue. They do not always represent a sufficiently recent time period or level of detail to be useful. They do not address changes in the reimbursement methodology of managed care companies. They may misrepresent aberrations in the data. And they do not address the lack of comparability between charge and payer data. These limitations make it difficult for a clinical department to develop and implement meaningful business plans.

Clinical department administrators are thus faced with the challenge of projecting increases or decreases in clinical revenue on the basis of historical data relating to charge mix, volume and payer mix. Charge mix data, defined as the percentage of charges by insurer, is determined by the specific patients who seek care. Although AMCs are entering into greater numbers of contracts with insurance companies to increase the base of patients who may use the services of the medical center, typically the contracts are not exclusive. Thus the insurer does not guarantee any particular volume from which charges could be estimated. Additionally, most professional fee billing programs do not assign any charges to secondary insurers at charge entry. For example, for patients who have Medicare as their primary insurer and Blue Shield as their secondary insurer, 100 percent of the charges are allocated to Medicare at the time of charge entry because it is the primary insurer. Consequently, it is difficult to make accurate projections of payments in comparison to charges because the charge data are misleading.

To predict charge mix data for a business plan, it is helpful to identify the most specific, relevant data from which projections can be made. For example, the business plan may expand existing activities for which data are available. The business plan may represent the initiation of a new program at the home institution, but specific data may be available from another institution. (This other institution is frequently the institution from which the new faculty member was recruited. The program, however, may not be willing to share data if the proposed program is perceived as competing with its patient base.) Alternatively, data from a similar subspecialty should be used.

Volume is frequently calculated by using charges as a proxy such that higher charges are considered to indicate higher volume and hence higher productivity.[10] For both medical and surgical specialties, the term "total charges" obscures the fact that higher charges may mean more higher priced procedures are being done even though the total number of visits and procedures may be decreasing. Situations are also more frequently occurring when physicians' collections are decreasing despite stable or increasing charge levels (when the price for services has remained stable). An analysis of relevant data on a case-by-case basis indicates that in some cases changes in payer mix from indemnity plans to managed care products or plans is responsible for the decreased payments.[16] These analyses are time-consuming and retrospective in nature.

Relative value units (RVUs) serve as a better indicator of increasing volume than do charges, both because they measure work and provide comparability across specialties.[10, 11, 12] A limitation of RVUs for surgical specialties is that the use of increasing RVUs as an indicator of increasing volume and, therefore, increasing revenue is not accurate in and of itself. When multiple procedures are performed at a single operative setting, the RVUs must be discounted for all but the primary procedure. One approach for predicting revenue would be to reduce the number of RVUs in proportion to the insurers' discounts of the payments. Most insurers follow Medicare's methodology for handling multiple procedures when all procedures performed other than the primary procedure are discounted. For example, Medicare typically approves an allowance of 100 percent for the primary (first) procedure and 50 percent for the second, third and fourth procedures. The fifth and additional procedures are individually reviewed by Medicare for payment. Medicare has exceptions to these rules such as its decision to not discount a venous graft (CPT code 33519) when this is done at the same operative setting as an artery graft (CPT code 33533).

Some departments track the number of operative cases as a tool in projecting volume and physician revenue. An advantage of this method is the availability of historical operative case data at a physician level. However, because operating room scheduling systems do not interface with professional billing software, charge mix or payer mix data must be manually linked with the operative case data. This methodology is also limited by the wide variability in the types and complexity of operative cases, in the number of procedures performed as part of a single operative case, and in the insurance companies' reimbursement for procedures. For example, an operative case during which a hernia is repaired (a single procedure) might be reimbursed \$486; an operative case during which a kidney is transplanted \$2310; and an operative case during which cardiac bypass grafts are done (a combination of two procedures) \$3334.

To accurately predict volume, the sources of referrals for the new initiative must be identified. Referrals from institutional colleagues should not be taken for granted. Although most AMCs have a single group practice plan and one might think that most, if not all, of the referrals would be made to other physicians in the plan, this often is not true. A physician may refer to someone outside of the practice due to a prior relationship with that physician; e.g., a medical school classmate. An outside physician's timely feedback to and ongoing involvement of the physician who made the referral is likely to result in future referrals. The availability of an appointment in a shorter time period may also cause a physician to refer outside of the practice.

Although marketing studies can be implemented to determine if new sources of referrals might be feasible, administrators should evaluate historical sources of referrals and recognize that a new initiative will be most dependent upon these historical sources. New initiatives may, however, threaten historical sources of referrals if these sources think that the need for their services will be diminished. In developing volume projections for a business plan, it may be helpful to contact five-ten of the key physicians from whom referrals would be expected to ascertain their interest in the initiative and, if appropriate, to solicit their input to the development of the plan.

Payer mix varies from charge mix. Even when charges per visit or procedure are the same for all patient care rendered, the payments per visit or procedure differ because they are based on specific contractual agreements. As with charge mix, it is helpful to identify the most specific, relevant payer mix data from which projections can be made.

State and federal agencies differ in their stated requirements of attending physicians. The implications of these differences need to be understood to accurately predict revenue. An example of this is the different requirements of Medicare and Medicaid for a physician to render a billable service. Medicare requires an attending physician to be present for the key portions of an operative case in order to bill,[15] but Pennsylvania's Medicaid requirements state that the physician must personally perform the surgical procedure.[16] Sometimes such differences are viewed as merely semantic differences. But at other times such differences are viewed as exact and specific and directly affect the physicians' ability to generate revenue.

In addition to developing projections of physician revenue for a business plan, the clinical department administrator may be expected to develop projections of hospital revenue also. The typical hospital indicators of revenue are listed in Figure 7.3. These data are historical revenue data and as such share the same limitations as historical physician revenue data. Also, these hospital data are seldom available at subdivision, physician or diagnosis levels. It is difficult to develop and monitor the implementation of a business plan which focuses on a single programmatic element; e.g., number of patients admitted to the hospital with inflammatory bowel disease, when specific data are not available.

Projecting revenue for a business plan is somewhat like trying to hit a moving target. Even within a five-year period, some diseases will be managed differently than had been projected or the incidence of a disease will dramatically increase or decrease. Insurers will delay payments beyond what one would consider reasonable. As with most predictions, it is best to be conservative, note the original assumptions, monitor changes, and have contingency plans.

Independent versus interdependent business plans

A unique characteristic of an academic clinical department is that it is an entrepreneurial entity as well as a part of a larger institution. Unlike the subsidiary of a company, academic departments are not free-standing but rely on business services provided by other parts of the parent institution as well as external organizations. When completing a business plan for an academic practice, the administrator must consider the site(s) in which the new initiative will operate. The fact that these sites may not be owned or operated by the academic institution should also be taken into consideration. For example, the lease of a particular site may limit the hours of operation of a new initiative to weekdays even though Saturday hours may be desirable.

Figure 7.3

Hospital indicators of revenue

- Number of elective admissions
- Number of emergency admissions
- Number of discharges
- Average length of stay
- Patient days by major insurance classification
- Average daily census
- Case mix index
- Number of operative procedures

The business plan needs to address which business services will be provided by the department, the parent institution, and the leased facility as well as each entity's ability to commit the resources which are necessary to fulfill the academic business plan. Business services which should be addressed include human resources, purchasing, telecommunications, information services, environmental services, facilities management and finance. When possible, service contracts and contingency plans should be developed for each business service upon which the new initiative is dependent. Service contracts are particularly important in those areas which most immediately affect the day-to-day operations such as telecommunications and information services. If these two areas are not working well, they can cripple the department's ability to appropriately respond to referring physicians or patients. It is unwise for a department to assume a reasonable response time from repair people or to risk delays in obtaining loaner equipment.

Hospitals frequently provide leased space to academic clinical departments. To further complicate matters, an academic clinical department may have activities in multiple hospitals. Therefore, the department administrators need to coordinate the business plans with the requirements of each of the hospitals. Specifically, attention should be given to: the credentialing of physicians to obtain hospital privileges; securing funding through budgets which may span different fiscal years and which will usually require different review and approval processes; notifying insurers of additional practice sites so that physicians may be reimbursed for services; and complying with different medical record standards. The business plan should identify those persons which will act as the liaisons between the academic clinical department and the administrators of the hospitals.

Historically, business plans have generally been developed by a single department or one of its components. Although a clinical program may be interdisciplinary in nature, few academic departments have successfully developed joint business plans. This predominant and continuing isolation in the development of business plans stems in part from: a reluctance to reveal specific financial data such as salaries or revenues; an inability to negotiate shared control and leadership of the planning process and the program; an inability to resolve responsibility for the sharing of the initial losses and the eventual profits; and an unspoken constraint that if the department cannot get more people, space or money, the program is without merit.

During the past five-ten years, the research mission of the academic clinical department has been changing. Interdisciplinary research projects, projects relating to health policy, health economics, epidemiology, and clinical outcomes, and joint MD/PhD programs between clinical departments and basic science departments have been instituted alongside the traditional, single-focus programs. Interdisciplinary programs require that multiple departments coordinate their business plans. Spawned by the availability of specific funding mechanisms, program project grants (PPGs) and specialized centers of research (SCORs) bring together investigators from different departments to accomplish common research objectives.

The business plan for a research program is required to take into consideration the financial integration of the program with existing departmental and institutional components. For example, research initiatives which are externally funded typically require some level of departmental or institutional support either due to restrictions on the types of expenses that can be funded (e.g., advertising to recruit for human subjects may not be an allowable expenses) or caps on expenses such as the National Institutes of Health (NIH) salary cap.[17] Historically, an important source of these funds has been excess clinical revenue. At this point in time, however, excess clinical revenue is needed to reengineer clinical programs and renovate clinical space. In addition, the intra- and interdepartmental competition for monies to subsidize research activities can be fierce and counterproductive to the development of collaborative research programs or the sharing of research resources such as technicians, equipment or space. A business plan which assumes cooperation and, therefore, does not provide a contingency plan for the purchase of critical equipment could be doomed to failure.

Additional evidence of the interdepartmental coordination of research programs is the development of detailed institutional systems to ensure that all research proposals are carefully reviewed before they are submitted to the funding agencies. These systems are designed to ensure that the grant demonstrates scientific merit and that the resources required to accomplish the grant's objectives are or will be available. Typically, the review process is a formal one with a routing form that requires: the signatures of all the department chairs whose departments will be affected; an attestation by the home department that the grant demonstrates scientific merit and that adequate space and personnel exist or will be funded by the project; and signatures indicating that the application complies with all regulatory guidelines regarding the use of animals, radioisotopes,and human subjects.

Although the degree of prospective planning is not as strong as in the research arena, medical education has been marked by the reasonable coordination of business plans. This is mostly due to the centralized control that the dean's office exercises over the curriculum. The recent revision of medical school curricula has required some collaboration in the development of joint business plans. Specifically, the integration of clinical experiences into the first two years of medical school training has opened the dialogue between the clinical departments and the basic science departments. Additionally, the development of new courses that address the health of the public, health policy and health economics has required cooperation among different schools within the university,; e.g., the business school, the school of communications and the medical school.

In contrast, most academic institutions have no systems for approving or disapproving entrepreneurial ventures in the clinical arena. Clinical activities are regarded as being under the purview of the individual department or program. If a department has sufficient internal resources to fund the new initiative and provide appropriate space, then no formal approval by or notification of the dean's office is typically required. In fact, it is not unusual for one department to learn of another department's initiatives via a radio ad, an announcement about a recently recruited faculty member, or a new name on the building directory.

The evolution of academic medicine has resulted in discrete specialties in departments that are redundant at the institutional level. Figure 7.4 provides some examples of these redundancies. Although the blurring of these clinical boundaries could at times lead to the development of joint business plans drawing upon the complementary nature of these specialties, this is seldom the case. Business plans for these programs are typically developed by the individual department. This is undoubtedly due not only to departments' desires to protect their primary source of all revenue, but to protect in particular their clinical revenue which is their primary source of *discretionary* revenue.

Figure 7.4

Departmental programs often duplicated at the institutional level

Program	Departments performing or overseeing
Hand surgery	Orthopedics Surgery, Division of Plastic Surgery Neurosurgery
Vascular laboratory studies	Radiology Medicine, Division of Cardiology Surgery, Division of Vascular Surgery
Sports medicine	Medicine Pediatrics Orthopedics Rehabilitation Medicine
Craniofacial surgery	Otorhinolaryngology Surgery, Division of Plastic Surgery Oral and Maxillofacial Surgery
Treatment of back injuries	Orthopedics Neurosurgery Rehabilitation Medicine
Carotid surgery	Surgery, Division of Vascular Surgery Neurosurgery

An additional problem which occurs because of these redundancies relates to the recruitment of new faculty. Because departments are acting in isolation or in direct competition, two departments may each recruit a new faculty member to meet the same perceived clinical needs. The result is that the pool of patients which warranted the recruitment of one faculty member is insufficient to support two physicians. Additionally, the institution may lose credibility with the public because of its mixed messages about who the experts are. Also, unless new sources of referrals can be identified, it is likely that within a three-five year period one of the physicians will be asked to leave the institution or change areas of focus because of his or her inability to establish a viable practice in the field for which he or she was recruited.

A notable exception to the building of clinical "silos" is the interdepartmental collaboration required for an institution to become a designated National Cancer Institute (NCI) comprehensive cancer center.[18] These centers, which are funded by the National Institutes of Health, provide multidisciplinary clinics for the diagnosis and treatment of cancers. For example, a comprehensive breast evaluation center may be established which is staffed by medical oncologists, surgical oncologists, radiation oncologists and plastic surgeons. Also, institutional tumor registries are developed so that each department does not have to expend resources to collect and maintain these databases. Thus, the data are widely available, and the data represent the complete clinical picture on an individual patient. Additionally, NCI comprehensive cancer centers provide core support services such as biostatisticians.

The lack of institutional oversight and coordination of business plans among departments and the lack of institutional communication about the relative priorities of various plans can have negative short- and long-term consequences. In AMCs, typically an individual department's business plan for a particular intradepartmental initiative is not subject to review by the medical center's senior administrative staff if the department has sufficient internal resources to develop and implement the program. If the department wants to request medical-center funding to support the program, then senior administrative staff typically review the program's business plan. This review, however, may be more perfunctory than analytical. It may not take into consideration potential medical-center redundancies or even the impact of the program on other departments (e.g., the need for increased social services' support for outpatients).

A common example of the lack of institutional coordination and oversight involves faculty recruitment. In addition to the problem of institutional redundancy mentioned earlier, few AMCs have a well-structured process for determining the clinical, research or academic roles of new faculty and the institutional or departmental support of each of these efforts. The premium placed on intellectual freedom is frequently interpreted as the department providing the new faculty member with an environment in which there are a myriad of academic, clinical and research opportunities. It is then up to the faculty member to decide which avenues to explore and which skills to foster. This historical, hands-off approach to the development of new faculty is coming under scrutiny because of departments' and institutions' lack of discretionary revenue to subsidize these "exploratory" years.

A department may allocate resources to a program that is important to a few individuals within the department (e.g., to support a particular area of research), but these resources may be disproportionate to the priority that would be placed on the program by the institution. Consequently, the department may not have adequate resources to support the institutional priorities such as the development of a satellite clinical facility. As institutional priorities increasingly take precedent over departmental priorities, the department may be placed in the awkward position of having to renege on its internal commitments to meet institutional goals.

On a long-term basis, this lack of institutional coordination and oversight may mean that individual departments as well as the institution miss opportunities such as creatively marketing a range of services, extending hours of service, identifying sufficient numbers of patients for clinical protocols or research studies, and sharing on-call coverage. These are opportunities that might have resulted in greater patient and provider satisfaction as well as greater revenue.

Barriers to change

Business plans must also address internal and external barriers to change that will affect their development and implementation. Increased competition in the health care market means that organizations must act quickly to reduce costs, increase the quality of services, and provide a continuum of services. At the same time, however, institutions are constrained by numerous external factors such as governmental agencies, regulatory agencies, accreditation organizations and insurance companies.

Although most academic clinical departments depend upon government funding, governmental agencies often do not provide funding in proportion to the resources expended. Consequently, a department must subsidize these activities. However, it is difficult for a department to provide appropriate incentives for physicians to cover these additional expenses. For the business plan to have a sound fiscal foundation, it is critical that physicians' efforts be reported in proportion to their salary and fringe benefit expenses regardless of the specific details of their efforts. For example, a physician may spend 50 percent of his or her time on research activities, but may receive only 40 percent funding for this effort due to NIH salary caps. The business plan should address the funding of the 50 percent effort spent on research by designating that 40 percent will be funded by NIH and 10 percent by other departmental funds. The specific source of these funds should be noted.

Government agencies also vary in the amount of latitude they allow administrative personnel. Although Medicare is a federal health insurance program, it is administered regionally by contracted organizations. These organizations are referred to as intermediaries. The intermediaries have discretion in interpreting some of the Medicare regulations and thus these regulations are not uniformly applied. For example, Medicare rules state that a physician may not bill for a consultation of a patient if the patient was seen by another provider for the same problem or diagnosis on that day. This has made it impossible for physicians involved in interdisciplinary clinics to be reimbursed appropriately. If an oncologist, a surgeon, a plastic surgeon and a radiation oncologist provide consultative services for a single patient on the same day for her breast cancer, only one physician is allowed to bill Medicare. This type of restriction discourages the medical profession from forming interdisciplinary clinics. These clinics are preferred by patients because they can be seen in one day and because the specialists can discuss treatment plans on that day and recommend a course of action to the patient. Recently, the Medical Director of EXACT, the Medicare intermediary for southeastern Pennsylvania, gave approval for more than one physician to bill for services rendered to a patient on the same day for the same problem if the patient was seen in a particular multidisciplinary clinic. This decision, however, was not promulgated by Medicare, and thus is not universally applicable to Medicare providers.

Government programs are not often characterized by well-thought out, long-term strategies. The uncertainty of federal funding for particular research initiatives fails to provide a meaningful context for business plans. Federal grants are now typically funded for three years in contrast to the standard five-year period prevalent in the 1980s. Three years of funding requires the investigator to begin seeking sources of additional funding shortly after the first year of funding is completed. Because insufficient data may have been collected to allow reasonable analysis, the investigator is faced with the dilemma of needing to obtain funding for years four and higher, and yet not having adequate information on which to base a grant application.

Regulatory agencies require that certain standards be met regardless of the inefficiency or waste that this necessitates. For example, the Occupational Safety and Health Administration (OSHA) requires annual certification of all investigators who conduct or oversee experiments using hazardous chemicals. The same program must be attended by those investigators who are seldom in the lab and those investigators in the lab on a daily basis. Without OSHA's mandate of attendance at an educational session, an institution might choose to assess competency by using a written test. It might also allow a senior investigator to designate a person within the lab who demonstrated a core set of skills as the operational director of the lab, thus rendering the senior investigator exempt from attending the educational sessions.

Accreditation organizations can impede an institution's ability to respond quickly to market changes and to undertake new initiatives. For example, an institution might want to re-allocate the residency training positions among its various training programs. Intrainstitutional re-allocation is not permitted. Instead, requests for changes in the number of specialty training positions must be submitted to the Accreditation Council on Graduate Medical Education (ACGME). An institution may wait several years to receive approval from the ACGME for a request to re-allocate its residency training positions.

Conflicts exist between governmental agencies' support of residency programs and the specialty boards' requirements for training. Although Medicare caps the funding for residency training at the level of funding for the fifth, post-graduate clinical year, the American Board of Surgery requires more than five years of training for a physician to qualify to take the board-certification examination for any of the surgical subspecialties. Consequently, departments and institutions must identify funding sources for these expenses commonly referred to as the "resident differentials."

Insurance companies have varying requirements for processing claims. Some allow claims to be submitted electronically. However, many of the managed care companies lack sophisticated computer programs and thus require claims to be submitted on paper. This paper-processing is more labor intensive and thus more expensive. It is ironic that for a lower level of payment, greater inefficiencies are imposed on the physicians' billing staff.

Insurance companies also follow varying rules for approving payments. Some follow Medicare's rules, some most of Medicare's rules, and some devise their own rules. Payments may or may not be made for second, third or fourth surgical procedures done at the same operative setting. Payments may or may not be made for office procedures performed on the same day as an outpatient visit. Although Medicare pays for immunosuppression therapy during the global, post-operative period, many other insurers do not. Some consider certain procedures to be experimental and, therefore, will not pay for them even though other companies have paid for the procedures for years. Typically, Medicare is slower to approve reimbursement for new procedures than Blue Shield or managed care plans. As discussed previously, business plans must take into consideration the proposed mix of charges, the various rules affecting payments by the insurers, and the assumptions made in predicting revenue.

Most AMCs are undertaking reengineering initiatives to address important internal barriers such as those listed in Figure 7.5. The business plan needs to address the effect of these initiatives on the new program.

Figure 7.5

Key internal barriers to change[19]

- Overcommitment to individual operating entities
- Fear of change/comfort with status quo
- Desire to preserve autonomy
- Organizational history and tradition
- Lack of system perspective
- Aversion to economic and social risk
- Lack of understanding of environment, governance roles, and responsibilities
- Lack of trust among key constituencies of the system

A common business strategy is to take advantage of preemptive opportunities. Changes in state, federal or local regulations may create a situation well recognized in the industry as an opportunity. The objective of preemptive strategies is to do something well before the competitor can do it well. For example, a preemptive opportunity would entail starting up new operations before a competitor can begin its operations and thus building brand equity. In many cases, the system constraints of an academic health care institution as well as external constraints may not support the vigorous pace needed to achieve a preemptive objective.

Information systems

The development and maintenance of state-of-the art information systems is critical to institutions' and departments' ability to develop and implement meaningful business plans. Despite this reality, many academic institutions lack adequate information systems' infrastructure. Many institutions have not implemented electronic solutions to processes for which electronic solutions have been developed. For example, most institutions have staff who manually enter charge data into hospital and professional fee billing systems rather than optically scanning the encounter form or superbill. In part due to the historical existence of clinical silos, processes which are computerized often do not have electronic interfaces that allow the data to be passed from one system to the other. For example, radiology departments and pathology departments typically have totally independent computer systems for reporting results. If a physician wants to obtain clinical data on a patient, he or she must separately access each computer system.

This lack of infrastructure impedes the development of the business plan because data are not readily available to be used in the plan itself or to monitor the success of the plan. With the exception of a few AMCs such as the Mayo Clinic and Brigham and Women's Hospital, most AMCs lack electronic processes to collect, store, retrieve, analyze, and transmit data related to patient care, insurance information, clinical outcomes, or real-time resource utilization such as occupied beds or operating room usage. The labor intensive, manual process of collecting and analyzing data must be taken into consideration in the development and implementation of the business plan.

Integration of the business plan with various institutional components

The business plan needs to identify the person or group charged with making decisions about the new program, including securing the resources to successfully implement it. The relationship of the initiative to existing governing structures and the accountability of its leaders to department chairs, the dean, various administrators, and the directors of interdisciplinary programs or centers must be clearly delineated. In the academic health care industry, there are some dominant models of governance as described in a previous chapter.

Some governance decisions may be dictated by state and federal laws. An example of this would be laws related to the ownership of medical practices in certain states. Typically, however, the governance structure for a particular business plan is constrained less by external factors than by internal factors. In some AMCs, the chair is nearly always designated as the head of a departmental initiative or as the department's representative on an interdepartmental initiative. These assignments may occur even though the chair lacks interest or expertise in the particular initiative. For example, the dean may designate the department chairs as the departments' representatives in the development of a business plan for a multispecialty satellite even though some of the department chairs have minimal outpatient clinical activity. If the principles agreed to by the department chairs are further developed by task forces with strong clinicians from the departments, then the process can be an effective one. If, however, the planning process is quickly deferred by the department chairs to other players in the AMC, then the outcomes may be less than satisfactory. In the interest of multidisciplinary interaction, the medical director and site administrator may combine medical and surgical practices in a single area. However, they may not plan adequately for the support services which are necessary for a surgical practice but not a medical practice such as admissions' staff to facilitate patients' admissions for operative procedures.

Additionally, central administrative and finance staff who are charged with developing the satellite's budget and the methodology for reimbursing departments for physicians' efforts at the multidisciplinary site may not be aware of important concerns. They may assume that revenue will be generated for all visits. They may not know that post-operative visits are reimbursed $0 by insurers because the post-operative care is included in the surgeons' payment for the operative procedure. They may not understand that some insurers do not pay for both an office visit and an office procedure when they are done on the same day. This lack of knowledge can lead to overstated revenue and poor financial projections.

Alternatively, some initiatives may be planned too independently of the dean or department chair with equally poor results. For example, a faculty member may secure funding from a pharmaceutical company to develop a Web page. The Web page may be viewed by thousands of browsers before it is discovered that a group of physicians have designated themselves as an approved institutional center of excellence without securing this designation through the appropriate channels.

Even when departments or divisions create strong business plans, the institutional decision-making process can wreak havoc on the approval and successful implementation of the plan. An important concern related to governance is the confusion that results when academic clinical departments must seek approval of the business plan from both the senior manager responsible for operations and the senior manager responsible for finance as a prerequisite to receiving the dean's approval. The differing perspectives and political arenas of the chief operating officer and chief financial officer often lead to lengthy delays and missed opportunities in the approval and implementation of the business plan. Sometimes this historical segregation of responsibilities leads to the demise of the business plan because of the senior managers' failure to work through the compromises which are necessary to its success.

To be effective, planning demands participation. Thoughtful participation among the members of the governance group is critical to successful business planning; open discussion of potential problems and contingency plans is critical. However, open discussion can be thwarted by the pressure to find a quick fix or by the pressure to conform. Although looking for "quick and dirty" fixes or "quick strikes" can be a useful exercise in establishing priorities within a business plan, to be successful the business plan must address the more complex goals and processes for achieving them.

The pressure to conform in a group discussion may result from the influence of a dominant personality in the group or from status incongruity. Sometimes lower status participants may be pressured by higher status participants to "go along," even though they believe their own ideas are superior; or certain participants may attempt to exert influence based on the perception they are experts in the problem area. Situations in which these types of interactions may be observed in AMCs include Professors discussing new initiatives with assistant professors, those on the tenure track discussing ideas with those on a clinician-educator track, and physicians discussing initiatives with non-physicians.

Some academic clinical departments have had striking success in implementing business plans and capturing the dominant market share. One example is an academic ophthalmology department in the South which has become the largest ophthalmology practice in the state by carefully analyzing the market needs, anticipating legislative changes, and carefully planning its growth. Implicit in this department's success is the fact that the governance group endorsed the planning and committed the financial resources and facilities to fulfill the business plan.

In creating the business plan, the Executive Vice-president/ Chief Operating Officer evaluated the nature of the medical marketplace in his state. He identified the weaknesses in the state marketplace, matched them with the strengths in the academic practice, and narrowed the opportunities to produce a viable plan. Subsequently, he bought independent ophthalmology practices that fit into the market needs of the state and the business needs of the academic practice. This strategy was enhanced by the anticipation of some legislative changes in the state, which enhanced the referrals by optometrists to ophthalmology practices. Developing and executing the business plan required teamwork among the medical staff and the administrative/financial staff.

Human resources policies and procedures

Frequently, academic clinical departments have personnel who have been hired through different institutional human resource offices and thus are governed by the policies and procedures of that particular institution. For example, an academic department of medicine may have: research staff hired through the university; professional fee billing staff hired through a practice organized as a 501(c)(3) business; medical support staff hired through the hospital; and faculty hired by the medical school but who receive compensation through the university, the practice and the hospital. The business plan needs to address what personnel will be hired through which institution and the effect on the plan of the varying fringe benefits. Differences in fringe benefits may include: the number of vacation days; the number of paid holidays; the employees' share of health insurance costs; tuition reimbursement policies; pension eligibility and pension benefits; pay scales; and incentive programs. Depending on the department's space, individuals governed by different human resource policies and procedures may be sitting next to one another.

It is important to establish the business plan with clearly defined goals to help create a sense of unity within the operation despite these differences. For business plans which receive funding from two or more of the institutions, there could be a conflict in the priorities of expenditures; i.e., which money gets spent first or which money gets spent for what purposes. To address this, the use of resources needs to be determined prospectively. Any cross-subsidization needs to be delineated and explicitly approved by the governing group(s). The business plan then needs to be managed within these constraints.

Allocation and renovation of space

Academic clinical departments have historically been characterized by overcrowding and an overdue need for renovations. This has resulted from the departments' assigning a low priority to the adequacy of the physical space when funding is needed to subsidize research activities. In addition, the traditionally topsy-turvy nature of departmental growth has meant that space is filled on a first-come, first-served basis. Certain locations develop an inherent value based on the former or present occupants or their adjacencies. Moving the occupants from such locations is politically difficult, if not impossible.

The business plan must take into consideration the realities of space constraints. It should not be assumed that if the program grows, additional space will be assigned to it. The comprehensive business plan should take into account the current facilities and how they might be changed within the context of the plans and goals of the parent institution to accommodate the new initiative. Candid discussions need to be held with the governing group regarding the timing and the funding of renovations which are critical to the success of the initiative. Renovating space in any institution is a prolonged experience. Swing space (i.e., space which can be used during the period of renovation) needs to be explicitly identified in concert with the institution's overall facilities planning. Also, most states require that renovations bring the area into compliance with current facility codes or laws; the expenses for this must be incorporated into the budget for the business plan.

Projecting the cost of space for the program is often difficult. In one AMC, allocation formulas for rent are based on the relevant revenue of departments and not on the actual square footage occupied by the department. In another institution, space costs were always tentative until the end of the fiscal year and then any increases in expense were applied retroactively. In addition to the cost per square foot of the space, related expenses such as increased electrical, telecommunications, long distance, information systems, heating/ventilation/air conditioning (HVAC), and parking costs must be taken into consideration. A solid and well-developed business plan can mean the difference between getting what is needed and not getting sufficient space to implement a business plan.

Marketing

As noted in a previous chapter, marketing in the health care industry has become critical to the success of existing as well as new programs. Most AMCs have corporate-level marketing departments that oversee all marketing activities within the institution. It is critical to coordinate the marketing strategy necessary for the implementation of the business plan with other institutional initiatives. Funding for marketing expenses may need to be managed through a supplemental budget overseen by the marketing department and not the academic clinical department even though the funding is an approved part of the business plan.

Information systems needs

The division of responsibility between the academic clinical department's information systems' staff who provide on-site support for minor repairs and corporate-level information systems' staff who oversee networking, contract negotiations for equipment purchases, and systems' interfaces needs to be delineated in the business plan. Also, computers, printers, and ancillary hardware expenses need to be budgeted in accordance with the institution's determination of which items are considered operating budget expenses and which ones are considered capital expenditures. The frequency of system back-ups needs to be discussed with the corporate-level information systems staff and arrangements made for more frequent back-ups if needed to protect the integrity of the program's data.

Summary

As AMCs more frequently adopt a health system perspective as they become part of an integrated healthcare network (IHCN), then business plans will need to be developed in a collaborative manner within this context. In particular, those developing business plans will need to integrate the new initiative into the existing governance structure while recognizing that these structures will change as the health system matures. The heretofore independence with which many department chairs have operated will be diminished. Their compensation and re-appointments as department chairs will continue to depend upon traditional measures such as total research dollars or the ranking of the department in terms of NIH dollars. But they also will also depend upon their ability to promote and implement institutional goals. Department chairs may be required by the dean or their peers through a governing council to staff satellite clinics, extend the operating hours of the practice, or change departmental incentive programs to reward institutional citizenship versus individual productivity. Division chiefs and individual faculty members will also be expected to fall into line with the institutional priorities.

The leaders of the IHCN will need to make decisions which will further the systems' goals and objectives even if this means thwarting an individual department's or program's goals. As a part of the institutional oversight of the business plan, programmatic and financial performance measures are likely to be more closely scrutinized and monitored. The challenge will be for AMCs to retain their roles as purveyors of new ideas and innovative techniques in the highly competitive health care environment.

References

1. University of Pennsylvania Office of Public Affairs, personal communication, July 1997.
2. Levitt, Theodore, "Marketing Myopia," *Harvard Business Review Business Classics:* Fifteen Key Concepts for Managerial Success (President and Fellows of Harvard College), 1991, pp. 1-12. Article reprinted from HBR September-October 1975, Number 75507, 1975.
3. University of Pennsylvania, Marketing Department, Focus groups on Penn Medicine at Radnor, personal communication, June 1996.
4. Zuckerman, Alan M., "Strategic responses of academic medical centers to the growth in ambulatory care," *Medical Group Management Journal* (Medical Group Management Association), January/February 1994, pp. 62-67.
5. Mayo Clinic, Division of Communications, Rochester, MN, personal communication, July 1997.
6. Results of the Liaison Committee on Medical Education (LCME) as reported by Suzanne T. Anderson in "Practice Plan Management: Faculty Compensation--How is it Changing?" *GFP Notes* (Association of American Medical Colleges), December 1994, 7(4):11-13.
7. Brennan, Terry J, "Physician Compensation in the Academic Group Practice", Paper prepared for fellowship in the American College of Medical Practice Executives, 1992.
8. Ceriani, Peter J., "Compensating and providing incentives for academic physicians: Balancing earning, clinical, research, teaching, and administrative responsibilities", *Journal of Ambulatory Care Management* (Aspen Publishers Inc.), April 1992, pp. 69-78.
9. Isack, Arthur and Axelrod, Ruth H., "Practice Plan Management: Building Clinical Productivity Incentives into the Physician Compensation Plan at GWU," *GFP Notes* (Association of American Medical Colleges), Fall 1993, 6(4):10-14.
10. Murri, Mitchell H., "Plan Management: Utilizing RVUs to Measure Physician Productivity and Distribute Clinical Income", GFP Notes (Association of American Medical Colleges), Spring 1993, 6(2):15-19.
11. Wright, Robert and Williams, Scott, "A Medical Group Practice Imperative: The Practical Use of RVUs for Managing and Contracting", *Medical Group Management Journal* (Medical Group Management Association), September/October 1994, pp. 42-49,109.
12. Smith, Norman S. and Weiner, Jonathan P., "Applying Population-based Case Mix Adjustment in Managed Care: The Johns Hopkins Ambulatory Care Group System", *Managed Care Quarterly* (1994 Aspen Publishers, Inc.), Summer 1994, 2(3):21-34.
13. Dunlap, S. Thomas, "'Score Your Practice' or Making Accounts Receivable Analysis Understandable", Medical Group Management Journal (Medical Group Management Association), May/June 1993, pp.70-76.

14. Rhodes, Nancy, unpublished data, FY94 and FY95 Budgets, Department of Surgery, Georgetown University.
15. 42 Code of Federal Regulations 415.172(A), 1996.
16. 55 PA.Code Section 1141.53(f) and 1141.54(f).
17. US Department of Health and Human Services Public Health Service Grant Application, Form PHS 398 (Rev. 5/95), p.12.
18. NCI-Designated Comprehensive Cancer Center Guidelines, National Cancer Institute, National Institutes of Health, Department of Health and Human Services, 1992.
19. Alexander, Jeffrey A., Zuckerman, Howard S., and Pointer, Dennis D., "The challenges of governing integrated health systems," Health Care *Management Review* (Aspen Publishers, Inc.), Fall 1995, Vol. 20, No. 4, p. 78.

Chapter 8

Government regulation of health care and the academic medical practice

by Ronald J. Davis, JD, MBA

It is appropriate that I preface this chapter with the statement that it is intended for working administrators. It is not designed to be a learned treatise on the law and regulation of academic medical practice. This chapter is intended to alert the reader to some areas of regulation and law that have specific pertinence to the administration of the academic medical practice. It should not be considered as a comprehensive work and should not be relied on for specific legal advice. Each area covered would warrant volumes to reach a reasonable level of explanation. The laws and regulations referred to vary among jurisdictions. Also, laws and regulations are very dynamic, with changes occurring daily.

The normal approach to a written statement regarding an area of "the law" will reference conservative interpretations of statutes, regulations and established decisions of appellate courts. This provides an unbiased background to general legal principles. By following these principles it is expected that an activity can be conducted in a correct manner. An administrator soon learns, though, that in a legal matter the expense of proving you are correct can be as big a disaster as being wrong. An administrator must be able to weigh and adjust for the chilling effect of a threatened lawsuit – even if the law is on his or her side. The question is never whether to break the law or not, but is often how much regulatory compliance can we afford?

The impact of regulation and legal proceeding on the academic practice has grown rapidly over the past four decades. In a study of the 240 reported cases between 1950 and 1991 involving medical faculty and academic medical centers, this impact was clearly shown for this area of litigation.[1] For litigation involving general administration, clinical affairs and research issues, the cases reported in each time period were:

1950-1959	3
1960-1969	8
1970-1979	36
1980-1989	151
1990-1991	42

It should be noted that the 42 cases reported for 1990-1991 were for a period of two years. Of the 240 cases, 108 involved clinical activities and demonstrated similar explosive growth in the volume of litigation. While the increase is significant, it would appear that the total of cases for the entire country is relatively small. This study was based on the cases which were reported on the appellate level. It is safe to say that only one in 20 cases will progress from the lower court to an appellate level. It is also common for suits to be settled prior to a full trial at the lower court. The study is accurate in demonstrating the rapid growth of the number of cases; however, the full magnitude of the impact on academic practices is not fully evident. The frequency with which our society resorts to the courts to resolve matters has grown. But a large portion of this trend in academic medicine is due to the increased complexity within which it operates.

As with many other areas, in administration of the academic practice the impacts of statutes, regulations, ordinances and court decisions are often oversimplified. The most frequent reason is the underestimation of the complexity of the academic practice. It is very true that the same laws that govern the non-academic practice also govern the academic practice. But it is equally true that the laws governing educational institutions, research organizations, charities and governmental entities may also govern the academic practice in a particular instance.

In any well-ordered society, rules are developed to organize the relationships within the society. The more complex the society, the more complex the set of rules tend to be. These relationships are between individuals, between individuals and companies, and between the individual and the society as a whole. The more complex the relationships, the greater the number of rules that will affect the parties to the relationship. To simplify the academic practice by saying that the relationships are the same as in a group practice will underestimate the complexity involved in academic medicine. As an example, physicians in a non-academic practice in providing a medical service will normally have a relationship with patients, employers and with payers for the services rendered. The same service rendered in an academic practice will involve all these same relationships, but may also involve the physician as a teacher, a researcher and the representative of a governmental entity. As we interlace the practice of medicine (both academic and non-academic) with MSOs, PPOs, HMOs, capitation, leasing partnerships, interlocking corporations, and other innovative delivery and finance methods these relationships increase in both number and complexity. The more complex the relationships, the more likely that any unforeseen occurrence will have to be resolved in a court.

As health care delivery has become increasingly complex, it has become an essential function of the administrator to balance multiple complex factors in decision-making. Laws and regulation are frequently key factors which must be considered in the operation of an academic practice. It is unfortunate, but administering an academic practice is in some respects similar to the game of baseball. To those who are not familiar with the intricacies, there appears to be very little difference between the skills of the 12-year-old sandlot player and the big leaguer. The skills required of the administrator are often underestimated because, like baseball, a superficial inspection of the task makes it look far easier than it is. Laws and regulations are key testing areas of the administrator's professional judgment; they are vital elements in this league.

Sources of the law

In the United States of America there is not one, but 51 legal systems – the federal government and the 50 states. The primary sources of law for each of these legal systems is a constitution, a legislature and an appellate court, or courts. A matter may be governed by the state law, the federal law or both. Generally, laws and regulation derive from legislative enactments or court decisions.

Common law

With certain exceptions most states have incorporated the common law of England as part of their laws (except Louisiana, whose legal system is based on the civil law). The common law is the "body of law developed in England primarily from judicial decisions based on custom and precedent, unwritten in statute or code, and constituting the basis of the English legal system." [2] Churchill, in his *History of the English Speaking Peoples*, describes committees (half colleges and half law schools) which studied court decisions in all areas of the realm to discover the "natural law." It was believed that there were always laws of nature to deal with the problems of man.

From this discovered law, they produced annual yearbooks which were recognized by judges.[3] The courts then tended to follow these earlier decisions, which became the doctrine of *stare decisis*, which means "let the decision stand." This ability to use precedence is a fundamental concept within our legal system. If a court of competent jurisdiction has decided an issue, future questions on this issue will be decided with the same outcome. Oliver Wendell Holmes wrote, "The life of the law has not been logic; it has been experience." The doctrine of stare decisis guides the courts, but does not rule their decisions completely. In rare instances the courts have completely changed course by ignoring stare decisis. A Pennsylvania decision overruled previous case law where the court reasoned: "Stare decisis channels the law. It erects lighthouses and flys (sic) the signals of safety. The ships of jurisprudence must follow the well-defined channel which, over the years, has been proved to be secure and trustworthy. But it would not comport with wisdom to insist that, should shoals rise in a heretofore safe course and rocks emerge to encumber the passage, the ship should nonetheless pursue the original course, merely because it presented no hazard in the past. The principle of stare decisis does not demand that we follow precedents which shipwreck justice."[4]

The principles of the common law are still the predominate part of the law today. The essentials of land ownership, the relationship between physician and patient, the elements of contracts, the foundation of torts and many other legal areas are all based on the doctrines of the common law.

Statutes

The Constitution of the United States is the preeminent law of this country. All federal or state statutes, all administrative regulations and all local ordinances are subject to the provisions of the Constitution. In the 10th amendment of the Constitution, it is specified that "The powers not delegated to the United States by the Constitution, nor prohibited by it to the States, are reserved to the States respectively, or to the people." Since the Constitution does not speak to the matter of medical care or medical education, it is accepted that they are the responsibility of the separate states, to the extent that the states do not infringe on those areas of personal liberty protected by the Constitution. Notwithstanding this reservation of the governance of medical care to the states, the federal government has passed numerous statutes affecting medical care. Generally, these statutes are protections of individual liberties (i.e., the Civil Rights

Act) or functions of the federal government's spending powers (i.e., the Medicare and Medicaid amendments). It is evident that there is a trend toward the federalization of health care and medical education. Increasingly, this area, which is the legitimate business of the 50 states, is the subject of regulation at the national level. Whether you consider this trend good or bad, it is appropriate to recognize its impact on the administration of the academic practice.

Each state also has a constitution, which is the preeminent governing instrument for the state. Frequently, state constitutions deal with the same matters as the federal Constitution. As specified in each state's constitution, the state legislature may enact statutes. The state legislature has a great deal of power in the governance of health care delivery and education, with the only limitation on this power being the federal and state constitutions. The volume of this legislation is immense. As health care becomes an increasingly complex industry, the states will enact increasing amounts of statutes to provide a legal framework within which to operate.

In addition to the statutory enactments of the federal and state legislative bodies, the executive branch of the federal and state governments creates rules and regulations which have the same force and effect as statutes. This regulating power is delegated by the legislatures for the purpose of administrating the laws. Examples of federal administrative agencies include the Food and Drug Administration (FDA), the Health Care Financing Administration (HCFA), the Internal Revenue Service (IRS) and the National Institutes of Health (NIH). The administrative regulating authority is limited to that which has been validly granted to the agency within the statutory enactment, but broad delegation is permitted.

Local jurisdictions, such as counties and cities, have been delegated authority by the state to regulate certain local matters. These laws are normally referred to as ordinances. While much attention is given to the federal and state laws, it is frequently the local municipal government with whom a practice plan has the most interaction. In most states, important powers are granted municipalities by the state's constitution. It should be remembered that on any level, any ordinance, regulation or legislation cannot conflict with a higher authority.

While the judiciary is a product of the constitution, it is the body that determines whether statutes are consistent with the constitution.[5] The courts are the primary agent in the establishment of private law, especially the laws of contract and torts.

Civil liabilities and risks

Civil liability and risks are those areas of law governing, generally, the relationship between individuals. In this context, it is important to remember that under the law, corporations, and other business combinations, are considered artificial individuals. Civil liability is primarily based on contracts or torts, and is found in the common law, statutes, regulations or ordinances.

Due to the numerous roles that members of the academic practice occupy, it is important to realize that in addition to the relationships inherent to an activity, the courts also imply liability through the various theories of vicarious liability. Vicarious means one who acts for another, a deputy or substitute.[6] In this context, it is a means through which the courts attribute responsibility to someone other than the parties directly involved. For the academic practice the significant theories of vicarious liability are:

Captain of the Ship Doctrine. The captain of the ship doctrine indicates that the physician in charge of care delivery is responsible for all those involved in the care, whether or not they are his or her employees. The application of this doctrine has been significantly reduced by recent court decisions which recognize that each health care professional delivering care is independently liable if at fault. Also, through the theory of corporate negligence, the hospital has its own duty for the supervision of care.[7]

Respondeat Superior. Respondeat superior means "let the master answer." It is a doctrine which holds employers liable for the consequences of their employees actions within the scope of their employment. Liability under this doctrine is not contingent on the employer committing an error. Unless the supervisor is also the employer, he or she will not be liable under this doctrine. This theory is for the benefit of the injured person and not the employee. An employee can be independently liable. If a recovery is made against the employer under respondeat superior, the organization can seek payment from the employee. An employer can insure its own risks without providing liability coverage to its employee.

Borrowed servant and dual servant. In some instances an employer can delegate direction and control of an employee to another. Increasingly, the trend is to apply a dual servant rule where the injured party can recover for the injury from both the borrower of the employee and the employer. In light of the role of academic physician in multiple settings, directing other health care personnel who work for multiple employers, it is appropriate to consider this an area of significant potential liability.

Ostensible agency and agency by estoppel. Some courts have determined that the relationships within the health care setting should be viewed from the perspective of the patient. Whether or not someone is employed, or has been authorized to act on behalf of another, may not matter if the patient is given the reasonable belief that an agency, or employment relationship exists. As complex structures are developed, it may lead to increased application of these theories as courts are unwilling to make patients responsible for understanding the structure of an MSO, HMO or other hybrid entity.

Corporate liability for negligent utilization review. As competitive market pressures induce academic practices to enter into increasingly strict utilization review, either internally or externally, it should be remembered that a utilization review decision can result in corporate liability. "The patient who requires treatment and who is harmed when care which should have been provided is not provided should recover for the injuries suffered from all those responsible for the deprivation of such care, including, when appropriate, health care payers. Third party payers of health care services can be held legally accountable when medically inappropriate decisions result from defects in the design or implementation of cost containment mechanisms, as, for example, when appeals made on a patient's behalf for medical or hospital care are arbitrarily ignored or unreasonably disregarded or overridden."[8] It should be noted that the Employee Retirement Income and Security Act of 1974 (ERISA) preempts some aspects of the provision of benefits in covered plans. In some cases ERISA has preempted actions involving denial of benefits as a means to maintain the cost savings of managed care programs. "By its very nature, a system of prospective decision making influences the beneficiary's choice among treatment options to a far greater degree than does the theoretical risk of disallowance of a claim facing a beneficiary in a retrospective system. Indeed, the perception among insurers that prospective determinations result in lower health care costs is premised on the likelihood that a beneficiary, faced with the knowledge of what the plan will and will not pay for, will choose the treatment option recommended by the plan in order to avoid risking total or partial disallowance of benefits."[9]

Contracts

"One of the most important roles of a practice manager is to facilitate the negotiation and execution of contracts and to draft and negotiate contracts for the practice group."[10] Contracting has taken on a secondary meaning within the health care marketplace. When we speak of contracting, it is often in reference to negotiating to serve large groups of patients covered by some form of health insurance or managed care product. This type of contracting is definitely governed by the laws of contract, but the laws of contract cover much more than just this activity. Contract law can be very complex and many exceptions exist to the general rules presented here. When dealing with any contractual matter, administrative judgment should be exercised and assistance in the negotiation and execution of a contract should be seriously considered on any complex matter.

A contract is a legally enforceable agreement for consideration between two or more competent parties to do or not to do something. In this definition the consideration refers to the price (be it money, goods, an act, not acting or inconvenience). An administrator is expected to be a sophisticated business person, and contracts, which might not be enforced against a less sophisticated party, will be binding. While there are provisions in the law which tend to level the playing field, the laws of contract favor those who have bargaining power. "Society, when granting freedom of contract, does not guarantee that all members of the community will be able to make use of it to the same extent. On the contrary, the law, by protecting the unequal distribution of property, does nothing to prevent freedom of contract from becoming a one-sided privilege."[11] The appropriate delegation of authority to contract should come from the governing body of your practice. It is important to make clear who has authority to negotiate and execute a contract. If the governing body reserves the power to execute an agreement, this should be made clear at the commencement of negotiations.

We generally think of contracts as written documents, and while some agreements by their nature are required, by the *statute of frauds*, to be in writing, it is very important to remember that many contracts may be entered into orally. Great care should be exercised to avoid having negotiations or expressions of intent to negotiate become binding contracts.

When a contract has been reduced to writing, most jurisdictions will apply the *parol evidence rule* to exclude from consideration any oral promises or agreements which are not in the written document. It is assumed that the written agreement is the entire agreement and any items omitted were negotiated away.[12]

Particularly in the physician-patient relationship, the courts have been willing to imply a contract where conduct alone indicated there was a relationship. Any treatment is generally considered to be sufficient to imply a contract and some courts have extended this concept to even less contact. In the academic setting, there is frequently a distinction between the "teaching cases," who are patients of an intern or resident and the "private patients," who are the patients of an attending. This distinction should be made clear to the patients and well documented, since it is likely that in a court of law, clarifying this difference may be difficult before a lay jury.

Some contracts can be terminated at will. In the health care setting, the ability to terminate the relationship gives preference to the patient. Patients may withdraw at any time (so long as they are competent and are not a threat to themselves or others). The health care provider is required to assure alternate care or may be liable for *abandonment.* The contract between the physician and patient is independent of the contractual arrangement between the physician and an insurance company. The new health care financing mechanisms, and their impact on the contract, between the physician and patient, have yet to be fully tested in court, but the administrator should be wary of this area.

Torts

A tort is a civil wrong made actionable by public policy. Tort liability is almost always based on fault; that is, an act or a failure to act was done wrong. This fault can arise out of an intentional act or from negligence. In instances where parties are conducting certain inherently extremely dangerous activities, the courts have held the parties to a standard of strict liability. But this would be unusual in an academic practice. The purpose of tort law is to compensate the injured party, not to punish the person at fault. This fact is reflected in the significant number of tort recoveries which are paid by insurance carriers. "Tort liability no longer merely shifts a loss from one individual to another but it tends to distribute the loss according to the principles of insurance, and the person nominally liable is often only a conduit through whom this process of distribution starts to flow. This does not at all mean that the loss disappears and does not have to be paid for. But it does mean that you ought to know who is paying for it, and in what proportions, before you can really see and evaluate what is going on even in terms of the fault principle. And it does mean that when the courts talk and reason about a rule of law as though the judgment were to come out of the defendant's pocket, they are often thinking in terms of complete unreality." [13]

In health care, it has been suggested that the tort liability and insurance system operate as a social taxation to compensate those who have unfortunate outcomes. If you have had involvement with the litigation of tort claims, you will recognize that the concept of fault does still apply even when the compensation may be largely covered by insurance. In rare instances, where the conduct has been deliberately malicious or fraudulent, courts will allow awards beyond that necessary to compensate the injured party. These punitive or exemplary damages are intended as a punishment, and a deterrent for others, and are not normally covered by any insurance.

A key distinction made in the common law doctrine of torts is the intent of the party causing an injury. If this person acted with intent to do the action which caused the injury, then this could be actionable as an intentional tort. If the action was unintended, then the injury may be compensated under the doctrine of negligence. The definition of intent refers to the action the person is undertaking and not to the result. There need not be any conscious willing to injure, merely to do the action which causes the injury.

Intentional torts of concern in a medical practice setting are: assault, battery, false imprisonment, defamation, invasion of privacy and infliction of emotional distress. As a general rule, *consent* is an absolute defense to an allegation of an intentional tort. It is increasingly recognized that there exists an overriding duty to provide sufficient quantity and quality of information to patients so they can make an informed decision in consenting to medical care and procedures. "The ethical duty arises from the collective wisdom of the medical profession; mainly, that patients are necessary partners in the diagnostic and therapeutic processes, that physicians have an inherent professional duty to respect a patient's wishes to know about his or her disease, and that patients have a right to know what they need to know prior to making a choice about whether to follow medical recommendations. The legal duty arises from the common law, statutes and the U.S. Constitution, which recognize that patients have a dignitary interest that does not allow them to be touched in the absence of consent and that Americans have a right to privacy, a right to refuse treatment, and a right to be informed about the benefits and adverse effects inherent in proposed medical care."[14]

The physician has some degree of discretion in the specifics which must be disclosed to constitute informed consent. In the case of *Arato v Avedon*, the California Supreme Court when faced with this issue said, "The context and clinical settings in which physician and patient interact and exchange information material to therapeutic decisions are so multifarious, the informational needs and degree of dependency of individual patients so various, and the professional relationship itself such an intimate and irreducibly judgment laden one, that we believe it is unwise to require as a matter of law that a particular species of information be disclosed." [15] The allowance of latitude for professional judgment as to the degree of information needed to constitute informed consent has not gone uncriticized. It has been commented that in the real world of practice: "(1) 'Disclosure' does not typically occur. Rather patients learn various bits of information, some relevant to decision-making, some not, from doctors' and nurses' efforts to obtain compliance and form 'situational etiquette'; (2) 'Decisions' are not made by patients. 'Recommendations' are made by doctors to patients; (3) 'Consent' does not exist. Instead what we find is 'acquiescence,' the absence of 'objection' or occasionally a 'veto'."[16]

Assault: An assault is the placing of another in the apprehension of a harmful or offensive touching. To be an actionable assault, no contact has to be made – just a reasonable belief that contact is about to occur.

Battery: A battery is a harmful or offensive touching. A physician is guilty of a battery when he or she performs an operation to which the patient has not consented or that is substantially different from the treatment to which the patient consented.[17] The doctor is liable for any injury or disability that results from unauthorized treatment even though it was skillfully performed.[18]

False imprisonment: False imprisonment is the unlawful restriction of a person's freedom. Physically restraining, or restraining by threats of harm, can constitute false imprisonment. All states have legal procedures to detain those that are a threat to themselves or others for reason of mental illness, communicable disease or substance abuse.

Defamation: Intentional injury to someone's reputation, whether in writing (libel) or spoken (slander), may give rise to a cause of action for defamation. As a general rule, the truth is a valid defense to a claim of defamation.

Invasion of privacy: The consent to treatment gives the medical team the right to acquire and use that information necessary for the care of the patient. Recognize that this consent is limited in nature, and, unless so specified, it does not include the right to the use of the information in teaching or research. The use of patient information for teaching and research is an established practice. Normally, so long as individually identifiable information is not used, this is not actionable. It is advisable in any academic practice to include within the general consent process, information regarding the teaching and research orientation of the practice. Also, great care should be taken to avoid discussion of patients in non-clinical settings, such as elevators and cafeterias. The consent to invade the privacy of the patient does not include distributing the information to persons not on the medical team.

Infliction of emotional stress: Intentional infliction of emotional distress could be considered an emotional battery. If intentional conduct is so outrageous as to be considered emotionally damaging, it can be actionable. The role of the patient's family and loved ones in very stressful situations must be given appropriate consideration. Flagrant disregard of the emotional well-being of those closely associated with a patient could be considered a possible tort.

Negligence: A negligent tort is so frequently the cause of action in a malpractice case that malpractice has been referred to as negligence in a professional capacity. While in many malpractice cases this would be correct, many malpractice cases also involve breach of contract, an intentional tort or some statutory cause of action.

There exist several very good definitions of negligence. Generally these say that it is doing what the average reasonably prudent person would not have done under the same circumstances or not doing what the average reasonably prudent person would have done under the same circumstances. Negligence is the unintentional causing of injury to someone. If your actions were intentional, it was not negligence. However, you may then be liable for having committed an intentional tort. Liability for negligence exists only when you have breached a duty to the party injured. The duty owed is dependent on the situation of the parties. The existence of a physician-patient relationship, based on an express or implied contract, is usually a prerequisite to imposing the duty to use professional care, skill and knowledge.[19]

"The difficulty with the duty concept in torts is that the word itself tends to confuse the true objective of the law, which is to sensibly, practically, and wisely delineate those misdeeds for which a recovery of money damages will be allowed. In the moral sense, we all owe a duty not to ever do that which may in any manner injure or damage anyone else...But our judicial concern is with a legal rather than a moral duty. In truth the word is a misnomer; for when the appellate courts or the Legislature...recognize a right of recovery for an unintentionally caused injury, we declare that a duty exists; conversely where a right of recovery is denied, we find no duty. In neither case do we consider the word in its commonly understood sense."[20] Or as one of the most famous commentators on torts put it, "(T)he problem of duty is as broad as the whole law of negligence, and... no universal test for it ever has been formulated.... It is embedded far too firmly in our law to be discarded, and no satisfactory substitute for it, by which the defendant's responsibility may be limited, has been devised. But it should be recognized that 'duty' ... is not sacrosanct in itself, but only an expression of the sum total of those considerations of policy which lead the law to say that the particular plaintiff is entitled to protection... No better general statement can be made, than that the courts will find a duty where, in general, reasonable men would recognize it and agree that it exists."[21]

To "breach the duty" is merely to have failed to meet the standard of care owed in light of your duty. In most settings, the standard of care is stated to be a "reasonable man of ordinary prudence."[22] The standard of care in professional health care services is generally accepted to be a national standard of what the average reasonably prudent professional under the same or similar circumstances would do or refrain from doing. A physician is liable for injuries to a patient caused by failure to possess and exercise, in either diagnosis or treatment, reasonable degree of skill, knowledge and care ordinarily possessed and used by other medical doctors in similar circumstances.[23] "Faculty in academic health centers have the weighty responsibilities of both training the health care providers of tomorrow and ensuring that care of a nationally recognized standard be provided to all patients in their schools' clinics or hospitals."[24] Both the increasing need to improve clinical effectiveness and a focus on quality of care and cost control have resulted in a current and projected emphasis among health professionals to develop guidelines for the provision of appropriate health care.[25] If the breach of the duty is the direct and proximate cause of the injury complained of, then an award to make the injured party whole may result. Generally the plaintiff in a medical malpractice case must establish that some act or omission of the defendant was the proximate cause of an injury suffered by the patient.[26]

The trial process in a case involving the academic practice has some aspects which do not generally get reported in the law books. It should be remembered that most of these trials will be tried in front of a lay jury. Even if the court is diligent in explaining the standard of care, and expert witnesses establish what a reasonable national standard of practicing physicians is, does a lay jury consider a professor in a medical school to that standard? Will the institution's reputation for research be a non-evidentiary bias the jury brings with them? Does the teaching role of the institution create in the minds of jurors false expectations? It is good to remember that many of the things which we consider as indications of quality, are to the lay public threatening, and may even be indications of opportunities for errors. These biases are unacceptable in a jury, and could result in a ruling of reversible error on appeal. But the reality is that lay juries do have biases which slip by the most rigorous empanelment process.

Alternatives

As a general rule, the best method of handling civil liability is to prevent it before it occurs. It is clear that no matter how comprehensive the prevention program, accidents do happen and the best approach is to try to minimize their frequency and severity, and manage your risks in a prudent fashion. (See risk management chapter of this book.) If prevention is unsuccessful, then resolution of the matter with the least amount of involvement with the legal system is preferable. The use of alternative dispute resolution is an effective means to limit the fees that attorneys generate from the traditional litigation system.[27] Arbitration and mediation have become increasingly popular methods in avoiding the complexity, delays and expenses associated with judicial litigation. Frequently, in discussion of the high cost of health care, the cost of litigation is cited as a significant contributing factor, and alternative dispute resolution is seen as a means of lowering this cost. When compared with the use of a lay jury, arbitration can more readily resolve a complex and emotional issue. Arbitration can more appropriately assess the compensation warranted by the injury and it can serve patients whose loss may not be lucrative enough to interest a plaintiff's lawyer. In fairness, the right to a civil jury trial is a valuable component of the United States judicial system, but the availability of quality health care is to be valued as well.

Legislative statutes

Antitrust

Antitrust laws, at both the federal and state level, are designed to protect competition by prohibitions on activities considered to create a restraint of trade or are considered anti-competitive. It is a very specialized area of law, which can involve extremely high legal expenses if a practice is forced to resolve an antitrust issue. Due to the increasing complexity of health care delivery systems, and the rapid innovation of new combinations of providers and payers, increased scrutiny is being given to antitrust issues in health care. Today's innovative marketing strategy may be tomorrow's Federal Trade Commission or

Department of Justice investigation. Academic practice situations are complicated by the fact that teaching requirements tend to emphasize coverage of all services. Historically many academic practices have dominated certain markets because: there were no other qualified providers; they introduced the new procedure; or no other provider was willing to incur the expense of the service. A teaching program not only needs patients as a matter of business activity, patients are also the teaching material. Providing services to a rural population also can create significant antitrust issues.[28] If a minimal market size is needed to support specific services, it may be difficult to assure competition in a small market.

The primary federal antitrust laws are the Sherman Act, the Clayton Act, the Federal Trade Commission Act and the Robinson-Patman Act. The Supreme Court has clearly identified that the purpose of federal antitrust laws is to prevent anti-competitive conduct. "The Sherman Act was designed to be a comprehensive charter of economic liberty aimed at preserving free and unfettered competition as the rule of trade. It rests on the premise that the unrestrained interaction of competitive forces will yield the best allocation of our economic resources, the lowest prices, the highest quality and the greatest material progress, while at the same time providing an environment conducive to the preservation of our democratic political and social institutions. But even were that premise open to question, the policy unequivocally laid down by the Act is competition."[29]

Most states have comparable acts which cover those instances where proper jurisdiction is the state. These laws have provisions which cover both agreements between competitors, called "horizontal" relationships, and agreements between producers and distributors, called "vertical" relationships. Because many aspects of these antitrust laws could be interpreted to prohibit virtually any business agreement, the courts have applied a "rule of reason" to look at the facts of each action on a case-by-case basis. As a result, the majority of antitrust law is found in judicial precedent. As recently as 1988, the federal government's position on the antitrust exposure of physicians was fairly straightforward. This was fully demonstrated by the Assistant Attorney General, Antitrust Division of the Department of Justice, Charles Rule, when he said in a speech to the AMA House of Delegates. "I am confident that the vast majority of you in the medical profession genuinely wish to comply with the law. And an ounce of prevention is, as they say, worth a pound of cure. So let me tell you what you can do to avoid the risk of criminal investigation and prosecution.

"The antitrust laws should not be thought to create an inherently gray zone of danger any time you so much as glance at a fellow professional. Unlike in the area of civil antitrust enforcement, criminal violation can be rather easily avoided by following a set of basic, simple, and easy-to-remember rules:

"First, do not agree with competing independent doctors on any terms of price, quantity, or quality - including fee schedules and relative value scales;

"Second, do not agree with competing independent doctors on the patients that you are willing to serve, the locations from which you are permitted to draw patients, or where you will locate your offices; and

"Third, do not agree with competing independent doctors to refuse to offer your services to alternative delivery systems.

"There can be exceptions to these general rules, particularly when the agreement is in the context of participating in a legitimate alternative delivery system. However, you should never act as if an exception applies until after you have consulted an experienced antitrust lawyer or until you obtain adequate assurance that competent counsel has structured the system to eliminate antitrust problems."[30]

This rather simplistic view of the health care market has changed rather significantly over the past few years. On September 15, 1993, in a response to a request by the American Medical Association for guidance on physician networks, a joint statement was issued by the Department of Justice and the Federal Trade Commission. This document was entitled "Joint Statement of Antitrust Enforcement Policy in the Health Care Area." In this document the agencies set forth a statement of policy regarding mergers and various joint activities covering: 1) hospital mergers; 2) sharing of high tech and expensive equipment; 3) physicians providing information to purchasers of medical services; 4) hospitals sharing price and cost information; 5) joint purchasing arrangements; and 6) physician networks. The joint statement is "designed to provide education and instruction to the health care community in a time of tremendous change, and to resolve, as completely as possible, the problem of antitrust uncertainty that some have said may deter mergers or joint ventures that would lower health care costs." This joint statement did not change the general direction of the enforcement of antitrust regulation of health care, but it can be said that it provides assurance of the permissibility of certain activities. It further commits the agencies "to swift and certain expedited review in an effort to reduce antitrust uncertainty for the health care industry in what the Agencies recognize is a time of fundamental farreaching change."[31]

Any antitrust question requires detailed review of the individual facts. Some of the general questions which should be investigated when considering if an antitrust exposure exists are:

- Is there a *per se violation*? These are agreements which are not viewed as having any redeeming competitive benefits. The court is, in effect, declaring the agreement to be unreasonable on its face. Examples of the types of agreements which would be per se violations are boycotts, divisions of markets, price fixing and product tie-ins;
- How much market power does this agreement represent? If an agreement involves 1 percent of a product market, it is significantly different than if it represents 99 percent of a market;
- What is the product market? The product area for an invasive cardiologist is different from that of a general practitioner; and
- Does this agreement materially affect competition in this market?

If the answers do not clearly indicate that there is no material anti-competitive impact, then seek competent antitrust counsel. It is also important to remember that there is always some provision of the antitrust law which can be used as a reason not to enter into an agreement. A fear of antitrust exposure within your organization can have a serious chilling effect on innovation and competitive motivation. In the dynamic marketplace, in which academic practices must compete, this can be disastrous.

Civil rights

Access to medical care is not a right, although there is significant political support for the position that the health of the populace is a national resource and as such care should be a right not a privilege. But there are several statutes which prohibit discrimination in providing care. These include:

- *Title VI of the Civil Rights Act of 1964.* Title VI, as it is referred to, prohibits discrimination on the basis of race, color or national origin by anyone receiving federal financial assistance. Since 1988, this prohibition has extended not only to those activities supported by the federal programs, such as Medicare or Medicaid, but to all areas of an institution receiving these funds;
- *Americans with Disabilities Act.* Title III of the Americans with Disabilities Act (ADA) forbids discrimination based on disability

in the full enjoyment of goods, services, facilities, privileges and accommodations of any privately owned place of public accommodation. Hospitals and the professional offices of medical care providers are specifically included in the act. Title II of the act forbids discrimination by public programs and facilities. The courts have interpreted this act broadly. Some aspects of insurance underwriting have been exempted from coverage, but close scrutiny should be given in any service delivery program which mixes aspects of insurance underwriting of risks and the delivery of care. *The Rehabilitation Act of 1973*, in a general sense, extends these broad prohibitions unless it would require a "fundamental change" or undue burden on the provider;

- *The Age Discrimination Act of 1975.* Any federally assisted program is prohibited from discrimination based on age. A reasonableness standard has been applied where there is a legitimate application of an age criteria, even if it results in disparate treatment for people of different ages. Also, extending benefits to children or the elderly has been allowed; and
- *Federal Emergency Medical and Active Labor Act.* The governmental role in prohibitions against "patient dumping" due to lack of appropriate medical insurance coverage is being tested in the courts. Academic practices have historically tended to serve underinsured populations. As financial constraints emphasize the need to generate practice revenue, it is important to remember that discrimination based on ability to pay, if permitted at all, it is being limited.

An interesting development in the regulations prohibiting discrimination in the delivery of health care services are some recent steps to *require* discrimination. In 1994, California adopted a proposition requiring health care providers to refuse some types of care to individuals who could not prove they were in this country legally. The enforceability of this type of state law, under the US Constitution, is yet to be fully determined.

Medicare and Medicaid

Academic practice has been treated like the domestication of the cow. Universities initially just knew it existed and tried to ignore it. Then they discovered that the leavings could have a benefit so they tolerated it. Then they found that you could milk the cow, so they started encouraging it. Then they found that you could bleed it, so they started controlling it. Now they have decided they do not get enough from it, so they want to butcher it for the meat. The academic practice is now supplying 57 percent of the clinical science revenue in medical schools in the United States.[32] Academic practices have clearly been able to generate revenue, much of which has come through the Medicare and Medicaid programs. It is reasonable to say that some medical schools have come to rely on this source of income. It is hoped that the reliance is not so severe that academic practices are facing a butchering for the meat.

In 1965, Congress amended the Social Security Act adding Title XVIII, creating the program known as Medicare, and Title XIX, creating the program known as Medicaid. These programs provided governmentally supported health care insurance programs for millions of Americans. To prevent fraud and abuse of these programs, the federal government has developed a series of statutes and regulations. Penalties for violations of these statutes and regulations can range from warnings, requiring return of overpayment, to felonies with punitive fines and incarceration.

"Historically, the relationship between physicians and Medicare, principally through the local Part B carriers, was much more benign. With a few isolated exceptions, the worst thing that happened to a practice plan that misunderstood Medicare billing rules, or failed to adhere carefully to those that it did understand, was a visit from the carrier, advice on how to correct the billings, and in some cases a request for a limited amount of money back, with interest. Even five years ago, enforcement actions against physician billing entities were rare, and what little hardnosed enforcement took place in the Medicare program was largely focused on proprietary suppliers in the lab, DME, home health and similar businesses."[33]

In December 1992, the Health Care Financing Administration (HCFA) issued a memorandum to "clarify" issues related to payment for services rendered by an intern or resident under the supervision of a teaching physician. This memorandum, known as the Booth Memorandum, "reiterates" HCFA's "longstanding" policy of these services being billable only if the attending physician was physically present when the service was provided.[34] This policy is based on the fact that within the Medicare Part A payments to hospitals is compensation to cover the cost of the services of interns and residents to Medicare patients. HCFA maintains that a payment to a teaching physician and a resident for the same clinical service would be "double dipping" and would constitute a flagrant abuse of the system. It should be noted that other payers, including some Medicaid programs, do not directly support graduate medical education and would not be involved in this issue. Further regulations were issued

December 8, 1995, which cover all teaching physicians, full time or voluntary, who involve residents in the care of their Medicare patients. These new regulations focus on the requirement that the teaching physician must be physically present during the key portions of each service and it must be documented in the attending and/or resident physician's notes.[35]

These regulations, while not directly mandating the operational policies of the academic practice, will have a significant impact on the operation of many medical schools in the United States. It is the stated intent of the Office of the Inspector General of the Department of Health and Human Services to focus on compliance, indicating it "has initiated a series of nationwide reviews of compliance with rules governing physicians at teaching hospitals (PATH) and other Medicare payment rules."[36] It is important that the applicability of these regulations and audit procedures be evaluated in light of the individual practice organization's potential liability. The Office of the Inspector General is willing to negotiate the liability of academic practices which pursue their own audit program (under the strict protocols provided by the Inspector General).

Medicare and Medicaid are not merely insurers to which bills are submitted and payments are made. These programs are creations of the law and are conducted with the full force and authority of the federal and state government. Their rules are arcane, difficult and frequently changed, but there is the force of law behind them and they must be taken extremely seriously.

Other statutory areas of concern

Stark I and Stark II: Section 1877 of the Social Security Act, commonly referred to as the "Stark" law, provides for regulatory prohibitions against certain types of referral of patients which may result in a benefit to the referring physician. With the increased complexity of academic practices, this is an area of concern.

Occupational Safety and Health Administration (OSHA): OSHA promulgates regulations governing employee work setting safety. Recent proposals regarding the handling of risks from blood borne pathogens and tuberculosis in the ambulatory setting may impact many academic practices.

Clinical Laboratory Improvement Amendments (CLIA): Federal regulation of the operation of clinical laboratories, including services provided within a physician's practice office, was significantly increased by this legislation. The amendments set forth specific categories of laboratory providers, the type of quality control required in each level, and the qualifications of the personnel required for provision of the services.

Reforms, trends and influencing change

"The human condition surrounding the delivery of health care is the same everywhere in the world: the providers of health care seek to give their patients the maximum feasible degree of physical relief, but they also aspire to a healthy slice of the gross national product (GNP) as a reward for their efforts. Patients seek from health care providers the maximum feasible degree of physical relief, but, collectively, they also seek to minimize the slice of the GNP that they must cede to providers as the price for that care."[37] This dynamic tension within the health care delivery and financing system have resulted in the situation, within the United States, where there is a desire to increase access and reduce cost simultaneously.

Massive and comprehensive restructuring of the private health care delivery system is an objective of significant powerful political forces.[38] While the ebb and flow of the political system is difficult to predict, an apparent trend toward increased regulation of the system is evident. As of this writing, the reforms of the health care delivery and the health care financing system are not a comprehensive restructuring but are individual specific changes.

Health Insurance Reform: Legislation at both the state and the federal level is geared toward increasing the availability and portability of medical insurance coverage. Specific changes include:

- Guaranteed coverage in the individual insurance market based on previous group coverage;
- Guaranteed insurance coverage, regardless of health status, in group policies;
- Limit on pre-existing condition exclusions;
- Guaranteed portability of coverage from one group carrier to another;
- Increased tax deductibility for self-employed coverage;
- Assistance in formation of small group coverage cooperatives; and
- Tax-free Medical Savings Accounts (MSA), similar to an IRA, but which could be used to cover medical expenses.

Health Care Liability Reform: Means are being proposed, at both the federal and state levels, to control and reduce the impact of liability claims on the health care system. These means include:

- Limits on compensation awarded for noneconomic damages;
- Restrictions on the application of joint and severable liability for noneconomic damages;
- Application of a collateral source doctrine;
- Allowance of periodic payments for awards; and
- Lowering and stricter enforcement of statute of limitation rules.[39]

Medicare Preservation: The Medicare Preservation Act was enacted as a part of the Balanced Budget Act of 1995, and includes many provisions to enhance patient rights within a managed care environment. It can be anticipated that as steps are taken to preserve the financial viability of the Medicare and Medicaid programs, there will be included patient protections and enhancement of governmentally protected patient rights.

Peer Review: *Health Care Quality Improvement Act of 1986.* Under this Act Congress created a limited immunity for peer review, created a national practitioner data bank to track problem professionals, and put in place a system of discipline, due process and reporting. In interpreting the limits of the Act, the United States District Court indicated that: "The Health Care Quality Improvement Act was not intended to replace existing procedural safeguards already in place at public hospitals nor provide a disciplined physician with a private cause of action. Rather, the Act is intended to establish certain criteria by which to determine whether procedural safeguards adopted for peer review of health professionals are sufficient to cloak the individuals acting pursuant to those procedures with the immunity provided by the Act."[40]

Influencing Change: Health care and academic medicine are in a period of tremendous change. Since this change is taking a course that is uncharted, the process is very receptive to input from those with a positive constructive approach. It is important to individually and collectively be proactive in providing guidance to federal, state and local authorities who are charged with making regulatory decisions that impact on health care. Working within professional organizations, such as the Medical Group Management Association and its Academic Practice Assembly, to effect positive change, can directly benefit your academic practice.

Executive regulation and rule-making

Administrative law

There is another type of law created by federal and state agencies in addition to regulations. These laws are frequently referred to as administrative decisions. Disputes resolved through a hearing process may result in written decisions which may be used as precedence in future similar situations. This quasi-judicial power is subject to review by the courts, and normally, any party who is dissatisfied with an interpretation may appeal the decision to a court of competent jurisdiction for review. These hearings are often informal and willing to accept broad input from interested parties. To influence the enforcement of statutes and regulations, it is important for the academic practice to assure that proper information is provided for these types of hearing.

Rule-making process

State and federal agencies, when interpreting statutory enactments, will frequently provide for a period of public comment prior to the rule-making process. With federal agencies, these calls for public comment are published in the Federal Register. As a general rule, it is much easier to influence the agency rulemaking during this comment period than it is to change regulations after they are enacted.

Choosing and using legal counsel

The services of legal counsel, lobbyists or arbitrators should all be treated as you would any expensive critical resource. Professional judgment in determining when a need exists is a critical talent. If you do not seek appropriate assistance in a timely fashion, then your practice can incur significant liability. If you seek assistance too early and too often, then your practice will incur significant consultative expenses. It may be better to err on the conservative side, but as margins are squeezed and issues become increasingly complex, this could become costly.

You should always attempt to get the best value for the legal expenses incurred. Before seeking independent counsel, determine if the information you need can be provided as a portion of your existing risk management program. If an insurance carrier has a portion of the potential liability, it may be very willing to provide legal counsel.

Courts often interpret insurance coverage broadly based on conduct, so even if you do not have "antitrust" coverage, your coverage for "piracy, unfair competition and idea misappropriation" may be sufficient.[41] This, of course, must be managed carefully as outside parties will protect their own interests. You may be able to clarify questions of law without great expense, but if you need the interests of your practice protected, then that should be done by your private legal counsel. Also, as an academic practice you should consider the connection of your practice with its School of Medicine parent to determine the role of the university counsel. Depending on the structure of the institution, you may be required to work closely with its legal counsel, or you may be prohibited from doing so since the interests of your practice may conflict with the interests of the institution.

Don't reinvent the wheel. It is often preferable to pay a higher hourly rate to a firm that will not need to do extensive research in an area, rather than pay for your attorney's education in a specific area of law. If you have information on the law relative to the issue, give it to your attorney prior to the commencement of research. Frequently, a practice administrator may know more about a specific area of law than does their attorney.

Use legal counsel efficiently. Remember, lawyers generally charge based on the amount of their time you use. If you are sociable and talk of vacations and families, you may find that it is included on your bill. You have a right to an estimate of the cost of a project, regular billings and progress reports. Just like a construction project, a legal project will stay on time and budget much better if properly managed.

Remember, there is seldom an easy answer to health care legal questions. In most cases, the advice you receive will be an educated guess of what a court or regulatory agency would decide. The ultimate business decision should be the client's – not the lawyer's.

Conclusion

The academic practice has an inherent level of legal complexity which makes administration increasingly professionally challenging. Academic practices must compete in a rapidly evolving environment which will continuously be years ahead of the legal interpretations which govern how it must operate.

The administrator of the academic practice plays a pivotal role in the maintenance of the finest medical education system in the world. This system is increasingly dependent on the academic practice for financial resources. It is a business whose mission is often stated to be to keep faculty members' clinical skills current and assist in supporting the teaching and research activities of the parent institution. But to meet the financial demand increasingly shifted to it, the academic practice must innovate and compete aggressively. Combining this complexity with a need to innovate, in an industry which is outpacing the laws which govern it, is a dangerous combination.

"Staying up-to-date on changing legal issues related to the practice of medicine is necessary for all involved in health care management. When dealing with legal issues, the manager of an academic practice must keep in mind that the practice is part of, or integrally linked with, an educational institution. The academic practice must be concerned not only with the quality of patient care and the financial solvency of the practice but also with the teaching, research and service mission of the institution of which it is a part. The responsibility to provide undergraduate medical education, graduate medical education, community service, academic freedom for the faculty, and research opportunities are what makes this setting special.

"Practicing medicine as part of the 'citadel,' the locus of knowledge and learning , creates interesting twists to the issues customarily facing all practices of medicine. Understanding the governance of the institution of which the academic practice is a part and seeking competent legal counsel early will go a long way in assisting practice managers in handling the legal issues that face the academic medical practice."[42]

GLOSSARY OF USEFUL LEGAL TERMS

Acceptance: *(Contract)* The act of a person to whom a thing is offered, whereby he receives the thing with the intent of keeping it, such intent being evidenced by a sufficient act.

Action: A lawsuit. A right to bring a lawsuit.

Actual Authority: Such authority as a principal intentionally confers on the agent.

Agency: A relation, expressly or by implication created in law or contract, where one party delegates the power to act for him to another.

Agent: One who represents and acts for another through agency.

Apparent Authority: That which, although not actually granted, the principal knowingly permits the agent to exercise or which the principal holds the agent out as possessing.[43]

Appearance: A technical coming into court as a party to a legal action. An attorney may enter a party's appearance by submission of written pleadings, without the formal presence of the party.

Arbitration: The determination of a matter by a person, generally chosen by the parties.

Award: To grant, concede, adjudge to. Also a decision or determination.

Cause of Action: Matter for which an action may be brought.

Charitable Immunity: A doctrine that relieves a charity of liability in tort; this doctrine has long been recognized, but currently most states have abrogated or restricted such immunity.[43]

Civil: The private rights and remedies of a person, as a member of the community, in contrast to "criminal," which are public and relate to the government.

Code: A collection of laws as promulgated by legislative authority.

Color: An appearance as distinguished from a reality.

Committee: A phrase, in some states, indicating the guardian of an insane person.

Complaint: In most states, the primary pleading commencing a lawsuit.

Consideration: The inducement to contract. The cause, motive, price impelling influence that induces a contracting party to enter into a contract. The reason or material cause of a contract.

Damage: Loss, injury, or deterioration, caused by negligence, design or accident.

De Facto: *Latin.* In fact, in deed, actually.

De Jure: *Latin.* Of right, legitimate, lawful.

Deposition: Testimony of a witness taken not in court but intended to be used in court. Generally a portion of the discovery process prior to trial.

Estoppel: A bar under the law preventing allegations or denying of facts, as a result of previous actions or denials; or a bar as a consequence of a final judgment of a court.

Executed: Completed.

Execution: Signing of a contract. Also, doing the thing indicated in the contract.

Exemplary: Punitive, for punishment or to set an example.

Fraud: Deceitful practice or willful method used to intentionally deprive another of his rights.

Implied: This word is used in law as contrasted with "express." If the matter is not manifested by direct words but is determined by deduction.

Indemnity: Liability for loss shifted from one person held legally responsible to another person.[43]

Injury: Any wrong or damage done to another.

In Re: *Latin.* In the matter.

Judgment: The official final decision of a court of law.

Jurisdiction: The authority constitutionally conferred upon a court.

Malfeasance: The wrongful doing of some act which the doer has no right to do.

Malum in Se: *Latin.* Wrong in itself. The act by its very nature is wrong under principles of natural, moral and public law.

Malum Prohibitum: *Latin.* Wrong because it is prohibited. Not inherently immoral, but prohibited by law.

Misfeasance: Doing what ought to be done but improperly.

Misrepresentation: Intentional false statement of fact by a party to a contract.

Nominal Damages: A trifling award.
Nonfeasance: Neglect to do what should have been done.

Perform: An act of doing what is called for under a contract.

Plaintiff: A person who brings a lawsuit, the party who complains.

Plea: A pleading, any one in the series of pleadings in a lawsuit.

Procedure: The methods under which a court functions.

Process: The means of compelling a defendant to appear in court.

Recovery: The collection of a debt through an action at law.

Remedy: The means by which the violation of a right is prevented, redressed, or compensated.

Right of Action: The right to bring suit.

Risk: Exposure to occurrences that potentially could result in a loss financial or otherwise.[43]

Satisfaction: Paying what is due as an award from a lawsuit.

Sovereign Immunity: A doctrine that precludes a litigant from asserting an otherwise meritorious cause of action against a sovereign (state governmental agency) or a party with sovereign attributes unless the sovereign consents to the suit. Historically, the federal and state governments, and derivatively cities and towns, were immune from tort liability arising from activities that were governmental in nature.[43]

Statute of Limitation: A statutory time limitation to the right of action.

Ultra Vires: *Latin.* Acts beyond the authorized powers.

Venue: The particular county, or geographical area, in which a court with jurisdiction may hear and determine a case.[43]

References

1. Helms, Lelia B., PhD, JD, and Helms, Charles M., MD, PhD, "Litigation Involving Medical Faculty and Academic Medical Centers, 1950-1991," *Academic Medicine*, Vol. 68, Jan 1993, 7-19.
2. *Webster's Seventh New Collegiate Dictionary*, 1961.
3. Churchill, Winston S., *History of the English Speaking Peoples* New York: Dodd, Mead, 1956-58, Vol. 1, p. 224.
4. Flagielo v. Pennsylvania Hospital, 417 Pa. 486 (1965).
5. Marbury v. Madison, 5 U.S. 137 (1803).
6. *Bouvier's Law Dictionary*, Banks Publishing, New York (1928).
7. Darling v. Charleston Community Memorial Hospital, 33 Ill. 2d 708.
8. Wickline v. State, 228 Cal. Rptr. 661 (Ct.App. 1986).
9. Cocoran v. United Healthcare, Inc., 965 F. 2d 1321.
10. Bonham, Vence, JD, *Managing the Academic Medical Practice: The Two-Headed Eagle* (Denver: Medical Group Management Association, 1992) 47.
11. Kessler, Friedrich, *Contracts of Adhesion--Some Thoughts about Freedom to Contract*, 43 Colum. L. Rev. (1941) 640.
12. International Business Machines Corporation v. Medlantic Healthcare Group, 708 F. Supp. 417 (D. D.C. 1989).
13. Fleming, James, Jr., *Accident Liability Reconsidered: The Impact of Liability Insurance*, 57 Yale L.J. (1948) 549-50.
14. Harsh, Harold L., MD, JD, "A Visitation with Informed Consent and Refusal," *Journal of Legal Medicine*, 1995 (147-203).
15. 858 O. 2d 598 (Cal. 1993).
16. Lidz, C.W., and Meisel, A., "Consent and the structure of medical care." *President's Commission for the Study of Ethical Problems in Medicine and Biomedical and Behavioral Research. Managing Health Care Decisions:* Vol. 2. Washington, DC: Government Printing Office, 1982.
17. Cobbs v. Grant 8 C3d 229 (1972).
18. Berkey V. Anderson 1 CA3d 790 (1969).
19. Keene v. Wiggins 69 CA3d 308 (1977).
20. Brousseau V. Jarrett, 73 Cal. App. 3d. 864 (1977).
21. Prosser, W., *Law of Torts*, s. 53 (3d ed. 1964).
22. Prosser and Keeton, *Law of Torts*, 5th ed. St. Paul, MN: West Publishing (1984).
23. Landeros v. Flood 17 C3d 399 (1976).
24. Butters, Janice M., MPH, Strope, John L., JD, PhD, "Legal Standards of Conduct for Students and Residents: Implications for Health Professions Educators," *Academic Medicine* (June 1996).
25. Audet, A.M., Greenfield, S., Field, M., "Medical practice guidelines: current activities and future directions," *Ann. Internal Med.* (1990).
26. Frantz v. San Luis Medical Clinic 81 CA3d 34 (1978).
27. White, William F., "Alternative Dispute Resolution for Medical Malpractice Actions: An Efficient Approach to the Law and Health Care," *Journal of Legal Medicine* (1995) 299.

28. Saner, Robert J., Esq., *Medical Group Management Update,* April 1996 (15).
29. Northern Pacific Railway Co. v. United States, 356 U.S. 1 (1958).
30. "Antitrust Enforcement and the Medical Profession: No Special Treatment," Remarks of Charles Rule, Asst.Attorney General, Antitrust Division U.S. Department of Justice, before the American Medical Association House of Delegates, December 6, 1988.
31. Department of Justice and Federal Trade Commission, Joint Statement of Antitrust Enforcement Policy in the Health Care Area (1993).
32. Pope, Christina, *Medical Group Management Update,* Vol. 35, No. 7, July 1996 (1).
33. Saner, Robert J. Esq., "Academic practices under fire: a guide to audit and investigational issues," *APA Matrix Supplement,* Medical Group Management Association (Summer 1996).
34. Teach, Randy L., and Artist, Jane E., *Legislative and Regulatory Briefing Book*, Medical Group Management Association (April 1995).
35. Teach, Randy L., "Update: Medicare teaching physician payment policy," *Medical Group Management Update* (June 1996).
36. Brown, June Gibbs, Inspector General in letter to Frederick J. Wenzel, MBA, FACMPE, Executive Vice President/CEO Medical Group Management Association.
37. Reinhardt, Uwe E., "Reforming the Health Care System: the Universal Dilemma," *The American Journal of Law and Medicine,* Vol. XIX.
38. Clinton, William, "The Clinton Health Care Plan, 327 *New England Journal of Medicine* 804 (1992).
39. Teach, Randy L., *Medical Group Management Update*, May 1996 (1).
40. Caine, 715 F. Supp. at 170.
41. CNA Casualty v. Seaboard Surety Co. (1986) 176 CA 3rd 598.
42. Bonham, Vence, L., Jr., JD, *Managing the Academic Medical Practice: The Two-Headed Eagle,* Medical Group Management Association (1992).
43. Black, Henry Campbell, MA, *Black's Law Dictionary,* St. Paul, MN: West Publishing Co., 1979), as used in the first edition of this book.

Chapter 9

Demonstrating value and quality in an academic medical practice

by Sara M. Larch, MS, FACMPE, and Deborah L. Walker, MBA, FACMPE

It certainly would be appropriate to ask why academic medical practices need to demonstrate their value and quality. After all, are not academic medical centers (AMCs) known for their high quality? They are also known for their high technological solutions to complex medical problems, translating bench research into the latest and most advanced clinical applications, and charged with the important responsibility of educating future clinicians, researchers and health care leaders. Nevertheless, the focus on value and quality for academic medical practices is necessitated by the current health care market, where differentiation on cost, quality and service dimensions has become the norm. Ironically, too often it is the academic practice that fails to compete on cost, struggles to match the high level of service afforded private practices, and must, therefore, demonstrate its quality to patients, health plans, employers and the public alike.

Competition in health care markets is currently based on price, range of offered services, quality and access. It is, therefore, incumbent upon an academic practice to demonstrate its quality in a manner easily understood by patients, payers, the public and other interested parties. When your local medical society reports outcomes for local hospitals, how do you explain if your results are not as good? The traditional explanation is that patients presenting to AMCs are "sicker" or have a higher severity of illness. While it is true that the tertiary nature of the AMC generally attracts both higher risk patients and the indigent, is this really true for your practice? Does the public believe that? Do your neighbors believe that? What about your parents? Can you "prove" it?

What is value?

How do we demonstrate the "value" of our academic practice to the community? A didactic exchange might include the background and experience of our faculty, the high quality of medical students we attract to our residency program, and the cutting-edge research that we conduct to advance the health status of patient populations. Unfortunately, this definition does not relate value in a way that permits it to be objectively measured from one practice to the next.

A quantitative definition of value that has been embraced by many practices is:

$$\text{Value} = \frac{\text{Quality}}{\text{Cost}} = \frac{\text{Outcomes}}{\text{Cost}} + \frac{\text{Service}}{\text{Cost}}$$

The value of our academic practice thus includes demonstration of quality, both outcomes and service quality, and cost elements. What this means for the academic practice is that it is no longer sufficient to say we incur higher costs due to the tertiary patients we treat. Rather, we must demonstrate the quality, the outcomes and service levels we provide in relation to expenditures incurred. What this also means is that the physician who has developed a national reputation for the treatment of a particular disease process may not be viewed as providing high value if he or she fails to consider cost as an important element of patient care.

What is quality?

Quality of patient care outcomes is extremely difficult to measure. The patient's age, sex, disease state, underlying health condition, patient compliance, and a host of environmental factors contribute to morbidity and mortality outcomes. The hospital or outpatient ambulatory care environment, its staff, its policies and procedures, tests and treatments, as well as clinical skills, all contribute to make the causal relationship for morbidity and mortality difficult to measure. The reliability and validity of comparative quality data across practices and physicians are thus difficult to assess without including "measures both of patient health outcomes and of the degree which the processes that led to these outcomes are stable and conform to scientifically based knowledge."[9] Published studies often fail to address the measurement of antecedent processes when articulating patient outcomes.

Quality service, on the other hand, is vastly easier to measure. This measurement is typically performed via patient surveys, surveys to referring physicians, and focus groups. However, this type of reporting relies heavily on individual experience and perceptions. Additionally, care must be taken to administer the surveys and focus groups in a manner that will elicit full disclosure and feedback from patients, assuring confidentiality and the importance of this feedback to the practice.

While customers are becoming increasingly sophisticated in their assessment of service dimensions of medical care, they also evaluate service in terms of commodity purchases, cost, reliability, assurance, ease of access. In addition, empathy, compassion and courtesy continue to play an important role in their perception of service quality.

Dr. Laurence Beck, Associate Medical Director for Quality at Georgetown University Medical Center, has defined quality as follows:[13]

> "For an individual:
>
> *High quality medical care is care that is effective and appropriate, and results in patient satisfaction*
>
> For a population:
>
> *Delivery of optimal services for the greatest number of people within available resources*
>
> For a physician, quality might be defined as:
> *Returning the patient to a functional health status with expected outcomes based on interventionist strategies employed."*

Whatever definition is chosen, the authors contend that the important dimension of clinical outcomes and service is integral to the value equation for healthcare.

Quality improvement programs

There are two fundamental types of quality improvement (QI) programs conducted by academic medical practices. The first is a formal program designed to monitor and evaluate appropriateness and outcomes of care, and to pursue opportunities for improvement. The second type of quality improvement program is designed to evaluate and improve service levels, focusing on the underlying processes that contribute to patient satisfaction. Written quality improvement plans are recommended for both types of QI programs. A common methodology is employed for each of these programs. However, the tools and measurements vary based on the underlying focus: outcomes versus service. The overall objective of QI programs is to reduce variation in services and processes. Other important objectives are found in Figure 9.1.

Figure 9.1

Objectives of QI Programs

To continuously improve patient care outcomes;

To develop effective and efficient processes in all areas that contribute to patient care outcomes; i.e., governance, management, clinical and support services;

To optimize resource utilization;

To compare patient outcome data and resource utilization with peer providers;

To provide routine reports to leadership;

To maintain records that will substantiate the effectiveness of the overall program;

To monitor and evaluate the populations served in terms of age groups, disease categories and special risk status;

To ensure that each clinical department has quality initiatives with measurable outcomes underway and being measured;

To actively support the enhancement of the information systems from a financial focus system to an integrated clinical information system.

The basic methodology for quality improvement programs involves the following steps:

1. Assume a process focus;
2. Assess customer needs and/or desired outcomes;

3. Analyze the current process;
4. Plan process changes;
5. Implement process changes; and
6. Measure process performance and outcomes.

QI program: clinical outcomes

Quality improvement programs focused on clinical outcomes involve the use of clinically relevant guidelines for the prevention, diagnosis, treatment and management of care. Practice guidelines are "systematically developed statements to assist practitioners' and patients' decisions about appropriate health care to be provided for specific clinical circumstances."[9] Basic quality evaluation tools include medical review criteria, performance measures and standards of quality. Process analysis includes prevention, diagnostic testing and treatment and is often documented via an algorithm or flowchart. Outcomes measures include such indices as: morbidity and mortality; immediate, intermediate and long-term health status; evidence-based outcomes; cost/quality analyses; quality of life; and patient satisfaction.

QI program: service

The second type of quality improvement program relates to the business and administrative processes within an academic medical practice that contribute to the perception of service/satisfaction. The key objectives of quality programs for service delivery are to: 1) reduce variation in process performance; and 2) reduce the number of process steps, decision points, waiting intervals, hand-offs, approvals, and cycle time for service delivery. Customer needs and wants are assessed by employing a number of tools including written surveys, focus groups and community forums. The current process is illustrated via a flowchart to document the process steps, hand-offs, waiting/delay points and approvals, and is then measured to determine the cycle time to deliver various steps. Analytical tools to assist with process improvement include brainstorming, nominal groups, structured discussion, cause-and-effect diagrams, force field analysis, run charts, control charts, Pareto charts and histograms.

The basic methodology for QI programs is found in Figure 9.2.

Figure 9.2

Methodology for QI programs

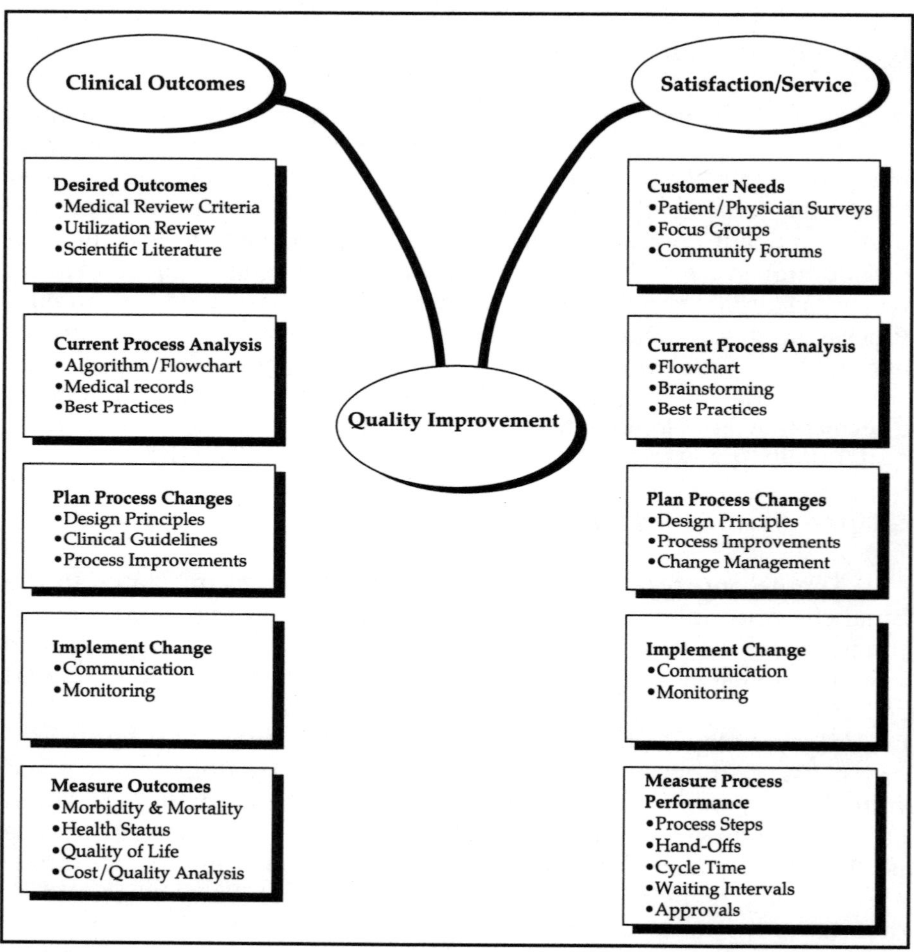

Cost

We have discussed the numerators in our value equation: Outcomes + Service. The denominator, Cost, continues to be an important factor in determining overall value of the services rendered by academic practices. It is imperative for academic practices to reduce costs in order to effectively compete with community practices.

At the same time, this area tends to be more difficult for the academic practice, due to human resources regulations and other business practices prevalent in the large university setting.

A systematic method to evaluate cost of care should be developed by the academic group practice. Cost factors should then be compared with published benchmarks and other "best practice" designations to determine targeted areas for improvement. Cost-related indices to be regularly monitored include:

Expenditures per RVU;
Cost per visit;
Cost per case;
Cost per covered life;
Utilization of preventive services; and
Staffing ratios by specialty.

Who determines value and quality?

Many individuals and agencies have recognized the importance of value and quality as differentiators of academic practice performance and have embarked upon efforts to define, quantify, and compare and contrast quality. A few examples are explained below:

Providers: Clearly, providers have a vested interest in evaluating the quality of care they render. This is typically conducted in a peer review fashion involving practice plan, clinical department and hospital representatives. Providers are now also paying increased attention to the notion of value, and thus resource utilization, cost of care parameters and satisfaction/service are receiving added focus.

Payers: Payers want high value at low cost. They have become relentless in pursuit of data to quantify the value of a physician or the practice. Their current focus is on cost and service. However, once cost of care in a particular market becomes flat (at the margin), and practices have improved their service dimensions, quality is expected to achieve prominence in the evaluation of practices and physician performance.

Patients: Patients have increasingly been involved in assessing quality for themselves and their families. Historically, patients have tended to evaluate quality of medical practice based on service delivery, as they would evaluate other service industries with which they come into contact. Service was assessed based on a practice's cost, assurance, reliability, compassion, ease of access and courtesy. More recently, patients have become active "shoppers" of quality with a shift in focus from an evaluation of service to outcomes. An example of this is found in Figure 9.3, depicting an actual patient experience.

Figure 9.3

How Do Our Patients Measure Quality?

- Mother of pediatric patient calls wanting information to decide where (which hospital) her son's elective procedure will be performed;
- Physician has privileges at two hospitals;
- Mother asked us:
  What is the complication rate for that procedure?;
  What is the post-surgery infection rate for that procedure?;
  What is readmission rate for that procedure?;
  How many of these procedures are performed by that physician per year?; and
  What is the nurse/patient ratio on the floor?

Could you answer these questions today about your institution?

Employers: Employers have a vested interest in value and quality, specifically as it relates to the cost of health care provided to their employees. Their search for high-value, low-cost services has led them to define certain quality parameters expected for their employees. For example, Rockwell wants its payers to demonstrate specific clinical indicators; e.g., What is the percentage of diabetic patients who received eye examinations in the last two-year period? What percentage of two-year-olds have received all of their immunizations? Similarly, Xerox provides incentives to employees to select plans rated by the National Committee on Quality Assurance (NCQA). As an incentive, employees selecting NCQA-rated plans pay $10 less per month for their health insurance premium.

Media: The media also has entered into the value/quality debate by publishing health-related outcomes data, report cards, clinical trials, clinical studies and providing this information to an even greater segment of the population. It is not unusual for the media to report the latest findings of popular health care journals; e.g., The *New England Journal of Medicine* or *The Journal of the American Medical Association*, before copies of the publication have been delivered to their physician subscribers.

The August 1996 *Consumer Reports* featured a 14-page report, "How good is your health plan?". This article was based on more than 20,000 responses from their subscribers about experiences in HMOs. Though the familiar *Consumer Reports* rating chart makes it easy to find the plan with the highest overall satisfaction score, it also leaves the reader with more questions than answers. A plan could receive good grades from NCQA, but patients be less satisfied because of their relationship with their physician or not getting the care they felt they needed.[3]

Government: Both Medicare and Medicaid have documented quality indicators required of providers of care. As more Medicare and Medicaid recipients move into HMO settings, we expect the data requirements to increase.

Professional Organizations: Lastly, professional organizations have become a major player in defining quality by seeking to establish their own quality initiatives. The American Medical Association, for example, proposes a single quality measure for all payers. It is based on credentialing (not unlike that performed by hospitals), personal qualifications, evaluation of the care environment, clinical performance, patient results and patient satisfaction. A five-year program, this measure would result in awarding of the AMA "Good Housekeeping Seal."

Provider credentialing

Historically, provider credentialing has been a "behind-the-scenes" activity performed by hospital medical staff offices as they appoint, recertify, reappoint and issue temporary privileges. The credentialing process has recently been raised to the forefront in an effort to ensure "quality" providers of care, both in ambulatory care settings as well as in hospitals. Verification through documentation efforts is performed to confirm medical licensure, education and experience history, hospital privileges, DEA licensure, malpractice history and professional liability claims. Data typically researched include the National Practitioners Data Bank, the Board of Medical Examiners and any government sanctions; e.g., Medicare or Medicaid.

The credentialing process has extended beyond this usual "background" check to include investigation of the physician's quality improvement activities, risk and utilization management, and patient satisfaction survey results. The credentialing process may include a site visit to the physician's primary practice site to obtain a general impression of overall satisfaction/service indices, medical records documentation and other related areas.

A new challenge for the academic group practice leader is deciding how to handle the percentage of physicians who do not meet established quality criteria. Could they be deselected by your managed care organizations? Could referrals diminish? How will the practice support their salary? What role should this play in academic personnel decisions related to merit, promotion or retention?

Service standards

At the present time, quality service is the differentiating factor among medical group practices. High quality clinical care is assumed and increasingly cost is at the margin, with practices unable to successfully negotiate higher reimbursement. Thus, differentiating the academic group practice on service quality has become a highly desirable strategy. Service strategies require investments in process design, support technology and human resources to ensure maximum effectiveness.

Indicators for satisfaction/service that need to be measured and monitored include the following:

Patient waiting time;
Frequency of physicians canceling office hours;
Results of patient satisfaction surveys;
First available appointment;
Patient complaints;
Member disenrollment;
Service to referring physicians;
Service to payers; and
Service to employers.

Health care reporting

A number of formal reporting mechanisms assessing health, value, quality and outcomes have emerged. These fall into two main categories: health care report cards, including formalized reports, consumer surveys and corporate purchaser ratings, and preventive care records. Academic practices need to establish mechanisms to independently capture the data reported via these formats. Knowledge of this data also permits the academic practice to differentiate its services when entering into managed care contracts and as part of its own marketing strategy.

The most prevalent report card format uses the Health Plan Employer Data and Information Set (HEDIS). HEDIS criteria were established to give employers a way to evaluate quality of care provided by HMOs and an incentive to offer only those plans that performed well on those measures. Critics state that the HEDIS data may be misused and that it tells us little about health outcomes. To others the HEDIS data offers some meaningful patterns that may show wide variation in managed care practices. A favorable performance on HEDIS criteria is desirable to effectively position the academic practice.

HEDIS measures include preventive care, access, membership and utilization of clinical services based on certain age groups and risk factors, and other descriptive measures. This data set includes benchmarks similar to those defined by the U.S. Public Health Service's Healthy People 2000 goals which the nation is to achieve by the year 2000. It is necessary to implement a number of administrative mechanisms to track, record and monitor practice performance related to these and other measures including:

Define IS reporting requirements;
Devise implementation work plan;
Define database requirements;
Design collection tools; and
Begin data tracking.

Preventive care records also are being developed to permit comparison of active approaches to health maintenance and prevention. Included in the preventive care records are a number of indices that must be tracked and measured by the academic practice and processes established to ensure effective measurement outcomes.

Measurements included in preventive care records include:
- percent primary care and specialists board certified;
- immunization rates;
- mammogram screening (age 52-64 yrs, in past two years);
- prenatal care in lst trimester;
- cholesterol screening (age 40-64, in past five years); and
- diabetic eye exam (in past two years).

Accreditation

The Joint Commission on Accreditation of Health Care Organizations (JCAHO) is a private corporation, but it operates as a quasi-governmental regulatory agency. Its "seal of approval" is used by hospitals to help qualify for Medicare and Medicaid reimbursement. JCAHO has expanded its breadth of responsibility to include ambulatory practice sites which have traditionally been run by clinical departments within an academic medical center campus. Trying to meet JCAHO's physician ambulatory care standards may be difficult.

The National Committee on Quality Assurance (NCQA), an independent nonprofit institution reviews and accredits managed care organizations. Its mission is to "promote improvements in quality of patient care provided through managed health plans."[8] Its formal review process consists of a pre-assessment survey, on-site survey and post-survey, with evaluation of health care delivery systems provided by those with whom they contract; e.g., physicians, hospitals and other agencies. The seal of approval by NCQA is viewed by many as an essential first step in documenting quality of care and service delivery: "Employers do not believe NCQA accreditation guarantees standards of care, but failure is a show-stopper."[2]

NCQA reviews the following areas as part of its accreditation process:

Quality improvement;
Physician credentialing;
Member rights and responsibilities;
Preventive health services;
Utilization management; and
Medical records.

As of this writing NCQA has reviewed 216 of the 500 HMOs with the following published results:

13 percent	Failed to pass;
12 percent	Received provisional accreditation;
39 percent	Received one-year accreditation; and
36 percent	Received three-year accreditation.

In all likelihood the reasons for failure will be attributed to particular providers, hospitals and other services involved in the assessment process, with the potential result of contract termination extended to impacted parties. NCQA began selling a CD-ROM that tracks quality data on 200 health plans nationwide in September 1996. Margaret Kane, NCQA president, said "The reports will make it possible for thousands of key decision-makers to compare hundreds of health plans in a way previously unthinkable. That provides a powerful incentive for plans to improve and compete on the basis of quality."[11] This increased intensity on health plans will translate to increased oversight of physician practices including the academic group practice.

Thus, a number of agencies now are interested in ensuring quality health care delivery. The "right care at the right time, in the right place, with the right providers, with the right outcome – no more, no less" is the clear expectation for medical practices, academic and private alike.

New quality initiatives

New quality initiatives continue to be developed, reflecting the high level of interest in this area. Two recent initiatives include life care planning and the Foundation of Accountability.

Life care planning

Life care planning encourages the patient to plan his or her own care by reviewing information specific to a disease process. For example, the patient is in need of hip replacement surgery. Life care planning provides bids to the patient including fixed price, mortality/reoccurrence rates by provider, names of 25 patients to survey, and warranty for a set number of years (similar to service warranty for manufactured goods).

Foundation of Accountability (FACCT)

Founded in 1995 by consumer groups and large private and public purchasers of health care, FACCT published its first five sets of measures last June for diabetes, breast cancer, major depression, patient satisfaction with health plan service and health risks.[12] Leaders in FACCT state they are not directly competing with NCOA, but now instead of one data set, there are two.

It is expected that the interest and attention to quality will continue. As clinical pathways, outcomes studies and comparative data become more sophisticated, quality of clinical care as opposed to quality of service will emerge as the differentiating factor in health care delivery. This would obviously be advantageous for the academic group practice.

As clinical administrators and practice plan leaders of academic practices, it is incumbent upon us to: develop appropriate quality improvement programs to evaluate and improve both clinical outcomes and service; continue to strive to reduce and evaluate costs; and develop the infrastructure and support services to measure and evaluate both processes and specific care indices that will differentiate and market our academic group practice.

References

1. Balestracci Jr D, Barlow JL: *Quality Improvement: Practical Applications for Medical Group Practice.* Center for Research in Ambulatory Health Care Administration, Englewood, Colorado, 1994.
2. Barron's, 3/4/96.
3. *Consumer Reports,* "How Good is Your Health Plan?", August 1996, pages 28-42.
4. Field MJ, Lohr KN (eds), Institute of Medicine (IOM), Committee on Clinical Practice Guidelines, National Academy Press, Washington DC, 1990.
5. Healthcare Forum Journal, 3/4/96.
6. Medical Group Management Association Journal. January/February 1996.
7. Sackett DL, Haynes RB, Guyatt GH, Tugwell P: *Clinical Epidemiology: A Basic Science for Clinical Medicine,* 2nd Edition. Little, Brown, and Company, Boston, MA, 1991.
8. *Standards for the Accreditation of Managed Care Organizations,* National Committee on Quality Assurance, 1995.
9. *Using Clinical Practice Guidelines to Evaluate Quality of Care.* Vol 1: Issues. U.S. Department of Health and Human Services, Public Health Service, Agency for Health Care Policy and Research, Washington DC, March 1995.
10. Using Clinical Practice Guidelines to evaluate Quality of Care. Vol 2: Methods. U.S. Department of Health and Human Services, Public Health Service, Agency for Health Care Policy and Research, Washington DC, March 1995.
11. *Washington Business Journal,* "CD-ROM takes guesswork out of HMO comparisons," September 6-12, 1996.
12. *California Medicine,* June 1997, p. 25-27.
13. From presentation to Clinical Quality Council, Georgetown University Medical Center, 1994.

Chapter 10

Measuring productivity in the academic setting

by Lindy Kirkpatrick, MBA, MS, and Robert B. Jones, MD, PhD

Historically, evaluation of faculty productivity in academic departments of medicine has been based on similar measures to those used for faculty in non-clinical departments. As such, it has focused on scholarly activity and, to a lesser extent, teaching. Demonstration of productivity in these areas has been necessary for academic advancement; i.e. promotion and tenure. Delivery of clinical care also has been recognized by some institutions as a component of service to the school or department and some credit has been given for this factor. However, in general, excellence in quality or quantity of clinical care provided has not been strongly rewarded.

A formula for faculty advancement in use in many universities and medical schools has required excellence in one of three arenas, and adequacy in the other two; the arenas being defined as research, teaching and service. Widely accepted measures of excellence in research have included federal support for research activities covering all or most of a faculty member's salary, ample publications in respected peer-reviewed journals, and a national or international reputation in the chosen field of scientific endeavor. Criteria for excellence in teaching have been less well defined, but have included the development of innovative new courses, direction of research by advanced students, or receipt of outstanding evaluations and awards from students and colleagues. Service activities which benefit the institution, local community or larger community have been recognized. These have included such activities as committee work, service on advisory panels, or establishment of new service programs. At Indiana University, excellence in service at present is recognized as "a major contribution to the welfare of the university (which) must be achieved and maintained..." (IU Faculty Handbook).

Promotion and tenure policies vary considerably among institutions, but one format commonly used allows tenure-track faculty a seven-year probationary period in which to develop their area of excellence and to demonstrate they have the professional characteristics that will allow them to continue to serve with distinction. Promotion from assistant to associate professor frequently occurs at the same time as tenure is granted. Promotion to full professor may occur at some time later and generally reflects attainment of international recognition in research or recognition as a truly outstanding and dedicated teacher. At Indiana University, promotion of tenure-track faculty based on service has been fairly infrequent. When it has happened, it has required a fairly unique contribution, such as the establishment of a successful transplant program.

Prior to 1970, most academic medical centers (AMCs) did not derive a significant proportion of their financial support from the clinical activities of their faculty, [1] and clinical productivity was not a significant factor in the promotion and tenure process. Consequently, little effort was expended to measure or reward it. However, with the development of faculty practice plans in the 1970s and the evolution of government health care programs, clinical activities now have become a major source of revenue. By 1995, they accounted for 57 percent of revenues supporting U.S. medical school programs and activities.[2] These additional revenues not only allowed the incomes of academic physicians to rise, but they also provided funds which could be used to develop research programs and to support medical education.

With this increased importance of clinical income to the budgets of academic departments has come increased interest in measuring clinical activity and in developing incentive programs for the most productive faculty members. Initially, measurement amounted to little more than keeping track of charges or collections and patient visits. In an indemnity market where all charges were paid for covered patients, this data provided a reasonably accurate measure of activity. Care given to patients not covered by an insurance product was considered charity and was regarded as part of the mission of an academic institution, particularly if there was associated teaching of medical students or residents. Concurrently, programs such as Medicare and Medicaid began moving more patients from charitable to reimbursable categories. As a consequence of these trends, the revenues available to institutions serving large economically disadvantaged populations increased dramatically until the 1990s.

However, in the past several years there have been vigorous attempts to control health care costs in both the private and public sectors. Utilization of services has been limited, leading to reduced hospital occupancy and attendant reduction in physician hospital visits and procedures. At the same time, reimbursement for each unit of service has been reduced through negotiated discounts in fees and increased use of capitation as a payment mechanism. As a consequence, practice income either has declined or has been maintained by a provider increasing the number of units of service generated. These trends are clearly having a major impact on academic health centers.

In response, many departments have attempted to increase their volume of clinical work by adding clinical faculty and by expanding services into surrounding communities. To some extent this strategy has worked. The average practice revenues received by US medical schools were still increasing as of the 1994-1995 academic year, although the rate of increase was declining.[2] Moreover, when practice revenues were calculated in constant dollars on a per faculty member basis, they had declined at 55 of 125 US medical schools surveyed. With declining utilization and reimbursement rates has come a realization that economic survival requires an atmosphere that encourages an efficient, cost-effective practice style for academic physicians — at least for the time they are engaged in the delivery of clinical care. In turn, this has led to attempts to determine the amount of clinical work done by individual physicians. One of the most popular systems which has evolved is the measurement of relative value units.

Relative value units

Clinical relative value units (RVUs) were designed as measures which would simultaneously take into account: a) the time involved in performing a clinical service; b) the skill required to deliver the service; c) the severity of the patient's condition relative to the service; d) the risk to the patient; and e) the medico-legal risk to the physician.[3] The most widely used relative value unit system is the Resource-Based Relative Value Scale (RBRVS) developed by Dr. William Hsiao of the Harvard School of Public Health.[4] Every service provided by a physician for which a fee can be charged has a current procedural terminology (CPT) code assigned to it. This is true for office visits, hospital visits and for procedures. Relative value units are assigned to each CPT code based on three components (work, practice expense,and malpractice) and are adjusted for various geographic locations. Geographic Practice Cost Indices (GPCIs) are printed each year in the Federal Register. The RVUs for each component are then summed to get total adjusted RVUs for a given CPT code. The formula is:

> (work RVUs x work GPCI) + (practice expense RVUs x practice expense GPCI) + (malpractice RVUs x malpractice GPCI) = total adjusted RVUs

The total adjusted RVUs are the basis for Medicare payment rates to physicians and other professionals under Part B of Medicare. To calculate the Medicare fee for a given CPT code, the total RVUs are multiplied by a conversion factor which is adjusted each year by Congress acting on the recommendation of the Secretary of Health and Human Services. The conversion factor is different for primary care services, surgical services and non-surgical procedures. RVUs have been used not only to determine Medicare payments, but also to set practice fees, determine costs in capitation rate negotiations, determine physician compensation for medical services, and measure physician productivity.

Physician productivity in academic vs. other practice settings

In a traditional solo or group practice, a physician's income is simply net revenue less expenses. A common arrangement is for everyone in a group to be allocated their own net revenue or collections, from which shared fixed expenses and each physician's variable and personal expenses are subtracted. The remainder is his or her income. Fixed expenses are either allocated based on each physician's charges or patient volume or they are divided evenly among the members of the group. Such an arrangement clearly provides a direct link between a physician's income and his or her clinical productivity.[5] In academic practices the relationships between revenue generated, expenses associated with that revenue generation and net income to the practitioner are often obscured by the administrative structure. For example, some or all of the practice expenses may be borne by the hospital or department, and compensation may be independent of, or only partially tied to practice revenue generated. In addition, practice revenues are usually taxed either explicitly, or implicitly by providing compensation below what physicians would receive if their income were just based on the revenue generated less a fair allocation of associated expenses. The proceeds from such taxes are used to support other activities of the school including research and education.

This lack of a clear relationship between clinical productivity and either personal income, or academic advancement, often leaves academic physicians with little incentive to practice in an efficient or cost-effective manner. As long as total practice revenues were rising, this did not cause great concern. However, now that revenues are actually decreasing, the efficiency and cost-effectiveness with which academic physicians deliver clinical care has become an issue of great concern for the schools and departments in which they work. Hence, a desire to accurately measure clinical productivity.

In the past, assessments of clinical productivity usually were based on gross charges, collections, or in an ambulatory setting, the number of patient encounters. In recent years there has been a move toward the use of RVUs as a means of measuring clinical productivity. In part this has been based on of the need of academic departments to determine clinical productivity in the context of other work being done by a particular faculty member; i.e. research and teaching. It also gives them a means by which they can use national survey data to compare the performance of their faculty to that of faculty at other institutions and to private practitioners.[6] While private practices still tend to use dollars earned per provider or visits seen per provider as their primary measures of productivity, academic departments also evaluate extramural funding support for research, scholarly articles published, and objective measures of teaching such as awards and student and resident evaluations.

Because of their different reimbursement structure, staff model HMOs use measures to evaluate physician performance which are different from those employed in the typical fee-for-service practice model. Parameters may include the number of members each physician manages, the per member cost of providing care, member satisfaction with that care, member access to the physician, rate of transfer of members off of physician panels, and the results of medical record audits. Since the HMOs are reimbursed on a capitated basis, they do not want to encourage excess patient visits, but they do want patients to be satisfied with the care they receive. This frequently leads to use of criteria such as those previously mentioned to measure and reward physician productivity.[7]

Research productivity

In academic institutions, research productivity is usually measured by publication of original research in peer-reviewed journals and by one's ability to secure extramural funding to support research activities. This includes salary support for the involved investigators (faculty members). Secondary measures of research productivity might include national awards, elected membership in national societies, invited lectures at national scientific meetings, participation in journal editorial boards and federal or foundation advisory panels, and leadership roles in national societies or meetings.

New physician faculty who have just completed postdoctoral training frequently are provided research support for a period during which they are expected to establish an independent research program. Typically this period is two to three years and by the end of that time they are expected to have secured extramural funding for part of their salary and most of their other research expenses. More senior investigators are expected to secure sufficient outside funding to cover all their research expenses and some or all their salary for that part of their time which they devote to research.

When an academic department includes research effort as part of its bonus system, it is usually only the funded research that counts toward the bonus. In response to the question "How Do You Reward Research?" in a survey of departments of internal medicine, responses received included:[8]

- Bonus of $0.25 on a dollar above goal level for funding;
- 80 percent of "funded" salary is matched by the department;
- 50 percent of indirect costs are refunded to division or principal investigator;
- 15 percent of all extramural funds paid as bonus; and
- Between 20-30 percent of base salary based on amount of publication and funding.

In addition, most academic institutions have a formula by which they return a portion of any funds generated by licenses or patents to an investigator either as personal income or as support for their research activities. Thus, rewards for research productivity usually are fairly closely linked to revenue generation. Examples of how this is done at a few institutions follow.

In the Duke University Department of Medicine, each faculty member's individual salary, supporting staff, other expenses and overhead are tracked.[9] The faculty members' expenses then are subtracted from the funding they generate and it is determined whether their research activity results in a net surplus or deficit for the department. This is calculated for each faculty member within a specialty division and for each specialty as a whole. If the division is generating a surplus, it may then receive a bonus from the department.

In 1991, the University of Alabama at Birmingham Department of Medicine decided to change its method of allocating funds.[10] The new allocation system was designed to accomplish four things: 1) provide funds for a reward system; 2) allow for individual and divisional entrepreneurism; 3) increase extramural funding; and 4) relate clinical costs to patient care revenues. The intent was to provide rewards, incentives and recognition for faculty contributions. In this system, research productivity is calculated based on the amount of faculty salaries and benefits paid from externally sponsored grants and contracts. The department rewards each subspecialty division by matching the salaries paid by grants and contracts in the preceding fiscal year. This money goes to the division for use by the division chief. The department also measures individual research productivity based on the number and dollar value of awarded and pending grants and contracts.

The Department of Medicine at Indiana University measures research productivity based on the proportion of the faculty member's salary and research infrastructure covered by extramural funding and the leadership that faculty member shows in mentoring junior faculty or fellows.

The University of Pittsburgh Department of Anesthesiology and Critical Care Medicine system was described in an article in 1991.[11] A point system is used in which clinical activities are worth a maximum of 3,000 points; administration = 2,000 points; education = 2,000 points; and scholarship = 3,000 points. The scholarship section is further broken down into three areas with points assigned by the number of papers, abstracts, chapters or grants from 0 - 5 and whether the faculty member was a first author or other author. The three categories are publications in peer-reviewed journals, published abstracts and book chapters, or external grant applications. When scores from all sections are added together, the faculty member with the highest score is given the largest portion of the bonus pool, and the faculty member with the lowest score receives the smallest bonus.

The Internal Medicine Department of the Ramsey Clinic in St. Paul, MN, has developed a compensation system which measures faculty productivity using an in-house system of weighted RVUs.[12] Weighting factors are assigned by a compensation committee according to the perceived difficulty or the value to the group. Tasks judged especially difficult to accomplish are assigned weights greater than 100 percent, while those judged easier to accomplish receive weights less than 100 percent. All recognized effort receives RVU credit. Research productivity is measured by the amount of funded revenue times a weighting factor of 118 percent. All weighted RVUs are totaled and compared to the department standard, which in 1995 was 4,500 RVUs per physician per year. They also have a quality adjustment factor which can positively or negatively affect an individual's RVU total by 10 percent.

The Louisiana State University School of Medicine also has developed a school-wide method of assessing physician productivity.[13] The departmental chairmen were charged with these tasks: 1) to list all activities a faculty might undertake; 2) to assign a relative value (RV) to each activity; 3) to develop a time component for each activity; 4) to develop a profile of a hypothetical faculty member; and 5) to test the system on selected faculty. The research component was broken into three areas: grants, abstracts and manuscripts. Within the grant category, RVs ranged from 2-6; 2 for a written, not funded or renewed grant and up to 6 for a funded national grant. Abstract values ranged from 1-3; 1 for an abstract presented at a local meeting or published with the faculty member as other author; to 3 for one presented at a national meeting as the first author. Manuscript relative values ranged from 1-4; 1 being assigned for being a contributing author on a reviewed manuscript and 4 for being a first author on a peer-reviewed manuscript in a prestigious journal. Study section participation is worth 3 RVs in this system.

Teaching productivity

In academic medicine, faculty teaching performance usually is evaluated in terms of teaching awards, recommendations of peers, and student or resident physician evaluations. Student evaluations have been the main quantitative measurement tool. However, as pressures increase to hold faculty accountable for other components of their work, pressure also will increase to measure teaching efforts accurately and to hold faculty accountable for their cost-effectiveness. However, the necessity of doing this is something that is just beginning to be widely appreciated. In a recent national survey of how departments of medicine,[8] reward teaching, the most frequent responses were:

- annual dollar prizes for top educators; and
- assume teaching is addressed in "base compensation" with teaching incentives used only for exceptional effort.

One approach has been to assign weights to different types of teaching activity as a rough reflection of the perceived difficulty. For example, the Department of Medicine at Cornell University has developed a relative value scale which is applied to all teaching activity undertaken by clinical faculty.[14] Weights range from 1 to 4 with attending at an outpatient clinic being assigned a weight of 1.0 and being the course director for a medical school course a weight of 4.0. Teaching hours are the number of hours actually spent teaching and do not include time spent in preparation, grading or meetings, because these have been factored into the weights. Each faculty member's teaching hours are multiplied by the weight of the activity.

This provides an overall measure of teaching activity. These data then are used in consideration of promotion and tenure, faculty compensation levels and in distribution of teaching assignments among the faculty.

Some schools set a standard number of teaching hours for which each faculty member is responsible. The amount of time a faculty member should spend teaching during any assigned activity (e.g. ward attending, outpatient, noon conferences, student courses, etc.) is set and the amount of teaching then can be calculated from the rotational assignments. The obvious disadvantage of this approach is that it does not make allowances for differences among faculty in levels of effort. Also, simply meeting a minimum standard does not motivate faculty to place a high regard on this activity.

In the University of Pittsburgh Anesthesiology Department compensation plan,[11] education is assigned a maximum point value of 2,000 or 20 percent of the total possible. Points are earned for didactic lectures, grand rounds, good resident evaluation scores and a positive educational review.

At the University of Alabama Department of Medicine, value is assigned to specific educational activities such as clerkship director, house-staff program associate director, etc. Subspecialty divisions receive allocations in their annual budget for each of these positions, for individual teaching awards received, and for fellowship training awards or divisional teaching awards to a division from the house staff. Examples include: $20,000 each for undergraduate and graduate teaching awards; $35,000 each for clerkship or residency directors; and $5,000 for each fellow who receives outside funding for his or her fellowship over $20,000 per year. Use of these funds is at the discretion of the division chief.[10]

At the Indiana University Department of Medicine, teaching RVUs have been developed which are weighted heavier for working with medical students than residents and fellows. The amount of time spent in each teaching activity is multiplied by the weighted RVUs to determine total teaching RVUs. Teaching RVUs, along with medical student and resident evaluations, awards received, and evidence of initiative and commitment are used in determining faculty annual compensation and bonuses.

At Louisiana State University, relative values (RVs) are assigned for component activities in teaching, research, administration and patient care in such a way as to reflect departmental values.[13] An appropriate amount of time for each activity is also determined along with the number of times a given faculty performs each activity. These RVs/activity, the time/activity and number of times the activity is done are then multiplied to give a global RV number for each activity. The global RVs for each of the activities are summed to give each faculty member a total score for work done in global RVs. This becomes a measure of that faculty member's productivity. Teaching is assigned RVs in one of two categories; classroom and clinical. Classroom RVs range from 1 to 10 with 10 being assigned for a grand rounds presentation. Clinical teaching RVs are either weighted 3 or 4. A month of general medicine ward attending is given 4 teaching RVs; a month of a consult service, 3 teaching RVs; and attending for 12 months in a half-day day clinic equals 3 teaching RVs.

The Department of Medicine at Columbia-Presbyterian Medical Center in New York City, surveyed its faculty in an attempt to determine: (1) the distribution of the teaching load among the faculty; (2) any variations in teaching based on sex, faculty rank, etc.; and (3) the extent to which physicians were compensated for teaching.[15] The results indicated that the teaching load was spread fairly evenly across the department; however, senior faculty taught more than junior faculty, and women taught more than men. The level of financial support for teaching was on the order of $15/hour, substantially less than most faculty are paid.

Clinical productivity

In some settings, clinical productivity is the easiest part of a faculty member's role to measure. In a single practice setting where each physician has the same patient mix and the same mix of other responsibilities, (e.g. teaching, administrative, etc.), a simple measure such as net revenue less expenses may suffice. The problem with this approach in more complex situations is that it unfairly disadvantages faculty assigned to sites with poor collections or high practice expenses. As a result, it may make it harder to find faculty willing to work at such sites. Thus, more complex situations necessitate more complex measuring instruments if fairness is to maintained. Again, some examples follow.

Until recently, Baystate Health Systems in Massachusetts used historical measurements of number of visits per hour, gross revenue and number of procedures performed to determine whether or not a physician or group practice was efficient.[16] However, because Baystate has multiple clinical sites in different geographic locations, differences in payer mix and charge structure made it difficult to accurately compare physician productivity in the different practices. As a consequence, Baystate developed a new system of tracking productivity which incorporated measures of revenue generation, practice expense, patient encounters, time spent with students, residents and physician extenders, and time spent on required supervisory and administrative duties. Physicians now complete time and effort reports and track hours spent as billable or not. In a given week of tracking 40 hours, only 20 may be billable. Billable hours include supervising residents, seeing patients, being on call, etc. Non-billable activities include administration and formal teaching. Monthly reports are generated for each facility, department and individual physician. An individual physician report will include the total number of patient visits, the number of unique patients, the average number of visits per patient, total charges, inpatient and outpatient billable hours, and RVUs generated per billable hour. The productivity of each physician is then compared to that of each of the other physicians within the same department and to the total group average.

The Southern Ohio Health Services Network in Cincinnati, OH, is a not-for-profit corporation employing physicians in a medically underserved area along the Ohio river. Annual salary increases are determined by physician productivity and quality assurance with the latter weighted heavier than the productivity.[17] Physician performance is audited throughout the year based on network quality assurance standards. If physicians achieve 80 percent or greater compliance with the standards, then they are eligible for 100 percent of the salary increase. If their compliance is 70 to 79 percent, they may receive only half the annual increase. If it is below 70 percent they are not eligible for an increase. Quality assurance makes up 80 percent of the decision on an annual increase and productivity accounts for the remaining 20 percent. To be eligible for a productivity increase, charges must exceed 75 percent of expenses. Bonuses are also based on charges exceeding a breakeven point. Since this system has been in place, productivity has increased and costs have decreased. Physician satisfaction with the plan has been high.

Another department of medicine located in the Midwest has set a productivity target for each half-day outpatient clinic of the RVU equivalent of 12 CPT code Level 3 follow-up visits. If a student is assigned to the physician, the RVU target is 25 percent less for that half day. There are also monthly RVU targets for each inpatient rotation. An interesting aspect of this plan is that individual faculty have a productivity target based on their own set of assignments. Thus, a faculty member can change his or her target by requesting a change in assignments. At bonus time, physicians are evaluated by how close they come to their target. If the target is exceeded, a greater than "one share" of the bonus pool is received.

The University of Virginia also has developed an incentive compensation system based on RVUs.[18] Clinical performance is evaluated in three areas and a substantial proportion of compensation is associated with achievement of preset goals in each area. The first area is productivity in RVUs compared using the median MGMA adjusted averages for each specialty as a benchmark. Increased compensation above base begins at 5 percent above the MGMA median with additional increases at 15 percent, 30 percent and greater than 50 percent. Also, if a physician achieves the MGMA RVU median, he or she then is entitled to 100 percent of incentive payments from contracted managed care contracts. Each physician is also evaluated for patient care satisfaction. Physicians must have at least 1500 active patients and achieve an average rating of 4.0 on a scale of 1-5, (5 = outstanding), on patient satisfaction surveys to get a monetary reward of $1,000. A score of 5.0 results in a $5,000 reward. The third area is HMO wellness. If annual physical exams are done on applicable patients, there is a financial reward for the physician. Quality in teaching is expected, but does not have specific incentives associated with it.

At the Indiana University Department of Medicine, the clinical component of faculty evaluation and compensation is based on both subjective and objective measures. Data are collected on: productivity (RVU generation for amount of time spent in clinical activity); proportion of clinical salary and overhead covered by clinical revenues; patient and referring physician satisfaction (determined from surveys); and staff relations. Program development and innovation, team play and administrative contributions are determined subjectively. Figure 10.1 shows sample clinical productivity tracking of a single specialty. The productivity of each physician in RVUs per unit of time is compared to the MGMA adjusted mean for a full time equivalent for his or her specialty and to the productivity in RVUs of the other physicians in their own division (specialty).

Figure 10.1

Indiana University Medicine Clinical Productivity Tracking

MD	Charges	Collections	Percent Clinical Effort	Total RVUs	RVUs Per 1% Effort	92 Division Target RVUs per 1% Effort	87.15 MGMA Target RVUs per 1% Effort	Variance to Division	Variance to MGMA
A	211,125	121,510	45%	3,248	72	4,140	3,922	-22%	-17%
B	533,865	281,221	60%	6,647	111	5,520	5,229	20%	27%
C	267,235	76,591	36%	3,519	98	3,312	3,137	6%	12%
D	456,119	259,174	36%	5,766	160	3,312	3,137	74%	84%
E	347,058	191,560	72%	2,874	40	6,624	6,275	-57%	-54%
F	501,028	314,759	60%	6,415	107	5,520	5,229	16%	23%
	2,316,430	**1,244,815**	**309%**	**28,469**					

In addition, the clinical revenue generated by each physician and the expenses (Figure 10.2) associated with each clinical practice is tracked. From these two figures the net profit or loss for clinical activities can be calculated. When these are summed up for a division (specialty), they allow a similar calculation for the entire clinical operation of that unit; i.e., whether clinical operations resulted in a profit or loss to the department for the period of time being examined.

Figure 10.2

Indiana University Medicine
Clinical Expense Tracking

MD	Clinical Sal/Fr	Staff	Malprac	Clinical Supplies	Billing Cost	Pagers Telep	Clinic Fixed Costs	Total Clinical Expenses	Amount Collected	Net to Clinical
A	58,523	14,238	1,430	4,500	12,151	924	17,324	109,090	121,510	12,420
B	84,285	15,899	1,430	4,500	28,122	1,380	11,549	147,165	281,221	134,056
C	74,605	12,789	1,430	4,500	7,659	1,944		102,927	76,591	-26,336
D	40,500	15,899	1,430	4,500	25,917	816	5,775	94,837	259,174	164,337
E	72,000	22,145	1,430	4,500	19,156	1,584		120,815	191,560	70,745
F	76,610	33,562	1,430	4,500	31,476	1,368	17,324	166,270	314,759	148,489
Total	**406,523**	**114,532**	**8,580**	**27,000**	**124,482**	**8,016**	**51,972**	**741,105**	**1,244,815**	**503,711**

Louisiana State University uses its own system of relative values as described earlier. The patient care relative values for half-day increments of clinics or procedures are valued at 2 RVs per year-long half day in clinic or performing procedures. A month-long ward attending rotation is also valued at 2 RVs. [13]

The University of Alabama Department of Medicine plan uses a responsibility-center system of budgeting with responsibility concentrated at a divisional level. Under this plan 57 percent of clinical collections are returned to each division (specialty) in the department. From the remaining 43 percent, practice expenses are paid by the department. The division has full discretion as to use of the collections it receives and thus it is primarily at the division level that the incentives operate.[10]

In the Ramsey Clinic model which uses weighted RVUs,[12] the conversion factor for inpatient care is 0.8; for outpatient procedures 1.0; for outpatient clinics 1.4; for supervising an extender 0.2; and for outreach 1.5. The differences in the conversion factors reflect differences in the perceived difficulty in generating RVUs in the different venues. These are then multiplied by the number of RVUs generated in each clinical activity to achieve the weighted RVUs generated by each physician in each activity. The weighted clinical RVUs for each physician are summed and added to the weighted RVUs generated by teaching, research and administration to yield a total productivity measure for that physician. This figure is used to determine compensation.

Where do we go from here?

Clearly changes in the health care market and the associated decrease in practice revenues will force changes in how medical school faculty function. They already have in most institutions in the United States, and the process is far from over. The time is rapidly drawing to a close in which a professor of medicine can consider as beneath him or her the contemplation of the source of funds used to pay his or her salary. Accountability will be the catchword for the future; accountability for quality of patient care, for cost of patient care, for practice expenses, for educational expenses, and for consumer satisfaction (patients, payers, referring physicians and society at large). Accountability requires accurate and equitable systems for measuring the different components associated with health care delivery and these, in turn, require sophisticated information systems.

Most academic departments of medicine by now have adopted some means of measuring clinical productivity or are moving in that direction. A common theme seems to be that simple measures such as charges or collections by themselves do not accurately reflect effort in the complex payer environment in which most academic centers function. Moreover, many centers need to identify and reward clinical care activities in populations where direct or indemnity reimbursement is poor. Consequently, something else is needed. For many, RVUs seem to be the answer, often with some system of weighting to reflect local values and unique circumstances. However, simply measuring and rewarding faculty based on the quantity of work done is not enough. It conflicts with traditional academic values and with patient expectations both of which emphasize other aspects of care such as quality and humanism. It also does not take into account the need to deliver care in a cost-effective manner and it is this more than anything else that is the driving force of the current revolution in health care delivery.

There seems to be an evolving consensus as to the other elements of health care delivery that need to be measured so performance can be enhanced. Often this is done through an incentive plan linked to compensation. The primary elements are quality of care, cost of care and patient satisfaction. However, quality of care is difficult to measure and quantify directly. Consequently, one approach which is increasingly being taken is to measure adherence to practice guidelines and other standards as a proxy for quality. Bohlman[19] suggests that future compensation plans at a minimum will have to take into account:

- Productivity measured by dollars and relative value units;
- Resource utilization measurements;
- Outcome or quality of service measurements;
- Patient survey responses; and
- Teamwork measured by the degree to which physicians participate in activities related to organizational goals.

In fact, University Mednet, a Cleveland group practice has developed a program for evaluating provider performance which contains the following elements [20]:

- Performance standards - procedures are defined for diagnosis and treatment of common medical problems, screening criteria for the healthy population, as well as standards for the appropriate use of inpatient and outpatient services;
- Customer satisfaction - patients are queried as to the services they want and surveyed to see if they are being provided;
- Marketplace comparison of physician compensation;
- Productivity - RVUs are assigned to each type of service and comparisons made between individual physicians; and
- Performance appraisal to assess physician compliance with standards.

All areas are linked to compensation. Many other institutions have developed similar programs.

One additional factor to be considered is the large and growing impact of Health Maintenance Organizations (HMOs). The cost-effectiveness of medical care is important regardless of payment mechanism, but the emphasis on it increases as the proportion of patients for whom reimbursement is capitated increases. Under capitation, payment is for total care and is made on a per member per month basis. Specialists no longer generate additional revenue by performing additional procedures. In fact, they, or the system, incur a non-reimbursed cost for every procedure they perform and for every extra diagnostic test they order. In this setting, the physician behaviors required for a successful delivery system are quite different and the incentive system likewise needs to be different. Parameters measured include access time to get an appointment, patient survey results, utilization (visits per member per year) and medical group profitability .[21] In addition, laboratory and radiology utilization as well as specialty consultation rates are measured and compared to historical practice patterns.[22] Performance standards such as those described are important tools for maintaining quality of care in a system where the financial incentives are directed at reducing utilization.

In addition to new and improved systems for measuring productivity, the increased emphasis on accountability will necessitate emergence of a new type of health care manager in academic medicine. These individuals will need to be capable of working within systems to effect necessary change without debasing those aspects of medical care associated with quality and compassion. They will need to understand the business aspects of health care delivery and to be in a position to inculcate business principles into the operational decisions of academic units. Among their many tasks will be adaptation and implementation of programs to measure physician productivity in ways that make sense for the unique circumstances at their own institutions.

References

1. Hoffstein PA. "The organization of medical schools." In: Nicholas WR, ed. *Managing the Academic Medical Practice: the Two-Headed Eagle.* Englewood, Colorado: Medical Group Management Association, 1992:1-27.
2. Krakower JY, Ganem JL, Jolly P. "Review of US Medical School Finances," 1994-1995. *Jama*, 276, 720-4.
3. Conomikes Special Report (1995). "Understanding and Dealing With RBRVS." Conomikes Report, Los Angeles, CA.
4. Berenson Robert A., Lieberman Richard N. "Special Report: Using Medicare's RBRVS to Evaluate Capitation Rates and Fee Schedules." St. Anthony Publishing, Reston, Va.
5. Azevedo D. (1991) "Can You Make Your Income-Division Formula Work Better?" *Medical Economics.*
6. Holets Thomas D. "Productivity Enhancement: Implications for Medical Group Management." *College Review* 1990;Fall 1990:22-36.
7. Schlackman Neil, MD. "Quality and Physician Compensation: Performance-Based Incentives in Managed Care," *The Quality Letter* 1994;March 1994:18-23.
8. Quinn James. "Faculty Incentive Programs: Where are we now... & Where are we going?" Workshop Session at AIM Sixteenth Annual Educational Meeting, October 30th, 1995.
9. Thacker, Paul A (1995): "Improving Faculty Productivity By Increasing Divisional Responsibility and Accountability and By Changing Resource Allocation Methods." Workshop Presented at AIM Sixteenth Annual Meeting, October 30, 1995.
10. Lewis James E., PhD. "Improving Productivity: The Ongoing Experience of an Academic Department of Medicine." *Academic Medicine* 1996;71 No. 4, 317-28.
11. Tkach David and D. Ryan Cook, MD. "Developing A Merit Compensation Plan in an Academic Setting." *MGM Journal* 1991;Sept/Oct 1991:32-6.
12. Spurrier Barb. "Summary of New Compensation System, Ramsey Clinic Department of Internal Medicine." Workshop Presented at APA Annual Conference April 29, 1996.
13. Hilton Charles W. MD, Lopez Alfredo MD, Fisher William PhD, Sanders Charles MD (1996). "A Relative-Value-Based System For Quantification of Faculty Productivity: A Simple, Adjustable, Weighted System for Calculating Faculty Productivity in Teaching, Research, Administration and Patient Care." Presentation at APM Winter Meeting, 1996.
14. Bardes C, Hayes J. "Are The Teachers Teaching? Measuring the Educational Activities of Clinical Faculty." *Academic Medicine* 1995;70:111-4.
15. Shea S, Nickerson KG, TemeBaum J, et al. "Compensation to a Department of Medicine and its Faculty Members for the Teaching of Medical Students and House Staff." *N Engl J Med* 1996; 334:162-7.

16. Lagasse P Jr. "Physician Productivity Measurement, Methodology & Implementation. Quest for Quality and Productivity in Health Services," 1995 Conference Proceedings. Institute of Industrial Engineers.
17. Wilhide, Stephen (1991): "Developing a Merit Compensation Plan in an Academic Setting." *MGM Journal* Sept/Oct 1991, 67-70.
18. Williams AS, Woodcock EW (1995): "The Practical Use of Relative Value Units." Workshop Presentation at the APA Conference, May 9, 1995.
19. Bohlman, Robert C (1996): "Physician Compensation in Transition." *MGM Journal* Jan/Feb, 9-15.
20. Henoch M M.D., "Compensation of Physicians in Group Practice," *Group Practice Journal* 1991;Sept/Oct 1991:46-50.
21. Erra RJ., "Compensating Physicians in a Mixed Fee-for-Service/Capitated Practice," *The Quality Letter* 1994;March 1994:12-7.
22. Lipsitz DJ MD, Nagler HJ MD., "A Physician Incentive Compensation Program in a Staff Model HMO," *HMO Practice* 1993;7 No. 2:82-6.

Chapter 11

Provider compensation in the academic medical practice

by Arthur C. Krohn, Jr., MBA, MS, FACMPE

In the past, academic medical centers (AMCs) appealed to a certain type of physician. These individuals were drawn by exciting intellectual surroundings, reduced administrative burden, the occasion to teach, and the opportunity to do research in an enlightened and protected environment. It was generally understood that in exchange for these benefits, the academic physician would usually receive less compensation than might be achieved in private practice. To those physicians who did choose to go into private practice, being an employee of an organization was totally unacceptable. However, with the decrease in revenues due to the advent of managed care and capitation and increased administrative burden due to changing regulations, many more physicians are looking for the security and peace of mind that being an employee rather than an employer brings. According to an AMA survey, 36.5 percent of physicians in 1994 described themselves as employees rather than self-employed or independent contractors as compared to 23.9 percent in 1989.[1]

Therefore, Health Maintenance Organizations (HMOs), hospitals and other health care organizations are now competing on a much larger scale for many of the same physicians who previously would have been interested in AMCs. Now more than ever, the ability to recruit and retain exceptional medical faculty is an issue for medical schools. Due to two disquieting facts, it is extremely important to have the best, most productive faculty available. First, according to the Association of American Medical Colleges (AAMC) Liaison Committee on Medical Education, clinical income as a component of total medical school revenues has grown from roughly 30 percent to more than 46 percent and, accordingly, the percentage from other

---

Written in fulfillment of the requirements for advancement to Fellowship Status in the American College of Medical Practice Executives, 104 Inverness Terrace East, Englewood, CO 80112-5306; 303-397-7869

sources has declined, notably for those schools with government support.[12] Second, an AMC, with its mix of tenure policies, teaching promotion stipulations, research grant requirements and administrative duties, presents a unique set of circumstances under which a physician must perform.

Given this environment, the determination of a total compensation package for physicians in an academic setting is an onerous, Herculean and sometimes, mystical task. However, it is usually a significant factor in determining which institution the doctor ultimately chooses as his or her employer. The provider's perception of such things as guaranteed salary, incentives and benefits (both the employee's share and Uncle Sam's share) will go a long way in determining the physician's final place of employment and how long he or she stay there. It is the authorís opinion that if physicians are fully satisfied with their compensation arrangement, they will then be able to devote that much more of their attention to providing the highest quality of patient care.

Historically, academic practice plans have provided a supplement to compensation provided by the medical school, which was usually lower than that available in the private sector. This allowed the school to recruit and retain quality faculty. A physician's compensation agreement with the medical school and/or the plan will usually include a guaranteed base salary and a package of basic fringe benefits from the medical school, supplemented by additional salary and/or an incentive payment, and an enhanced program of fringe benefits, all funded by practice plan clinical income.

For a clinical administrator at an academic medical center to be better prepared to handle the task of preparing a compensation plan, this dissertation will illustrate and comment upon the various salary components and benefits which have been used historically for physicians in general, and specifically, at AMCs. Methods of distributing physician compensation in an academic environment will also be examined. Furthermore, the methods of funding academic practices will be described. Since most academic medical centers are not-for-profit, the significance of specific regulations and regulators pertaining to compensation will be commented upon. Inasmuch as the Internal Revenue Service is always a part of any discussion of salaries and benefits, a section will be devoted to possible tax-saving or tax-deferring alternatives.

With the coming of managed care and capitation, historical methods of physician compensation will have to be reviewed and updated. Physician offices will no longer be regarded as profit centers, but must be treated as cost centers.[3] Therefore, a plan will have to be developed which rewards physicians who are able to cut costs and see fewer patients rather than those which compensate a physician in direct proportion to the number of patients seen or the number of Relative Value Units (RVUs) produced. Examples of compensation schemes which have been utilized under a managed care/capitation environment will be presented.

Salary components

To the majority of physicians, the most important elements of compensation, and the segments they are most likely to understand, are the various salary components. Salary usually contains one or more of these elements: a base, supplements, incentives and deferred compensation. Historically, physicians' salaries have consisted primarily of a base and an incentive, with the other components becoming definitionally blurred. However, with increasing pressure on tenure procedures and decreasing revenue streams, AMCs are beginning to reevaluate their salary plans.[4] Definitions of the primary salary components being used today are:

- Base salary - This is usually an amount set by the institution as a percentage of average salaries at that institution.[5] This is meant to cover the basic academic commitment to the university. This portion is usually guaranteed as part of tenure or if not tenured, for the life of the contract;

- Supplement or negotiated salary - This amount is usually determined upon renewal of the physicianís contract and is based on such things as seniority, contributions to the department, market factors, academic and scholarly activities, etc.,[6, 7] This segment is usually guaranteed for the term of the physicianís contract; and

- Incentive - This piece of the compensation is dependent on the physicianís contribution to the department over and above that which was expected or budgeted and the financial performance of the department.[8] This amount is almost never guaranteed.

This description is highly subjective and prone to a great deal of interpretation. Figure 11.1 summarizes some of the key issues involved in salary determination and offers a range of alternatives.

Figure 11.1

Individual Compensation

Characteristics	Range of Alternatives			
Determination of Base	Rank/Years of Service	Subjective	Specialty	Combination
Base Compensation Activities	Teaching/ Research	Administrative	Clinical	Combination
Directness of Incentive	Individual	Division/ Section	Department/ Clinical Units	Group
Activities to be Incentivized	Clinical	Administrative	Teaching/ Research	Combination
Method of Determining Incentive	Subjective Judgment	Objectively Measured Statistics	Revenue/ Income Production	Combination

It is now the task of the practice plan (both physicians and administrators working in concert) to determine a method of distribution which incorporates some or all of the components shown in Figure 11.1. In private practice, devising a salary distribution plan is rather uncomplicated. Basically, after providing for operating expenses, overhead and capital needs, the remainder is divided among the physicians, with seniority and productivity being the major determinants for base salary and incentive, respectively.[10] However, the academic practice plan, with its three-fold mission of patient care, teaching and research, has a daunting task in arriving at a plan which is fair and equitable.

Compensation design is an endless task. New physicians, new departments, new government regulations, and new ideas in the health care marketplace mean that changes are always necessary. [11] However, there are certain parameters which must be considered. Several of the most significant are:

- The first, and perhaps most important, criterion would be for an institution to formulate a mission and value statement that includes the principal goals of the organization. The income distribution scheme should then support this statement and goals. To illustrate, if one of the institutionís stated goals is to provide superior medical care at reduced cost, a part of the physicianís compensation formula would include an incentive for reduced costs while maintaining the same productivity and patient satisfaction;

- The institution must always strive to maintain equitable remuneration for teaching and research functions. A recent study at a major AMC showed that the teaching effort was poorly compensated. It is incumbent on the institution, in this time of declining revenues and over-taxed budgets, to maintain its focus in these two important areas. One way that many institutions support education is an assessment on revenues which is given to the dean's office for educational endeavors;
- When structuring a compensation formula, it is usually appropriate to incorporate a policy which will insure a solid financial base for the practice plan. This is accomplished by making regular contributions to designated reserve funds;[14]
- An income distribution formula must be objective and easy for the participants to understand. It also must be perceived as fair and impartial, carefully reflecting an individualís labor;[15]
- It is critical that the interests of the physicians be aligned with the interests of the institution. A very effective way of accomplishing this is through incentives. Incentives, if properly devised, can improve productivity, encourage support of institutional programs and improve the competitiveness of the salary program. At an AMC, it is also important that, if possible, incentives motivate accomplishments in research and teaching as well as patient care;[16, 17]
- A well-designed income distribution program must have the flexibility to allow for market factors. If a certain physician or specialty is needed to help ensure the success of the practice plan, then the plan must possess the ability to pay what is necessary, and still reasonable, to acquire and retain the necessary talent. Clearly, the plan must be able to do whatever is necessary to remain competitive.

Fringe benefits

In designing a compensation plan, the fringe benefits take on a very significant role. The U.S. Chamber of Commerce shows that in 1994, fringe benefits for the hospital category were 38.8 percent of salary (including paid time off). A hospital-based group practice and the mean for academic practice plans was 19.4 percent.[20] (The latter two surveys did not include paid time off.) Sometimes a unique or generous fringe benefit program will help to recruit and retain physicians who are looking beyond salary dollars to the peace of mind which a superior retirement plan or health insurance policy will bring.

There are many varieties of benefits available today. There are statutory benefits, regulated benefits and non-regulated benefits. Explanations and examples of the more significant benefits are now described.

There are three prominent statutory benefits mandated by the federal/state government:

- Social security includes retirement benefits, long-term disability benefits, survivor benefits and health insurance for those over 65 (Medicare). Financing for this program is provided by taxes levied equally on the employee and the employer, while self-employed individuals pay both the employerís and employeeís portion. Further details of this program can be obtained from the Social Security Administration, an agency of Health and Human Services;
- Unemployment insurance results from the Social Security Act and the Federal Unemployment Act of 1935 and is administered jointly by the federal and state governments. The purpose of this insurance is to financially aid those who are unemployed for limited periods of total or partial unemployment. Support for this insurance comes from taxes levied on the employer by both the state and federal government. The amount of taxes and benefits varies among states; and
- Workers' compensation is required by law in every state in one form or another. It is designed to provide health care costs and/or income replacement for employees who become sick, contract a disease, or die in the course of or because of their job. Since the amount of contributions and coverage varies so widely from state to state, it is beyond the scope of this exercise to delve into this topic any deeper. It is recommended that the laws of the individual states be consulted should there be a problem or concern.[21]

Many benefits provided as part of a compensation plan are in the form of insurance of one category or another. Some of the more significant and desirable varieties of insurance are:

- Health insurance is certainly one of the most popular and most frequently provided benefits. In a recent survey[22] by Sullivan, Cotter and Associates (SCA), 100 percent of the groups surveyed offered health insurance. Until the early 1980s, health insurance was offered through indemnity plans which contained deductibles and copayments. However, increasing medical costs have caused employers to look for other alternatives in an attempt to contain their rising health care costs. These alternatives have included HMOs, Preferred Provider Organizations (PPOs), self-insurance and managed care (including capitation) among others.

  A total analysis of the different kinds of health insurance available is beyond the scope of this document. Nevertheless, due to the mobility of academic physicians, there are several sections of a new piece of legislation which should be of interest. On August 21, 1996, the Health Insurance Portability and Accountability Act of 1996, was signed into law. This bill amends ERISA (Employee Retirement Income Security Act),[23] the Public Health Service Act and the Internal Revenue Code. Thus it applies to both private and government plans.

  The bill contains numerous provisions affecting various aspects of health care portability and renewability. Nevertheless, there are two sections, both effective July 1, 1997, which will probably have a significant effect on many participants of health insurance plans. First, nearly all employees will be able to change jobs and not be denied coverage because of preexisting conditions. Second, insurers must offer coverage to individuals who have lost group coverage, exhausted COBRA (Consolidated Omnibus Budget Reconciliation Act)[24] continuation, participated in an employerís health plan for at least 18 months, or do not have access to other group coverage or Medicare. Thus it appears that individuals will now be able to maintain their health insurance coverage, without interruption, throughout their entire life, assuming they are able to pay the premiums;

- Life insurance is also one of the most popular fringe benefits. In the SCA survey,[25] 99 percent of the groups surveyed offered life insurance as a fringe benefit. This benefit is usually offered as group term life insurance with no proof of insurability required and at no cost to the employee. The amount is typically a multiple of the employeeís base salary. In the survey, this multiple averaged 2.13. [26] Employers often amplify the value of this benefit by allowing employees to acquire additional life insurance at the employerís group rate. It should be noted that income taxes and FICA are required to be paid on the cost of coverage in excess of $50,000.

Nearly all groups offer the right to convert the group term insurance to an individual life insurance policy at termination of employment, again without proof of insurability. This becomes a valuable benefit to employees who, because of advanced age or poor health, would not otherwise be able to obtain life insurance.

- Malpractice insurance is often considered to be a cost of doing business since it is almost always required by hospitals and/or state law. Therefore, it is offered as a fringe benefit in most practices (98 percent in one recent Medical Group Management Association [MGMA] survey).[27] The premium for this coverage represents a national average of 7.34 percent of physicianís base salary.[28] It is not included in the previously cited data for fringe benefits as a percent of salary. This value continues a three-year trend of declining cost of malpractice insurance where the corresponding percentages were 8.2 percent in 1995 and 9.4 percent in 1994.[29]

  Two types of malpractice policies are generally employed. The first is a "claims made" policy which provides coverage "only if a claim arising from a hazard insured against is presented during the policy period."[30] Consequently, the insured is not covered against any incidents, no matter when they happened, once the policy lapses. This type of coverage requires "tail" coverage once the policy is terminated. Tail coverage is a policy protecting against claims which might be filed during the time following the termination of another policy. The second type of malpractice policy is an "occurrence" policy which provides coverage "if the event insured against takes place within the policy period, regardless of when the injured party makes a claim."[31] Therefore, a physician is protected permanently against all claims that might arise from events that occurred during the term of coverage. No tail coverage is required in this event. Due to the many state laws controlling malpractice insurance, extreme care should be exercised in this area, especially in determining adequate coverage for an arriving or departing physician;
- Dental insurance is usually designed to accomplish two objec-

tives: (1) to encourage participants to engage in preventive care; and (2) to partially offset the cost of routine and major dental work. These plans often have clauses to prevent adverse selection; i.e. only those people in need of significant dental work sign up for the insurance. The clauses include required minimum participation levels of the group and waiting periods before certain procedures are covered;

- Long-term disability insurance is designed to protect the physician against financial hardship resulting from extended illness or injury. In addition to Social Security and worker's compensation coverage, physicians will often enhance their employer's policy with one from a professional association. This insurance can be very complex and may require extensive analysis. When determining coverage for a group, an administrator should consider disability benefit, disability definition, benefit offsets, benefit duration, portability, survivor benefit and cost of living adjustments in the plan; and
- Accidental death and dismemberment insurance is usually provided at no cost to the participant as part of the group term life insurance. Consequently, if death or dismemberment occurs during an accident, this policy will pay an additional benefit distinct from the life insurance benefit.

The next major category of fringe benefits is retirement. This is also a popular benefit with 95 percent[32] of the SCA survey participants and 91 percent[33] of the MGMA survey participants indicating they offer this benefit. There are two major types of plans: qualified and nonqualified. Qualified plans are afforded special tax treatment both for the employer and the employee if they meet a myriad of requirements of the Internal Revenue Service (IRS) Tax Code. Nonqualified plans do not qualify for these special tax treatments.

Qualified Plans-ERISA became law on September 2, 1974. In an effort to safeguard the interests of retirement plan participants and their beneficiaries, this Act established a new set of participation rules, added mandatory vesting schedules, set minimum funding standards, established standards for administering the plan and dealing with plan assets, and established a method of insuring the payment of pension benefits (Pension Benefit Guaranty Corporation [PBGC]).[34] All of the ERISA regulations apply to qualified plans. A schematic showing various types of qualified plans, along with a comparison of the features of the plans, is shown as Figure 11.2. A short description of each type of plan follows:

- Defined contribution plans are those where specified contributions are made to the plan by the employer and/or the employee and usually designated to be invested as specified by the participant. Retirement benefits will be determined by the amount of these contributions combined with any gains or losses experienced by the investments minus the expenses of the plan. This type of plan shifts the risk of making appropriate investment decisions from the employer to the employee;
- Profit-sharing plans are defined contribution plans where the employer's contribution is discretionary from year to year. There are maximum amounts which can be contributed to each participant, as explained in the IRS tax code;
- Traditional plans are those where all employee contributions are made as a percentage of salaries. The percentage is the same for all employees;
- Cross-tested plans are those where the percentage of salary may be weighted for age, amount of compensation, etc. These plans are somewhat complex and care should be taken when they are written;
- Salary deferral plans are those where employees designate a portion of their salary, which is not taxed, to be contributed to the plan. The employer may or may not match a percentage of the employee's contribution up to certain limits specified in the tax code. A popular version of this plan is the 401(k) plan, referring to the section of the tax code which created it;
- Pension plans require a fixed commitment by the employer to contribute a certain percentage of salary to the employee's account. Again, there are maximums specified in the tax code for these contributions;
- Money purchase plans are an example of pension plans where again the employer puts in a fixed percentage of the employee's salary;
- Target benefit plans are pension plans which factor age, salary, and length of service into determining the percentage of salary which will be contributed on behalf of the employee;
- Defined benefit plans are retirement plans where the benefit is specified, usually by formula, and it is the responsibility of the employer to provide that benefit. The risk of pension investment performance rests entirely on the employer; and
- 412(I) plans differ from traditional, defined benefit pension plans in that all of the investments for these plans must be in insurance contracts, a type of guaranteed investment.[35]

Figure 11.2

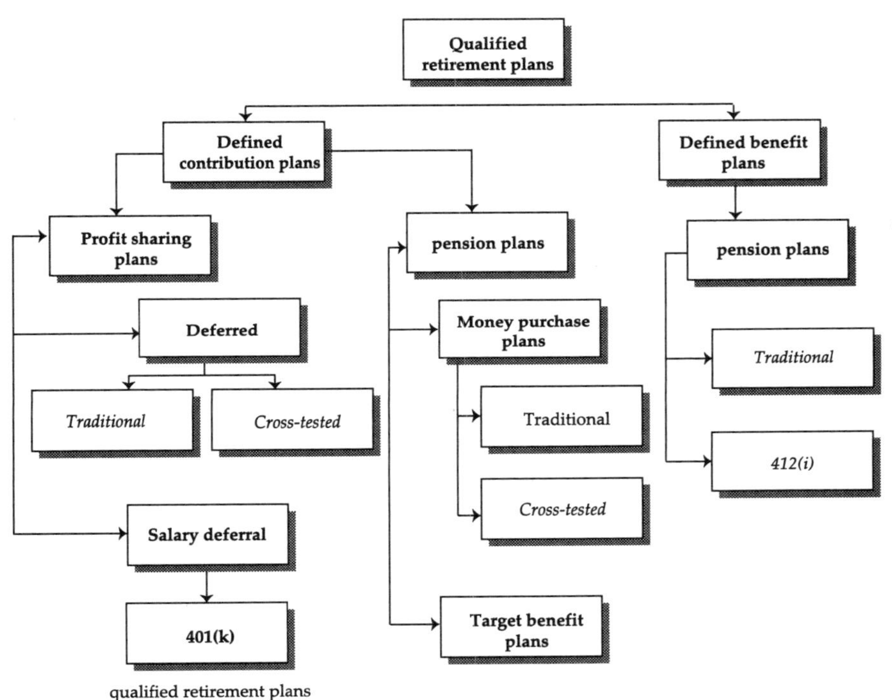

qualified retirement plans

Features of various qualified retirement plans

	Traditional Profit Sharing	Cross-Tested Profit Sharing	401 (k)	403 (b)	Traditional Money Purchase	Cross-Tested Money Purchase	Target Benefit	Traditional Defined Benefit	412 (i)
Flexible contributions	X	X	X	X					
Fixed contributions					X	X	X		
Participants share in gains and losses	X	X	X	X	X	X	X		
Salary Deferrals		X	X	X					
Predictable fixed contributions					X	X	X		
Predictable retirement benefits								X	X

Nonqualified plans are usually established to supplement the retirement of certain highly compensated employees or to avoid the complicated rules involved in operating and administering qualified plans. There are two types of nonqualified plans, funded and unfunded.

Funded plans allow an entity to make contributions to a trustee or an insurance company on behalf of an individual. To avoid immediate taxation on these contributions, there has to be a "substantial risk of forfeiture" surrounding these funds. When this risk is removed, the recipient is considered to be in constructive receipt of these contributions and is immediately taxed on the entire amount. Therefore, the physician always faces a dilemma; either the accumulating benefit is at risk or a significant tax bill is due. However, it is possible for the employer to gross up the recipient for the amount of the taxes.

The overwhelming majority of academic practice plans are not-for-profit entities.[36, 37] The Tax Reform Act of 1986 applied Section 457 to unfunded nonqualified plans for non-state tax exempt entities. The key change which occurred was that now, for virtually all academic practice plans, a recipientís nonqualified contributions would have to be combined with any 401(k) or 403(b) contributions to determine whether the $7,500 limit had been exceeded. This change in the tax law effectively eliminated any deferred compensation provisions because of the low dollar threshold.

A word should be said here regarding 403(b) salary reduction plans and their significance to academic practice plans. These plans involve two types of deferred compensation arrangements which are available only to employees of tax-exempt organizations: 403(b) pensions and 403(b) tax-deferred annuities (TDA). The employer makes contributions to the pension for the employee. This is usually based on a percentage of salary. There may be a requirement that the employee contribute up to 5 percent of his or her salary into the same plan. Voluntary contributions made only by the employee fund the TDA portion of the plan. There are, of course, maximums on both the employer's and employee's contributions which are contained in the tax code. Essentially all academic practice plan physicians participate in a 403(b) plan which is administered by the Teachers Insurance and Annuity Association (TIAA) and its partner organization, the College Retirement Equities Fund (CREF). Consequently, as individual and distinct as academic practice plans are, there is a common denominator which unites the physicians. This is the common pension plan which has assets of over $100 billion. In addition, this fact gave these physicians pension portability long before it became a national dilemma.[38]

As just described, the Tax Reform Act of 1986 (TRA 1986), virtually eliminated the ability of academic practice plans to provide any nonqualified deferred compensation plans for the physicians over and above qualified pensions and profit-sharing agreements. In addition, TRA 1986 also established a 15-percent excise tax on both excess distributions and excess accumulations attributable to all qualified plans, 403(b) plans and IRAs. The calculation and measurement of these excesses as prescribed by the tax code is beyond the scope of this document. However, it is very possible that a highly paid individual could lose more than half of his or her retirement accumulation to income, estate and excise taxes. Therefore, it is becoming very apparent that the highly paid physician needs to find a mechanism to accumulate both retirement funds and distributions to surviving beneficiaries.

It appears that the most likely candidates for this purpose are several forms of life insurance coverage. Life insurance is not considered a qualified retirement plan. It is also exempted from the nonqualified plans addressed in Section 457. In addition, proceeds from life insurance policies are not subject to income tax. Accordingly, if a reasonably priced enhanced life insurance product can be added to the fringe benefit package, then worries over excess accumulations and related excise taxes, additional employer provided retirement benefits and onerous income taxes on distributions will be greatly reduced. Two examples of these products are now described:

- Split dollar life insurance is an agreement in which the benefits and the costs of a life insurance policy are split between an employer and an employee. The plan can be used to provide life insurance protection currently and cash accumulation for retire-ment. Cash value life insurance rather than term insurance is used for this type of plan. Before implementing this type of plan, a careful analysis of the tax implications to the employer and employee should be undertaken.[39]

- Group Universal Life Plans (GULPs) provide a great deal of flexibility in retirement, life insurance and tax planning. This type of arrangement is able to link term insurance coverage with a tax-advantaged "side" investment fund. In implementing a GULP, the employer purchases either guaranteed issue or underwritten life insurance. Attached to this policy is a side fund to which contributions can be made by both the employer and the employee. This fund can be either fixed (invested in the insurance company's conservative asset base with a guaranteed minimum rate of return) or variable (invested in a variety of mutual funds selected by the participant). All funds deposited into the side fund would be after tax. However, the appreciation grows tax-deferred. This tax deferral can become permanent if the associated life insurance remains in place until the participant dies. This appreciation of the fund is then distributed as life insurance proceeds and is free of income tax. Access to this money during retirement would be through a loan arrangement. In addition, there is no restriction on access to the fund throughout the life of the participant, as there is with qualified retirement plans. Hence, this plan could also be used as a savings vehicle for educational purposes, a new home, etc.[40] This is not a widely used or understood plan at the present time. Due to the increasingly burdensome tax laws on retirement benefits, this plan provides a great deal of flexibility not currently available elsewhere.

There are many other fringe benefits which may be included to one extent or another by a particular institution depending on the cultural environment and the history of the fringe benefit program,. A list of these benefits, all of which are self-explanatory, is shown in Figure 11.3.

Figure 11.3

Other Fringe Benefits Available[41]

Vacations	Discounts	Health Care Promotion
Club Memberships	Adoption Benefits	Continuing Medical Education
Severance Pay	Parking	Prescription Drug Plan
Retiree Health Insurance	Sick Leave	Association/Society Dues
Vision Insurance	Other Leave (Maternity Funeral, Jury, etc.)	Financial Planning
Tuition (Employee& Dependents)	Licensure Fees	Subscriptions
Legal Assistance	First Class Travel	Tenure
Dependent Care	Executive Physical	Sabbaticals

Two fringe benefits which can be offered at no cost to the employer (except additional administrative expenses) are flexible spending accounts (FSAs) and cafeteria plan benefits (Section 125). FSAs represent individual accounts where the employee deposits pre-tax contributions and then is permitted to receive reimbursements from the account for certain eligible expenditures (health, dependent care or personal legal expenses). Thus, the federal and state governments are subsidizing these payments. The only drawback to these plans is that employees must specify at the beginning of the year how much to allocate for each purpose as a pre-tax reduction of their salary. If the employee does not use all the money for the intended purpose, it is forfeited ("use it or lose it").

In recent times, the work force has undergone a great change in composition with the advent of the dual-income family. Now individual employees have far different benefit needs than they did in the past. Implementation of a cafeteria plan of benefits helps to solve this problem. Under this design, an amount is designated by the employer as to how much the employee can spend on a prescribed set of benefits. Consequently, the employee whose spouse has a very adequate health insurance plan can direct his or her funds into retirement or added life insurance, while the single employee can reduce the life insurance component and purchase more vacation. Naturally, the plan must allow these options. However, if offered, a cafeteria plan can be a valuable benefit.[42]

There is one last benefit that is not widely offered in the academic practice plan, but could prove to be extremely valuable, especially to the less financially sophisticated employee. This is a benefit statement listing all of the current salary and benefit information pertaining to the employee. In addition, it may show such things as asset holdings in retirement accounts, value of fringe benefits, current projection of retirement income, etc. Two pages from a sample statement are shown in Figure 11.4. Along with being very informative and providing the physician with some peace of mind concerning his or her benefits, this statement can prove invaluable in dealing with a personal financial advisor. Usually it is necessary for financial advisors to perform an analysis of all assets, sources of income, etc. Depending on how organized a person is, this may result in several hours of work for the advisor. Given the hourly rates charged for this service, it is not too difficult to see that a benefit statement will more than pay for itself by allowing the physician to present this analysis already performed for, in many cases, the majority of the his or her holdings. It should be noted that this benefit is relatively standard for senior executives in private industry.

Figure 11.4

This statement has been prepared for:

**William H. Doe, M.D.
Endocrinology**

This statement summarizes your total compensation from the University of Virginia and the Health Services Foundation for the fiscal year beginning July 1, 1992 and ending June 30, 1993.

The information in this statement is based on the following data bout you:

Date of birth: **March 27, 1947**
Hire date: **July 1, 1978**

Summary of Compensation

Total Negotiated Compensation	$ 114,200
1992 Incentive Payments paid in 1993	19,760
Value of university and Health Services Foundation benefits (see page 2 for details)	23,910
Total Compensation	$ 157,870

Retirement Income
(see pages 8-9 for details)

Current Retirement Savings

TIAA/CREF	$ 316,142
Other University Retirement Plan Savings	15,378
BEST Plan Cash Value	1,589
Other Supplemental Tax-Deferred Savings Plans	52,220
Total Retirement Savings as of Jun3 30, 1993	$ 385,329

Projected Retirement Income at age 65 on March 27, 2013

Annual annuity from retirement savings	$ 118,984
Annual Social Security benefit	14,796
Estimated Total Retirement Income	$ 133,780

Figure 11.4 (continued)

**Your Total Compensation . . .
The Details**

The first table on page 1 includes a total for the annual value of your University and health Services Foundation benefits. The table below indicates the plan-by-plan components of that total

Total Negotiated Compensation			$ 114,200
1992 Incentive Payments paid in 1993			$ 1 9,760
Value of Benefits	University-Paid	HSF-Paid	
Health Care Benefits	3,888		
Value of tax savings in the:		–	
• Medical Reimbursement Account	–		
• Dependent Care Reimbursement Account	–		
TIAA Total Disability Benefit Plan	141	–	
HSF Long-Term Disability Plan	–	230	
TIAA Basic Life Insurance	180	–	
BEST Program Life Insurance	–	991	
University Retirement Plan Contributions	11,500	–	
BEST Plan Contributions	–	1,000	
Clinicians Retirement Plan Cost	–	489	
Social Security taxes*	3,989	1452	
Miscellaneous benefits	100	–	
Total, Benefits Value			23,910
Total Compensation			$ 157,870

**These amounts are estimates.*

The Total Negotiated Compensation shown above and on page 1 reflects your negotiated University compensation rate as of June 30, 1993, and your fiscal year 1993 actual HSP compensation.

Sources of funds

Figure 11.5 shows the sources of revenues for 126 academic practices in the United States and the trending of these funds for three years. It is these funds which eventually go to support the compensation plans derived by AMCs. Although the trend shows that funds supporting academic medicine are on the increase, challenges posed by the growth of managed care and pressures for reduced medical spending at the federal and state level call into question the continued growth of academic medicine. A recent article by the AAMC indicated that average faculty salaries for 1994 and 1995, by region, rank and department, declined in dozens of instances from the prior year. After adjusting for inflation, this figure more than doubles. If this trend continues, then the clinical base supporting medical school programs will be reduced. In addition, federal support for graduate medical education appears to be a target for material cuts. As these challenges are presented, academic health centers are considering crucial structural changes to try to strengthen their financial position. As the struggle continues, it is evident that the financial methods used to support academic medicine may undergo unprecedented change.[43]

Figure 11.5

Table III-U.S. Medical School Revenues[44]

Amount of Revenue, $ Millions

	Fiscal Years		
	1991-1992	1992-1993	1993-1994
Federal Appropriations	105	106	110
State and local government appropriations	2680	2719	2781
Practice plans	7505	8291	9120
Tuition and fees	955	1048	1130
Endowment	401	431	436
Gifts	508	534	579
Parent university support	198	205	188
Hospitals/medical school programs	2662	2964	3659
Miscellaneous sources	952	1118	1097
Research	3705	4014	4287
Teaching and training	533	568	564
Service and multipurpose	761	873	928
Research and teaching/training at affiliated institutions	688	742	864
Recovery of indirect costs	1516	1639	1768
Total Revenues	**23169**	**25253**	**27509**

Regulators

There are several divisions of the government which seem to be taking an ever-increasing role in physician compensation. The two most significant agencies are the Department of Health and Human Services (DHHS), through the National Institutes of Health (NIH) and the Health Care Financing Administration (HCFA), and the Treasury Department in the form of the Internal Revenue Service (IRS).

The NIH controls many research and training programs which are supported by the federal government. This agency is able to determine the level of salary and benefit support provided to a physician to conduct specified research or training. NIH sometimes imposes maximum salaries which can be paid under a grant.

HCFA is primarily responsible for administering the Medicare program. With increasing budget pressures and public opinion against expanding medical costs, this department is taking steps to reduce its expenses by implementing new fee schedules based on Resource-Based Relative Value Units (RBRVU), and implementing managed care programs throughout the country for Medicare and Medicaid.

Furthermore, this agency is actively enforcing fraud and abuse laws. Paying or receiving compensation for referral of patients in either of these two programs is considered a criminal offense. Thus, any incentive or salary components which reward physicians for referrals are illegal. In answer to perceived problems with this fraud and abuse law, Congress has passed two clarifying measures labeled "Stark I" (1989) and "Stark II" (1993) in reference to their originator, Fortney "Pete" Stark (Democrat, California). Both of these laws clarified and expanded the definition of referrals. Stark I prohibited referrals to laboratory services in which the physician had a financial relationship. Stark II expanded the list of prohibited referrals to 11 "designated health services," including inpatient and outpatient hospital services.[45]

Of much greater importance to academic practice plans is the investigation currently being conducted jointly by the Department of Justice and the DHHS at AMCs throughout the country regarding the legitimacy of Medicare claims submitted at these institutions. The investigation has resulted in a $30-million settlement[46] at one institution and a $12-million settlement[47] at another. These investigations center around first, IL-372 guidelines where the government says that claims have been filed on behalf of faculty physicians for services performed by residents and there was an absence of documentation indicating the involvement of the attending physician. Also, claims were allegedly coded at higher levels than the services represented by the documentation as completed by the attending physician.[48] The government has stated publicly that this investigation will eventually extend to every AMC in the country. If it does, and the results continue in the same order of magnitude, this event may have more of an effect on physician compensation than any other single force.

Unquestionably, the IRS is the government agency which has the greatest effect on providersí compensation and benefits in an academic group practice, as it does on almost all other people in this country. Distinct from the code sections which have already been mentioned in connection with several benefits, and the fact that most practice plans are tax-exempt entities, the IRS also maintains an overseer status on two very important issues. Subsequent to 1991, the IRS has maintained that a 501(c)(3) tax-exempt entity must comply with Medicare fraud and abuse laws to maintain this status. Second, the tax code obligates a 501(c)(3) organization to function for charitable and/or educational purposes. It also prohibits any surplus earnings inuring to private individuals. Therefore, a practice plan must be very careful when structuring physician compensation plans so that it does not appear that any of the physicians are receiving an inordinately large salary, incentive or even recruiting bonus, as defined by the IRS. Several suggestions which appeal to the IRS include: putting a cap on incentive compensation in relation to base salary; basing incentives on patient satisfaction, cost containment and quality of care; and ensuring that incentives are approved by a board of directors consisting of outside directors.[49]

Tax-saving opportunities

Inasmuch as the importance of the IRS as a regulatory body has just been examined, it is necessary at this juncture to summarize those benefits which provide significant tax saving opportunities. These are as follows:

- Deferred tax-savings plans like a 401(k) or a 403(b) are the most powerful tools an individual currently has to provide for retirement and, if a borrowing option is attached, a new house or an education for dependents. Since the contributions and the earnings are tax deferred, the amount grows much larger than it would in a bank or mutual fund outside the plan. These plans demonstrate as well as any, the immense power of compound interest;

- Salary reduction plans allow an employee to pay for various qualified benefits such as health insurance, dental insurance, etc. ,with before-tax dollars. In this way, the actual expense is being reduced by the amount of tax savings;

- Flexible spending accounts allow employees to segregate part of their salary before taxes and reimburse themselves for health care expenses not covered by insurance, dependent care and legal expenses. Even the "use it or lose it" penalty should not be enough to dissuade people from taking advantage of these tax savings; and

- Insurance arrangements allow a great deal of flexibility combined with the opportunity for some significant tax savings. The variable group universal life plan, described previously has the advantages of: unrestricted access to the investment account, either through loans or withdrawals; deferred tax or tax-free accumulation of interest on the investments, depending on whether the participant keeps the life insurance active until his or her death; and significant additional contributions by the employee outside the plan agreement with the employer and income-tax-free distributions of the insurance proceeds to the estate of the insured. None of these restrictions is subject to ERISA discrimination or cap requirements.

The changing environment of provider compensation: the appearance of managed care and capitation

For years, the two most prevalent physician income distribution methods were sharing surpluses equally and rewarding the "big producers" with incentives based on productivity.[50] As long as fees and revenues continued to rise, these methods appeared to be appropriate. This was especially true in academic health centers. The expansion of staff and facilities could be warranted when the associated clinical practices were generating large surpluses. An example of this expansion is reflected in the significant increase in medical school professors over the past 30 years. Medical students have risen from 32,835 in 1965 to 66,970 in 1995, while the number of full-time professors rose from 17,118 to 90,017[51] during the same period of time.

However, with the public outcry against rising medical costs and the development of managed care, the medical community in general and AMCs specifically, are beginning to see revenues diminish. It is quite possible, given the data, that there may be an excess of faculty. Accordingly, it will be even more imperative to formulate a compensation plan which rewards behavior that is aligned with the goals of the institution in order to recruit and retain faculty which will help to bring the practice plan through this fiscal crisis.

In the past, the physician has always been rewarded for productivity. The more patients seen, the more procedures done, the more ancillaries ordered, the more revenue that was generated. This revenue led in turn to higher compensation for the physician. However, managed care and capitation now stress cost control, quality of care and access. The physician must now focus on controlling costs rather than being a revenue producer. It is now necessary to begin to transition from fee-for-service revenue toward capitation. Geoffrey T. Anders of the Health Care Group suggests that a review of this transition process begin immediately because managed care is moving fast, and it takes time to develop and implement a new formula. He suggests that waiting until the current plan is truly ineffective may be too late.[52]

During this transition period, it is necessary to develop a plan which adapts to the fixed payment of capitation and still provides high quality care, customer service and access. In arriving at such a plan, there are several factors which must be considered in trying to determine an incentive. These are:[53]

- A strong group commitment and the promotion of the managed care entity;
- Number of new patients;
- Appropriate utilization;
- Patient satisfaction and complaints;
- Ability to meet quality standards;
- Necessity of providing for a reserve for future purposes;
- Cost control; and
- Seniority.

Since a fixed payment encourages physicians to reduce costs and see fewer patients, the development of the bonus must be done very carefully so that the patient still receives the highest quality of care available. In fact, the 1990 Medicare Amendment placed the following restrictions on any prepaid plan which contracts to enroll Medicare beneficiaries:

- No specific payment may be made under a physician incentive plan as an inducement to reduce or limit medically necessary services to a specific individual enrolled in a prepaid health care plan;
- If the physician incentive plan creates a substantial financial risk for a physician, the plan must provide stop-loss protection and periodically survey enrollees to ensure adequate access and quality of care; and
- Prepaid plans that contract with HCFA are required to provide sufficient information to determine compliance with these rules. Violations can result in fines of up to $25,000 and suspension from the Medicare program.[54]

A search of the literature indicates that compensation plans are being developed in a capitation environment. The three that follow are only meant to be examples. Each practice plan will have to formulate its own scheme taking into account the culture and environment existing at each institution. As a wise man once said, "If you have seen one compensation plan, you have seen one compensation plan."[55]

The following compensation formulas all assume a transitional market where both capitation and fee-for-service revenue exists.

Plan #1

Capitated Revenue plus
Fee-for-Service Revenue minus
Direct and Indirect Costs equals
Total Physician Compensation[56]

Plan #2

Base Salary (25%) plus
Seniority Factor (5%) plus
Production (50%) dependent on:
Utilization-refers to a physician's referral patterns
Cost per patient
Fee-for-service equivalent which prevents penalizing the physician with high volume and difficult caseloads
Patient service credit determined by surveys
Case management credit plus
Performance Credits (15%) for such things as:
Continuing education
Board Certification
Administrative Duties plus
At Risk portion (5%) awarded when group objectives have been accomplished for such things as number of patient encounters, number of referrals, appropriate use of ancillaries and overall financial performance equals
Total Physician Compensation[57]

Plan #3

Productivity (50%) based on number of patients seen compared with peers plus
Utilization Management (20%) depends on appropriate use of resources; i.e. per patient cost, length of stay in hospital, etc. plus
Patient Satisfaction (12.5%) using surveys plus
Citizenship (7.5%) administrative duties, participation in professional organizations, etc. plus
Practice Efficiency (7.5%) punctuality in seeing patients, ability to keep staff functioning, etc. equals
Total Physician Compensation[58]

It should be noted that these formulas are only for the distribution of clinical revenue. Research and education should, obviously, be factored in.

Summary and conclusions

The intent of this activity was three-fold. It was first to show that in the past and into the future, the circumstances surrounding compensation plans are dynamic and constantly changing. Regulations, environmental considerations and public opinion are just three factors which dramatically affect physician compensation and which can change from day to day. In view of this situation, it will always be necessary for an administrator to know the current trends in physician payment. Figure 11.6 is a list of ten organizations which survey and report this data.

Furthermore, an effort was made to expose the reader to the many types of salary distribution and benefits available. In their attempt to produce compensation formulas designed to recruit and retain the highest qualified faculty, administrators should be aware of the many weapons in their arsenal. As revenues from all sources begin to decline, a real challenge will exist to create a plan which will appeal to the academic physician and still be affordable.

Finally, in this world of change, one of the most extensive examples of change is now upon us, in the form of managed care and capitation. The physician's world has been turned upside down. Instead of seeing as many patients and performing as many services as possible, the effort is now directed toward controlling costs and seeing fewer patients. Therefore, compensation distribution has to reflect this change. The three compensation plans presented, attempted to show how some practices are initially dealing with this situation.

The current atmosphere of change in which medicine exists cannot be over-emphasized. It is very difficult to create a plan to distribute salaries and benefits that will satisfy the physicians when almost daily HCFA, the IRS, Congress or the general public change the rules. However, a constant effort must be made to keep updating the compensation plan to measure up to the goals of the practice plan and the external surroundings.

References

1. Collins, H. and Buntz, D., "Effective Income Distribution for Employed Physicians," *Health Care Financial Management*, 49(9) September 4, 1995, 26.
2. Anderson, S. T., "Practice Plan Management: Faculty Compensation-How is it Changing?",*GFP Notes*, 7(4) December, 1994,11.
3. Washburn, E. R., "Budgeting for a More Likely Future," *Medical Group Management Journal*, 42(4) July-August 1995, 74.
4. Anderson, S. T., op. cit., 11. Excerpted from the AAMC Symposium entitled "Tenure, Compensation and Career Pathways," February 4-6, 1996.
5. Ibid.
6. Ceriani, P.J., "Compensating and Providing Incentives for Academic Physicians: Balancing Earning, Clinical, Research, Teaching, and Administrative Responsibilities," *Journal of Ambulatory Care Management*, 15(2) April, 1992, 71-72.
7. Ibid.
8. D'Antuono, R., "Income Distribution, Physician Compensation, and Aligning Incentives," *Academic Clinical Practice*, 8(8) November, 1995, 2
9. Ceriani, P. J., op.cit., 69.
10. Collins, H. and Buntz, D., op.cit., 27.
11. Ceriani, P.J., op.cit., 70.
12. Shea, S, M.D., Nickerson, K.G., M.D., et al, "Compensation to a Department of Medicine and its Faculty Members for the Teaching of Medical Students and House Staff," *The New England Journal of Medicine*, 334(3) January, 1996, 162.
13. Isack, A.G., and Axelrod, R.H., iBuilding Clinical Productivity Incentives into the Physician Compensation Plan at GWU GFP Notes, 6(4) Fall, 1993,11.
14. Ibid.
15. Cotter, T.J. and Bonds, R.G., "Structuring Competitive Physician Compensation Programs," *Health care Financial Management*, 49(12) December1995, 55.
16. Isack, A.G. and Axelrod, R.H., op.cit., 11.
17. "Beyond the Fringe" A Study of Benefits Practices and Costs of a Cross Section of American Firms published by the U. S. Chamber of Commerce, 1995, Table 6.
18. *1996 Physician Salary Survey Report, Hospital-Based Group Practice and HMO*, published by Hospital & Health Care Compensation Service, John R. Zabka Associates, Inc., 350 Ramapo Valley Road Oakland, N.J.,
19. *1995 Financial Survey of Faculty Practice Plans Data* produced by the Association of American Medical Colleges.
20. *Doing business in the United States* published by Price Waterhouse, 1994, 112-117

21. *The 1996 Physician and PhD Compensation and Productivity Survey* conducted by Sullivan, Cotter and Associates, Inc.(SCA) which polled 192 health care organizations covering 14,000 physicians, PhD's and mid-level providers.
22. Employee Retirement Income Security Act of 1974 which completely overhauled federal pension law.
23. The Consolidated Omnibus Budget Reconciliation Act of 1985 which essentially required employers to provide health insurance coverage for a specified period of time after termination for employees and dependents.
24. The 1996 Physician and PhD Compensation and Productivity Survey, op.cit.
25. Ibid.
26. *MGMA Information Exchange, Salaries and Fringe Benefits-Physicians,* March 1993.
27. *1996 Physician Salary Survey Report, Hospital-Based Group Practice and HMO,* op.cit.,20.
28. Ibid.
29. Long, R.H., LL.M., *The Law of Liability Insurance,* Volume I, published by Matthew Bender & Co., Inc., New York, New York, 1996, 1-99.
30. Ibid.
31. *The 1996 Physician and PhD Compensation and Productivity Survey,* op.cit.
32. MGMA Information Exchange, Salaries and Fringe Benefits-Physicians,op.cit.
33. Krass, S. J. Esq., *The Pension Answer Book,* published by Panel Publishers, Inc., New York, New York,1990, 1- 4-5.
34. Prince, A.P., Phillips, E.K. and Apolinsky, H.I., Physician Financial Planning, Published by McGraw Hill Health care Management, New York, New York,1996, 135-143.
35. *1995 Financial Survey of Practice Plans Data,* op.cit.
36. *Faculty Practice Plans: The Organization and Characteristics of Academic Medical Practice* published by The Association of American Medical Colleges,1991,10.
37. *Managing the Academic Medical Practice: The Two-Headed Eagle,* edited by W.R. Nicholas, published by Medical Group Management Association, Englewood, Colorado, 1992, 188-190.
38. Smith, H.A., Esq., Downey, B. K., Esq. and Connors, M. P., Esq., *Nonqualified Deferred Compensation Answer Book,* published by Panel Publishers, Inc., New York, New York, 1994, 6-1.
39. Nordyke, C.K., "Group Universal and Variable Life Programs," *Medical Group Management Journal* 41(6); November/December 1994, 56-61.
40. Managing the Academic Medical Practice: The Two Headed Eagle, op. cit. 193.
41. Gifford, D. L. and Seltz, C. A., *Fundamentals of Flexible Compensation,* published by John Wiley & Sons, New York, New York,1988.

42. Ganem, J. L., CPA, Beran, R. L., PhD and Krakhower, J. K., PhD, "Review of U S Medical School Finances, 1993-1994," *JAMA*, 274(9), September 6, 1995, 723-730.
43. Ibid. 724,
44. Dieck, E. S., Heisen, P. R., M.D. and Laarman, L. M., J.D., "Physician Compensation: Driving Critical Behaviors through Incentives," *The Marsh & McLennan Companies Quarterly*, 23(4), Fall 1994, 40-41.
45. Information released by Ernst & Young, LLP.
46. Information released by MGMA
47. Ernst & Young, LLP., op.cit.
48. Dieck, E. S., et. al., op.cit.40-41.
49. "Does Productivity Income Division Still Make Sense?" *The Physician's Advisory*, 94(1) January 1994, 1.
50. Mangan, K. S., "Medical Schools are Reining in the Salaries of Faculty Members," *The Chronicle of Higher Education*, 42(46) July 1996, A16.
51. "Does Productivity Income Division Still Make Sense," op. cit. 2.
52. "Living With Managed Care: A View From the Front," The *Proceedings From the Managed Care Sessions* of the Medical Group Management Association's 69th Annual Conference, published by The Medical Group Management Association, Englewood, Colorado, October, 1995, 69.
53. Hirsh, B.D., JD, "Risky Business," *Texas Medicine*, 90(12) December,1994, 30-31
54. Erra, R.J., "Compensating Physicians in a Mixed Fee-for-Service/Capitated Practice," *The Quality Letter*, 6(2) March 1994, 12.
55. Hunter, A., "How to Maximize Doctors' Productivity and Profitability in the Shift to Capitation," *Medical Staff Strategy Report*, 4(2) February 1995, 9.
56. McCally, J.F., Lewin, J.A., and Miskowic, A., "Capitated Income Distribution Systems: They're Better with a New Approach," *The American Group Practice Association/Group Practice Journal*, 43(5) September/October 1994, 50-51.
57. Jaklevic, M.C., "Groups Experiment to Find Best Formula for Doc Compensation," *Modern Health Care*, 25(29) July 17, 1995, 41.

Chapter 12

Managed care contracting in an academic medical practice environment [1]

by William R. Beekman, JD

The test of a first-rate intelligence is the ability to hold two opposed ideas in the mind at the same time, and still retain the ability to function.

— *F. Scott Fitzgerald*[2]

The American medical school is in the midst of a revolution. Not since Abraham Flexner's report on the status of medical education in 1910[3] has medical education been faced with such tumultuous times. In Flexner's time, the revolutionary changes principally involved the quality of medical education,[4] and thus the quality of medical care. Today, the revolution surrounds how Americans finance their medical care.[5]

"Managed care" is fast becoming the only type of health care available in the United States.[6] Even traditional indemnity plans are now often "managed" to some degree. At the center of this revolution is the academic medical practice. In this revolutionary time, academic practices are faced with all of the issues that their colleagues in the private sector face, but they must also consider a host of issues unique to academia. In particular, the academic principles of tenure and academic freedom discourage, or at the very least do not facilitate, the organization of the practice into a cohesive group, poised for financial success in a private sector where the market rewards efficiency at the expense of traditional academic values. It is the ability to assimilate the two divergent goals of academic and business success into a cohesive and progressive medical practice that marks the successful academic practice manager.

While a patient coming in for a check-up may not recognize any difference between an academic physician and a physician in private practice, the management of the academic medical practice often bears little resemblance to private practice management. Certainly, many issues that the two practices face will be identical: each must negotiate with payers around participation in managed care products; each must circulate the resulting contracts through the appropriate administrative and legal channels; and each must ensure that it has in place the administrative and information systems to monitor contract compliance, both internally and externally. It is in the details of how these functions are carried out, however, that the academic medical practice presents unique circumstances. Some of these unique circumstances are assets to the practice; for example, the ability to market the practice under the university name. Other unique characteristics of academic practice are liabilities. For example, the academic practice administrator must not only manage a medical practice, but must, of necessity, do so within a university structure ill-suited for business management. The successful academic practice administrator will recognize and capitalize on the strengths of the academic medical practice while, simultaneously, accepting and compensating for the liabilities inherent in academic medical practice.

While managing an academic medical practice is assuredly not an easy task, the academic practice does maintain certain substantive advantages over a private medical practice–particularly when contracting with managed care organizations. The academic practice administrator must come to the negotiating table prepared to utilize those assets, as the strength of the practice is on the "front end," or the negotiation stage, of the managed care relationship. While at the negotiating table, the administrator is typically negotiating on behalf of the largest, or one of the largest, multispecialty practices in the community. Often, the academic practice will include sub-specialists not found elsewhere in the region, potentially maintaining a monopoly of sorts on certain specialty services within the community. The administrator must utilize those and similar practice strengths when negotiating the relationship because the academic practice's Achilles heel is in the "back end," or operation and implementation stage, of the managed care relationship. The academic practice's greatest challenges are created by its size and its diverse, multilayered governance structure as well as the organizational and communication challenges inherent in such a structure. Thus, normally simple tasks such as ensuring to whom various reports and payments should be sent, determining which physician's practices are open or closed to new patients, and making sure that credentialing documents and information are forwarded to the appropriate academic manager can all become daunting tasks. In short, for the academic medical practice "the devil is in the details." The academic administrator must work at the beginning of the relationship, when the managed care organization is likely to be most flexible, to negotiate terms that are as favorable as possible, facilitating the operation and implementation of the contract.

While a myriad of treatises, books, articles and periodicals addressing managed care contracting have been published over the past decade, there is little, if any, literature specifically addressing managed care issues *particular to the academic medical practice.* The goal of this chapter is to fill that void. This chapter addresses the issues affecting the academic practice as it grapples with managed care and negotiates managed care contracts. This chapter is in four sections, beginning with this Introduction. The second section asks the reader to analyze what form his or her academic practice should take to most effectively contract with managed care entities. Third, a host of issues specific to managed care contracting and the academic medical practice are addressed. Finally, this chapter addresses the future of managed care contracting for the academic medical practice.

Structuring the academic practice to succeed in managed care

Perhaps one of the most fundamental rules of contracting is that an entity must take great care analyzing its own needs and wants before attempting to negotiate for those desires. Stated in the vernacular, "If you don't know what you want, no one else will." This is particularly true for the academic medical practice. Because the academic practice has multiple priorities and a multitude of parties whose needs must be met, the practice must use great care to determine precisely what objectives it wishes to achieve when entering into a relationship with a managed care organization. For example, if an academic practice has decided that its mission includes delivering primary care within its community, it might be completely logical for that practice to engage as a partner a managed care organization that provides a group model HMO.[7] The practice might negotiate to provide all of the HMO's primary care needs at a single practice site. Conversely, assume that the practice exists solely to provide opportunities for a medical school's physician faculty members to maintain their practice skills. A more logical relationship might be for the practice to contract to provide services to a more limited pool of patients, allowing the physicians to close their practices to new patients as necessary.

While this process of internal prioritization before contracting might seem second nature to the private practice physician, it is a much more difficult, and hence, a much more important, task for the academic medical practice. Consensus around the priorities of the academic medical practice must be sought among the medical school's various departments, as it is likely that the various departments will have competing, or at least different, goals. But the practice must also seek consensus among the faculty members within each department. Academic "practice" is only one of three (or more) tasks commonly ascribed to the faculty of a medical school. In addition to practicing medicine, most faculty members must also teach students and conduct research. Those responsibilities are often in addition to administrative roles and community service responsibilities. By way of example, the department of physical medicine and rehabilitation may have student instruction and faculty practice as its mission. Conversely, the department of radiology might focus almost exclusively on research. In this example, it would be foolhardy for the practice to commit both departments to a managed care contract requiring an extensive practice commitment.

What structure for the practice?

The academic medical practice can take any one of several forms – each one potentially successful depending on the needs of the practice, the medical school and the university. The first and most fundamental rule when determining what structure an academic medical practice should take is that a structure should not be created merely for the sake of having structure. The creation of an organizational structure for the practice will only be of value to the extent that it directly and specifically serves the practice's goals, as they relate to contracting with managed care entities and other needs. Depending on the goals of the practice, there are a number of organizational options. Of course, the permutations of those options are limited only by the creativity of the practice's management.

In the academic setting, the managed care options available to the academic practice depend primarily on the practice's organizational structure. For example, a true academic group practice will probably find it easier to contract with a group model HMO than would an academic practice where the providers/faculty members[8] function as the group's primary decision-makers. Thus, the academic practice must recognize and understand its academic governance structure; it must be able to translate that structure into a roughly equivalent organizational structure; and it must, finally, work within that structure to solicit and contract with the appropriate managed care organizations, payers, third parties, hospitals and other appropriate entities.

Managed care contracting in an academic environment

An academic medical practice can take many forms. The structure of the academic medical practice can be thought of graphically as a continuum as shown in Figure 12.1. On one end of the continuum, the providers can make decisions together as a group with a group governance structure. On the opposite end of the continuum, the providers can be permitted to individually choose the payers and products with which they wish to associate.

Figure 12.1

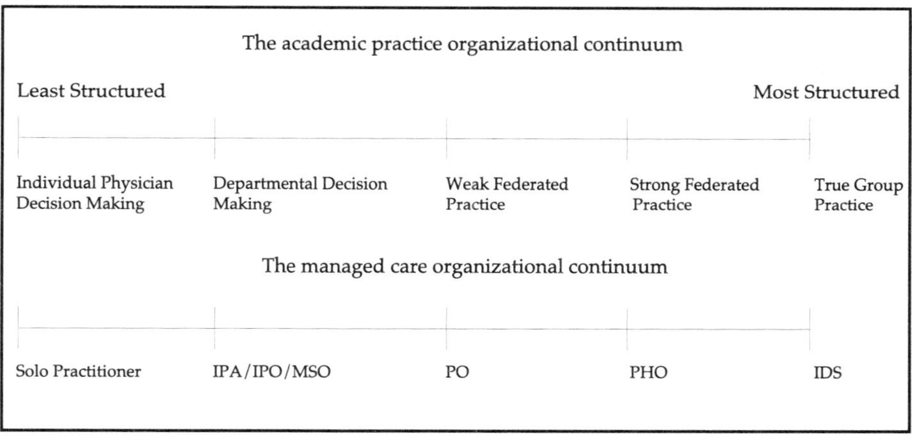

The most common organizational options available to the academic medical practice are described in the next section. In addition, the managed care organizational structure most suited to each academic practice organization is also analyzed. Finally, the form of the academic practice will dictate the parties and managed care organization with which the academic practice can most successfully contract. Those entities are also briefly considered.

The provider as decision-maker. When organizing the academic practice, one option is to allow each individual provider/faculty member to determine the managed care products with which that provider wishes to participate. This option is fraught with problems and should not be utilized to any significant degree. Obviously, each provider in the practice must have the opportunity to participate in the decision-making process, either directly or via a representative, and must be comfortable with most of the decisions made by the group. There are simply too many weaknesses in this structure, however, and too many strengths in the other options, to make individual decision-making a viable option.

Virtually every weakness inherent in this approach can be solved by utilizing a more structured approach. By way of example, in this model it is possible that physicians in the same department will not all participate in the same product. This presents problems when those same physicians are required to provide call coverage for each other. It also confuses the patient who might have chosen a particular product because it has marketed its relationship with the academic practice, or even with a specific department or specialty area, only to discover his or her physician does not participate with that particular product – even when other members of the department do. Additionally, this structure is detrimental to the provider, the practice and the medical school to the extent that the bargaining power of each entity is, in all likelihood, directly proportional to the ability of the practice's providers to work together, presenting a united front and strength in numbers.

Conversely, there is virtually no benefit to this structure. Only the individual provider has the opportunity to benefit when that individual is, without limitation, the master of his or her own fate. There are probably only a few providers in any given practice whose specialty or reputation are so unique as to allow an individual to bargain with the strength that would otherwise be available only to the practice. For example, if the academic practice's pediatric pulmonologist is the only pediatric pulmonologist in the practice's geographic region, he or she will likely be able to negotiate favorable relationships with most payers. Both the practice and the institution are better served by leveraging the pediatric pulmonologist's bargaining power for the benefit of the entire practice.

The academic practice forced to utilize this structure can be equated with the solo practitioner and is not in actuality equivalent to any managed care organization or other organized delivery structure. Rather, each sole practitioner has the autonomy to make independent practice decisions regardless of the objectives and goals of the other academic practitioners.

The department as decision-maker. Because the department is the primary organizational unit in most medical schools, it is only natural that the department act as the primary organizational unit in most academic practices. Many of the problems inherent in the individual decision-maker structure are not present in this structure. Call coverage issues, for example, are more easily resolved when the department, as a group, decides which physicians will participate with a particular payer product. While all physicians may still not participate, the department is at least aware of that fact and can account for it as necessary. In addition, utilization of this structure will begin to allow the physicians to share information about their practices and patient populations. The larger the pool of data available to the practice, the easier it will be for the practice to make rational, informed decisions about managed care.

The most substantive detriment to the departmental decision-making approach is that it does not go far enough. Provider/faculty members are unlikely to raise substantive complaints about this model largely because it is identical to the organizational structure that they must work within as academics. All of the positive attributes of a departmental decision-making model are all the more true in a federated practice model. The exchange of information and the communication that exists within the departmental model is strengthened in the federated practice model where the various departments communicate with each other and make joint decisions in some form.

The department, acting as the decision-maker, can be equated with either the Independent Practice Association (IPA)/Independent Practice Organization (IPO) structure, the Management Services Organization (MSO) structure, or the Physician Organization (PO) structure. The IPA (or IPO) is typically defined as a group of physicians (or, in the academic practice, departments) affiliated with one another for the purpose of contracting on behalf of the group's physician members. The physicians provide their own malpractice coverage, maintain their own offices and support staff, and are responsible for their own billing and collecting. The physicians are typically not equipped to accept risk as they generally do not share substantive practice or financial information across practices, and they do not share practice revenues.

The success of the IPA depends upon the ability of the departments to cooperate with one another and to collectively utilize the IPA only for the purpose for which it was created. IPA member departments must be able to share information sufficient to ensure success in their managed care relationships and to ensure that all participating departments are aware of any expenses shared by the departments. For that reason, a group of departments that agrees to create an IPA for the purpose of negotiating non-capitated managed care products and that can work together to accomplish that specific goal has the greatest opportunity to enjoy a successful IPA relationship.

However, if the departments wish to negotiate capitated products or otherwise share in risks and opportunities, they should avoid the IPA structure in favor of a more structured and integrated relationship.

The MSO acts to centralize certain practice expenses, creating economies of scale, while allowing the member physicians (or, again, in the academic practice, departments) to retain their individual revenues to the extent that those revenues exceed their share of the MSO's expenses. Thus, MSO-affiliated departments can be described as a group when analyzing practice expenses, but as a collection of individual departments when analyzing profits. In an MSO, the departments may organize themselves collectively to utilize shared facilities, staff, billing and collecting arrangements. They may share the same name. Alternatively, the MSO may be a separately organized, non-provider group that provides management services to the various departments. The MSO affiliated department will presumably be better equipped to undertake managed care contracting than will an IPA because, by virtue of centralized billing, collecting, information systems and recordkeeping, the MSO is better equipped to interpret and understand managed care utilization and payment data.

The PO, however, may be the best organizational structure by which the academic practice, at the department level, can negotiate managed care contracts. The PO is very similar to the IPA, but is typically thought of as being more structured, usually, but not necessarily, with a defined corporate or partnership structure. The PO is a collection of providers (or, for the purposes of academic practice, departments) who have united for the purpose of negotiating managed care contracts. Like the IPA, the PO does not require that departments share revenue, nor does it require that each department participate in each product for which the PO contracts. The success of a PO, like that of an IPA, will depend on the PO's ability to negotiate relationships within the restrictions imposed by its structure.

While the IPA and MSO are not the best organizational structures from which to negotiate managed care contracts, they may be acceptable means to the practice that has no other alternative as a result of its academic structure. As noted before, however, any negotiated relationship beyond a standard, discounted fee-for-service contract, should be analyzed carefully by each provider as the IPA or MSO may have difficulty successfully negotiating such a relationship on behalf of a group about which it may not be able to obtain solid statistical information either as to the patient population or the services rendered by any given provider.

The PO structure allows the department to negotiate managed care contracts from a position of greater strength than the IPA and

MSO models allow. Working together, the departments can exchange physician utilization information, as well as patient utilization information that can be obtained from the department's billing and collecting information. Because the departments utilizing the PO model can begin to obtain the information they need to successfully negotiate managed care contracts both with and without capitation, the PO is an effective model for the academic medical practice.

The federated group practice as decision-maker. The federated group practice is the best decision-making structure for most academic medical practices. The federated model can be either strong or weak depending on the amount of authority relinquished to the practice by the academic structure (the university, the deans, the departments and the individual providers). The benefits of this structure include the ability to utilize many economies of scale, such as: centralized credentialing; maintaining centralized medical records (at least within the same physical structure); and pursuing centralized quality improvement initiatives. More important, however, this structure allows the practice to engage in centralized decision-making around the various managed care products with which the practice might choose to contract. In addition, this structure allows the practice to more easily obtain and analyze the information necessary to successfully enter into managed care contracts. For example, a centralized practice can collect and analyze capitation-related data across primary and specialty care practices. A centralized billing and collecting function is also essential if the practice is to analyze its managed care relationships. Without centralized billing and collecting, it is difficult to obtain the information necessary to effectively analyze managed care contracts and to improve physician performance under managed care.

Unlike the previously described models, the detriments to this form of practice are more likely to be detriments as perceived by the medical school's academic structure rather than its practice structure. While the federated group practice model provides the practice with a sound business model, it does so at the expense of the traditional academic structure and, perhaps, traditional academic values. Inherent in the creation of a federated group are restrictions on departmental authority and control. The same department chairperson who manages the academic unit of the college may be required to relinquish control of his or her faculty to the extent that those individuals are health care providers. The strength or weakness of the federated model is directly proportional to the degree of control over the practice relinquished by the dean and the department chairs.

This control may include control over: the revenue generated by the faculty; the percentage of that revenue retained by the department; the managed care products with which the department participates; and even, perhaps, the hiring of additional clinical practitioners. Thus, the viability of the federated model is dependent upon the dean and each department chairperson believing that he or she will receive value for the control ceded to the practice.

A federated group practice may organize itself as an IPA, as a PO, or through an MSO, depending upon the degree of management control that the various departments are willing to release to the group's management. A weak federated practice may be required to structure itself as an IPA, while a stronger federated practice will be able to utilize strong, centralized management to function as a PO. Generally, the success of an academic practice that falls within this model is directly proportional to the willingness of the practice's departments to forego autonomy for the greater good of centralized practice management. As noted, resistance to a centralized structure will most likely come from the department level because of the autonomy typically afforded the university or college department. As a result, the practices that function within this model are those that carefully balance the academic providers' roles as teachers with their responsibilities as providers of care. Where each academic practice falls on the academic and managed care organizational continuums is simply evidence of how the institution has prioritized its various missions, as well as its success in operationally implementing those missions.

The true group practice as decision-maker. The true group practice, while ideal from a business perspective, is difficult to achieve in an academic setting. The true group practice is governed centrally with a single business plan. It utilizes central registration, scheduling, collection and billing systems, as well as centralized cost and quality measures. Perhaps, most importantly, the practice also maintains a central account of revenues and expenses. The true group practice ignores most academic considerations, maintaining that academic issues are the responsibility of the medical school's governance structure, a group that is likely different than the governance structure of the practice.

While this structure is ideally suited to negotiate and manage managed care, it is ill-suited to the academic environment. It is, in fact, the antithesis of the academic environment – a pure business enterprise, identical to a private, community, multispecialty group. For that reason, it is inappropriate for an academic medical practice to find itself at this end of the organizational continuum – for when it does, it is likely that the group has lost focus of its primary mission, the dissemination of knowledge through the education of medical students and research. Rather, the ideal medical practice will be organized so that it is sufficiently united to effectively negotiate and monitor its managed care relationships while, at the same time, recognizing that the focus of the academic medical practice must be its academic mission.

Continuing down the managed care continuum, the true group practice has a variety of managed care options. Of course, the true group practice can effectively utilize a PO structure, creating an academic physician group actually structured as a group. The practice can also pursue organizational models that would be difficult for all but the true group: participation in, or creation of, a Physician/Hospital Organization (PHO) or an Integrated Delivery System (IDS). A PHO is an organization jointly owned and controlled by a PO and a hospital. The organization is almost always incorporated. The PHO allows a hospital and a PO, typically comprised of the providers affiliated with that hospital, to negotiate jointly around managed care products. For the many medical schools that hold an ownership interest in an academic medical center, the ability to contract jointly with the hospital may provide the academic practice with a strong incentive to utilize a PHO structure. But even community-based medical schools can utilize the PHO structure with affiliated hospitals in much the same way that a provider participates in an IPA. The PO can participate in the PHO around certain managed care relationships while reserving the right to opt out of any managed care relationships where the PO has the ability to negotiate its own relationship.

Finally, the academic medical practice may wish to create, or affiliate with, an IDS. An IDS is an organization that provides a full range of health care to the payers with which it contracts. Unlike the PHO, which typically provides physician and hospital care, the IDS may also provide additional health care services and facilities, including but not limited to: hospitals, skilled nursing facilities or nursing homes, durable medical equipment suppliers, home health agencies, free-standing outpatient facilities, emergency care facilities, physicians and management services organizations. The academic practice can either join a preexisting IDS, or it can create an IDS of its own in conjunction with, or apart from, an academic medical center and other university-owned organizations and facilities.

The principal advantage of the IDS structure is that it allows the physician significantly greater bargaining power than might otherwise be available, even in the PO structure. In addition, expenses may be reduced due to economies of scale around billing and collecting, information systems, and the like. The academic practice's most significant problem with participating in an IDS structure is simply that it forces the academic medical practice to function as a true group, requiring the participating providers to surrender departmental autonomy and to develop a business (rather than an academic) attitude toward providing medical care, In short, the true group practice model (and, in all likelihood, the IDS) requires the academic physician to forgo those values that likely were factors in the physicians' decisions to practice in an academic environment: flexibility, a reduced practice schedule, and the opportunity to conduct research and teach students. Thus, while the true group practice and participation in an IDS can be successful, the academic practice must be aware of the "cost" of the venture in terms of reduced provider teaching time and an increased emphasis on the "business" of the practice.

In sum, the organizational models for the academic medical practice are limited only by the creativity of the practice's management. Typically, however, academic practices can be distinguished by the degree of autonomy afforded the academic provider. The continuum ranges from a model where individual provider decision-making is permitted, to a true group practice where decision-making is centralized at the expense of individual and departmental autonomy. The academic practice's organizational continuum loosely mirrors the managed care organizational continuum, ranging from the IPA to the PO to the PHO and IDS. Each place on the continuum may be appropriate for any particular academic practice; there is no one correct organizational structure. Rather, each academic practice must consider its goals and its institutional requirements and must select whichever organizational structure will be best suited to meet those objectives. Once the practice has determined its structure in managed care terms, it is ready to begin negotiating with payers around managed care contracts.

Critical issues in the academic contract

Perhaps the greatest asset of a managed care contract, or any contract, is that it requires that each party clearly articulate its understanding of the relationship. The contract provides a mechanism by which individuals can discuss, agree upon and memorialize in writing, the terms and conditions of their relationship. While the typical managed care contract may run for a period of one or more years, most contract manuals encourage the parties to include a "without cause" termination provision in the contract, typically between thirty (30) and one hundred eighty (180) days. Assuming a ninety-day without-cause termination clause when the parties sign the contract, they are committing to a legally binding contractual relationship for only ninety days. Thus, the end result of the contract is not the creation of a legally binding, long-term relationship. Rather, the creation of a contract serves two purposes. First, it allows the parties the opportunity to reach a clear understanding of the parameters of the relationship at its inception. Second, it creates legal enforcement mechanisms should either party fail to uphold the terms of the contract. Therefore, the managed care contract negotiator should be able to affirmatively answer several questions:

- Does the contract clearly articulate my goals and objectives for the relationship? Have I deleted any provisions that are unclear to me or may be unduly detrimental?;

- Do I understand both the letter and spirit of the provisions that the other party wishes to include in the contract?; and

- Am I comfortable with my ability to terminate the contract should there be a misunderstanding of the terms of the contract or should the other party breach the contract?

One means of ensuring that these questions can always be answered affirmatively is through the utilization of a contract checklist.

The managed care contract is often a complex document. The contract may run from only a few pages to 20 pages or more. But regardless of length, managed care contracts are often drafted using legal terminology that is difficult to understand and fine print that is difficult even to read. There exists today a multitude of commercially published checklists that review those issues most pertinent to the negotiation and operation of a managed care contract.[9] This section is designed to serve as a supplement to those checklists. It examines those portions of the managed care contract that the academic medical practice will most likely find unacceptable and will, therefore, most likely desire to change.

Preliminary issues

The academic medical practice faces a number of unique issues before negotiations with the other party around the contractual relationship are even considered. These issues, which the academic practice must resolve before it even steps up to the bargaining table, include: 1) Is the particular managed care organization an appropriate organization with which to contract? Has the practice conducted a due diligence review of the organization? 2) Who will be on the negotiating team: management staff, physicians or both; specialists, primary care physicians or both; individuals who will represent the different needs of Ob/Gyn, pediatrics, subspecialists, surgeons, lab and radiology; other providers such as physician assistants and nurse practitioners? 3) Who has the authority to sign the contract?

Conduct a due diligence review of the other party. Every medical practice should perform a due diligence review of any managed care organization with which it wishes to contract. This due diligence review typically includes a review of:

- The financial viability of the organization;
- Its track record in managed care; and
- Its ability to make money, and thus, stay solvent, over time.

If the organization is publicly traded, some obvious sources of valuable information are its Form 10-K, its prospectus, its annual report, or even anecdotal evidence available from local brokerage houses. Additionally, larger entities should have a Dun and Bradstreet report. The academic practice should also attempt to utilize any assets that might be available from the larger college or university. For example, the institution's business school may maintain a file in its business library on the company. Often these files contain prospectuses, Form 10-Ks, annual reports and other relevant financial information. The academic practice should also utilize the information available from national organizations such as the Medical Group Management Association (MGMA), the American Association of Medical Colleges (AAMC), the American Medical Association (AMA), and the American Osteopathic Association (AOA). Finally, the academic practice's faculty members/providers often have ties to providers at academic practices across the country who may be able to provide valuable information, anecdotal and otherwise, about organizations established in their geographic region that are moving into the practice's service area.

In addition to the due diligence data that may be derived from various external sources, it is also important to make inquiries directly to the organization, seeking information about the organization's present business as well as its future goals. Specifically, the organization should be able to provide detailed information about its current pool of covered lives, how that pool has increased (or decreased) in the past, and how the organization expects to ensure its growth in the future. Also, the organization should disclose which of the area's major employers have purchased the plan. Of course, if the medical school, the practice, or the larger university has purchased the plan, it will be of value to discuss the organization with the benefits office. Finally, review the organization's provider directories. An academic practice will often have a larger and more diverse group of specialists and subspecialists than the typical community-based practice. Among that group are likely to be unique providers not otherwise represented in the organization's provider pool. As a result, the organization may be more flexible when negotiating for their services.

Determine who will negotiate the contract. When developing a negotiating team, the practice must consider two issues: 1) What is the appropriate size of the team? and 2) How can the practice ensure that the team reflects the diverse interests of the primary care physicians, specialists, diagnostic practitioners and others who make up the academic practice? There is no standard number of individuals who should participate in managed care negotiations. Rather, the practice should ensure that the selected individuals adequately represent the interests of the entire group. For providers, this will usually require that they put aside individual and departmental biases, advocating only as representatives of the group. To ensure that the views of all departments are represented at the table, the academic practice may be best served by relying on its professional management staff. Those individuals not only possess professional, legal and financial management skills, but also should be capable of providing objectivity internally, when analyzing the contract's impact on the various departments, and externally, when negotiating for the services of the practice's providers.

Thus, the ideal negotiating team will consist of those members of the practice's management staff responsible for the practice's external relations and contracting as well as the practice's finances and operations. Provider participation in some form, however, is also critical. Therefore, the practice should appoint one or more providers to serve as either members of, or advisors to, the team. The team must be small enough to effectively negotiate, yet large enough to encompass the varying concerns and issues raised by the academic practice; typically a large, multispecialty group practice. Of course, it is also critically important for the team to regularly seek advice from and report results to the practice's governance structure. One of the most common roadblocks to an operationally sound contract is the practice's, and the university's, structure and size. Before entering into a contract, the team must consult not only with the relevant academic departments or units, but with the appropriate administrative units that will be responsible for the operational aspects of the contract. Every managed care relationship will inevitably involve the billing office, the registration area, information systems, quality assurance, and probably many other administrative offices. Only by consulting with all of these units will the team be able to negotiate the contract with an understanding of all relevant operational issues. The discussions should occur prior to the negotiations, and should continue through the conclusion of negotiations as operational issues occur. For example, the registration manager should be consulted about what information should appear on the plan's identification card while information systems should be consulted if the plan and the practice anticipate a computer interface. Finally, as capitation plays a larger role in the market, or to whatever degree the contract is not a pure fee-for-service relationship, the role of the practice's various data and information gathering units will be critical.

Ensure the appropriate parties receive and review the agreement. Presumably, the contract will be signed by an individual representing the practice as well as, where applicable, an individual representing the university. A common but complex mechanism requires the signature of the department chair, as well as the head of the practice and an official representing the university. The academic practice would be better served, however, by creating a coordinated governance and sign-off structure so that decisions can be made and implemented in a timely, expedient manner – the ideal would be a one person sign-off.

The most fundamental, and the most important, action that any practice must undertake before signing a contract is reading the contract. Ensuring that the contract has been received and properly reviewed by all relevant individuals is of critical importance to the academic medical practice. Because the academic practice falls not only under the authority of a medical school, but also a larger college or university, the negotiating team must be in contact with all relevant internal parties, including both the appropriate practice and university officials, as the contract is being negotiated. Of particular importance, of course, are any individuals whose signature is required on the contract. These parties may include, but are not limited to, the following:

At the university:

- The president's office
- The provost's office
- The contracting office
- The office of the general counsel
- The risk management office

- Other necessary university signatories

At the medical school:

- The dean
- Relevant chairpersons and/or unit managers
- Physicians who will participate with the organization
- Other necessary medical school signatories

At the practice:

- The chief executive officer
- The chief financial officer
- The billing and collecting officer
- Registration personnel
- The medical records officer
- The credentialing officer
- The quality assurance officer
- The managed care officer
- The contracting officer
- The information systems officer
- Relevant nurse managers
- Physicians, physician assistants, nurse practitioners, physical and occupational therapists, psychologists and others who will participate with the managed care organization

At best, this contact will allow each academic unit the opportunity to apprise the negotiating team of any special concerns related to their practice area. At the very least, by providing every department with the contract and soliciting their advice, the negotiating team has put each department on notice and provided each department with the opportunity to provide comment and advice.

The various units of the practice must not only review the contract, but any other relevant documents as well. This includes documents incorporated into the contract by reference as well as any supplementary or explanatory materials that the organization can provide. It is, therefore, critical that the negotiating team select an individual who can act as a "clearinghouse" – sending the contracts and materials out to the various academic departments and administrative units and recording and evaluating the comments received in response. The diversity inherent in the academic practice makes this function particularly critical.

The agreement

Ensure the services to be provided are clearly defined. The fundamental distinction between fee-for-service and capitated payments is that a capitated payment covers a specific, pre-negotiated "list" of services to be provided by the practice. In a fee-for-service arrangement the primary care physician's decision to provide a particular type of care may be made when a patient visits the physician's office. In a capitated payment structure, the physician commits to providing a specific list of services in advance of signing the contract. The physician is then bound to provide those services for the established, pre-negotiated fee over the term of the contract. Thus, establishing a clearly defined list of services to be provided by the physician is one of the most critical elements in a successful capitated relationship. These services are most typically defined by CPT coding. The practice must be careful to avoid phrases or qualifications in the contract that are ambiguous or unclear. For example, if a "routine annual checkup" is included in the capitation payment, it is important to determine precisely what the checkup includes. If the managed care organization interprets that language as including certain vaccinations in the capitation, the practice must be sure that those vaccinations are accounted for in the capitation payment.

Establishing the specific covered services by CPT code is particularly important to the academic medical practice. An example illustrates the point. The practice's management may negotiate a capitated arrangement around its primary care physicians. Those physicians may be internists in a department of internal medicine; they may be pediatricians in a pediatrics department; or they might include family practitioners in a department of family practice. It is likely that each primary care department, however, will not able to provide the exact same list of services. Family practice physicians might be very comfortable including a particular code in its capitation that the pediatrics department may not provide. While there certainly may be compelling reasons to enter into the contract even if all departments do not provide all capitated services, this scenario provides a very simple example of the importance of internal communication. All capitated practices within the group must carefully review the CPT codes covered within the capitation. Then, if the group chooses to participate, each practice will be aware of those areas in which it must use particular care when referring – as those referrals will likely penalize the primary care physician financially. To the extent that the managed care organization refuses to delete certain codes from the capitation schedule, the practice may be able to resolve the problem internally. It can refer those services to others in the practice who perform them; providing, of course, that at least one department performs every service on the capitation schedule.

Agree only to a standard of care equal to the accepted standard within the community. Occasionally, a managed care organization will attempt to include language requiring that the academic practice provide a standard of care greater than the accepted standard of care within the community; including, for example, language in the contract requiring that the group practice at the highest standard of care. Under no circumstances should the academic practice agree to language requiring that it provide a standard of care other than the accepted standard of care within the community. Agreeing to provide a higher standard of care is likely to create at least two critical problems. First, it will be more difficult for a physician to defend a malpractice claim when the physician has contractually agreed upon a standard of care higher than that typically provided by other physicians in the community. Second, the practice's malpractice coverage may prohibit it from agreeing to a standard of care higher than the standard of care that is prevalent in the practice's service area. Thus, any malpractice action for services performed under the contract may be excluded from coverage.

Ensure that the agreement is operational. Because managed care organizations and academic medical practices are both notoriously large and complex entities, one of the most common problems that the parties face is ensuring the agreement reached by the negotiating team is an agreement that can operate smoothly. One of the most common operational deficiencies is the failure to clearly define: the information that the organization will provide to the practice; the individuals at the practice to whom that information should be sent; when it must be provided; and in what form. One method of resolving any potential such problem is to add an exhibit to the contract that clearly establishes:

- What information the practice wishes to receive;
- In what form the information must be provided;
- To which individuals, departments or administrators the information must be sent;
- When the information must be sent;
- The specific information to be included in each report; and
- Any penalty that can be negotiated for failing to comply with the contract.

Finally, if the organization is providing regular reports, it may be possible to receive that information electronically. If so, can it be made available at any time that the practice wishes to download the information, or will the practice be restricted to receiving the information periodically? A similar exhibit may be established to cover any payments to be received by the practice.

The quantity or type of operational issues in any particular contract is impossible to predict. What follows are brief, but far from inclusive, examples:

Information systems
- To the extent that information can be transferred electronically, how will this be accomplished?
- Will either party need to bear any additional expense to electronically communicate with the other?
- Are systems compatible?

Billing and collecting
- Can the academic practice's billing staff meet any time deadlines imposed by the managed care organization?
- Are there any unique forms (other than the standard HCFA Form 1500) that must be used?
- Can claims be made electronically?

Medical records
- What type of release will the practice require before providing medical records to the organization?
- Does the organization require that any particular information be included in the record for quality assurance purposes?
- If so, can all departments comply?

Quality assurance
- Does the organization require on-site inspections?
- How much time do such inspections typically require?
- What information does the organization seek in its inspections? (The practice cannot pass a "test" if it does not know the material to be tested.)

Credentialing
- What information is required?
- Must the organization require primary source documentation or will it rely on state or other regulatory entities for certain information?

Review carefully all hold harmless and indemnification language. Hold harmless and indemnification provisions are, from a legal perspective, extremely important provisions in a managed care contract. These provisions speak to those situations in which a party agrees in advance to make the other party financially whole based on particular legal determinations. Some form of indemnification or hold harmless language will appear in the vast majority of managed care contracts. The academic medical practice should attempt, whenever possible, to remove this language from the contract. Mutual indemnification and hold harmless language often does little good – and in all but the most rare of circumstances, even mutual language serves only to the detriment of the provider.

Indemnification and hold harmless language may be even more dangerous, however, to the academic practice affiliated with a public college or university. Often, the actions of public officials are not subject to liability based on the principles of governmental immunity. While the law of governmental immunity varies from state to state, it is possible that the academic medical practice's providers may be immune from certain liability based on their status as government employees.[10] Whether the practice is private or has a public affiliation, it is critical that the practice seek the advice of its legal counsel before entering into managed care contracts that contain either indemnification or hold harmless language.

Verify that all providers who wish to participate with the managed care organization can do so. Because of the diversity inherent in the academic medical practice, it is not uncommon for the academic practice to utilize the services not only of physicians, but also of physical and occupational therapists, nurse practitioners, physician assistants, psychologists, and, of course, residents. To the extent that these individuals perform services for which the practice can bill, the practice must ascertain that the managed care organization will allow these individuals to provide services under the contract and that it is willing to pay for those services.

a. Physicians

A common example of problematic contract language is language requiring that all billable services must be performed by physicians who are "board certified." While this language obviously rules out the use of physician extenders, of greater importance to the academic practice is that it will in almost all cases prohibit the utilization of residents as well. If, in fact, residents cannot provide services under the contract, the practice will need to disassociate participation with the organization from its residency programs to some degree. To the extent that the practice wishes to utilize residents in the care of its patients, it must carefully negotiate language acceptable to the parties.

b. Other providers

Of equal importance to the academic practice are the practice's non-physician providers. Those individuals include, but are not limited to, nurse practitioners, physician assistants, physical and occupational therapists, psychologists and social workers. The academic practice must carefully analyze the managed care contract to determine whether the contract allows these individuals to provide services and to be compensated for those services. Some managed care organizations will create exclusive, "carve out" relationships around specialized areas such as physical and occupational therapy and mental health. As a result, the academic practice's physical and occupational therapists and psychologists may be excluded from providing services. This problem is most effectively solved by negotiating for providers to participate with the entity providing the "carved out" service. Of course, the best solution is simply for the academic practice to negotiate providing the carve out itself – by agreeing to provide all of the organization's physical therapy services, for example. While direct contracting may present a challenge to the academic practice, the "carrot" that the practice presents to the managed care organization is its ability to advertise its exclusive relationship with the academic medical practice of the university.

The academic practice must be able to quickly and accurately verify eligibility. The verification of patient eligibility is obviously a critical issue to any medical practice. The issue is of greater importance to the academic medical practice because of the diversity of the practice. Not only does the academic practice consist of multiple department-based units, but it is also common for the academic practice to be located at multiple sites that may be great distances from one another. The practice must attempt to ensure that the managed care organization can quickly and accurately communicate relevant information to all of the academic group's practices and practice sites. While eligibility verification is an excellent example of why good communication between the organization and the practice is critical, the practice must ensure that its various practice units can effectively communicate with the managed care organization for all other necessary purposes as well. A few examples are: the addition or deletion of covered services from the contract; the addition or deletion of providers from the plan; changes in billing procedures; and open enrollment marketing information.

Ensure the academic practice can comply with all contract provisions requiring that the practice notify the managed care organization of certain actions or activities. Again, because the academic practice is a large, diverse group practice, it is critical that the academic practice ensure that its internal channels of communication are sufficient to comply with any contract provisions requiring notice. Typically, the managed care contract will require that the practice notify the organization when certain events occur. Failure to provide this notice may constitute a breach of the contract. Those events might be practice-wide, or they may be specific to a certain individual provider. For example, the practice may be required to notify the organization when any of these events occur:

- A provider fails to maintain a required license or hospital privileges;
- the practice's, or a particular provider's, insurance is altered or terminated;
- a provider relocates an office location or changes a telephone number;
- a provider alters office hours;
- a provider changes his or her name; or
- a provider goes on sabbatical or is otherwise unable to practice for an extended time period.

To ensure that the practice can comply with its contractual commitment surrounding notice, the academic medical practice is well advised to maintain a central data bank and to require that the various providers and departments notify the keeper of the data bank when any changes occur.

A centralized database that includes this information flows naturally from centralization of the contracting and credentialing functions. By requiring that all contracts be created and administered centrally, the practice ensures that there is a centralized mechanism for monitoring compliance with the contracts' terms. By requiring that all of the practice's providers be credentialed through a central office, the practice ensures that all relevant information about the provider can be accessed by one centralized unit.

The practice must be able to monitor compliance. A centralized information structure is not only important to the academic medical practice in its efforts to ensure that it can comply with the contract, it is also critical to the practice if it wishes to ensure that the managed care organization is in compliance with the contract. The managed care organization should communicate with the practice for at least four purposes: 1) providing notice to the practice as required in the contract; 2) providing performance data to the practice on a regular basis, thereby allowing the practice to "manage" the care it provides; 3) responding to questions and concerns regarding the operation or interpretation of the contract; and 4) payment for rendered services. The managed care contract will usually state that notice will be provided to certain specified individuals or offices. Notice certainly may be provided to various departments, the dean, or others, depending upon the nature of the contract. But notice should always be provided to a central administrative office responsible for contract monitoring and compliance. This allows the practice to act expeditiously should problems requiring official notice occur. It also provides a simple mechanism for ensuring that important issues do not "fall through the cracks."

The practice will presumably receive certain performance data that will assist the practice in managing the care it provides. While this information may be analyzed and interpreted most effectively by personnel in the clinic, it is particularly critical in the academic medical practice that this information be sent to a central location. Sending the information to only one address serves several purposes. First, it avoids the inevitable confusion typical of the academic practice that has multiple providers, in multiple locations, with academic providers coming to or leaving the practice at a greater rate than is typical with multispecialty, community group practices. In short, it ensures that all of the appropriate information is received in the format that it should be received as required by the contract. Second, requiring the organization to provide data centrally allows the practice to collect and analyze data across the group. Group-wide data will help the practice determine whether the practice is appropriately managing care and will identify those departments or individuals that may be having a problem. This will allow the practice's governance the opportunity to assist those individuals in improving their management of managed care. In addition, group data will assist the practice as it negotiates future capitated relationships.

Finally, the managed care organization should be required to send all compensation to a single practice address. As noted before, this decreases the confusion inherent in a diverse academic practice. A central check clearinghouse also allows the practice to ensure that it is receiving all payments required under the contract and that payments are received within the required time periods. To the extent that payments are not received, the central office will be able to determine whether any delay is an isolated incident or is part of a pattern of noncompliance that may require the practice to reevaluate the contractual relationship. Finally, a central check clearinghouse allows the practice management to ensure that all checks are flowing through the practice plan in the appropriate fashion.

Expect the managed care contract to allow the practice to utilize ancillary, diagnostic and commonly "carved-out" services. A particularly unique attribute of the academic medical practice is its wide array of ancillary services, diagnostic services and other services not provided by the typical practice . In many cases, the managed care organization will carve out some portion of these services. For example, despite the ability of some primary care physicians to provide certain radiological services in their offices, the managed care organization may require all primary care physicians in the network to utilize the services of a radiology group with which it has negotiated a special relationship. In the typical private practice this means that the physician will generate less revenue from the product because he or she will not be able to bill (or receive an additional capitated amount) for a service that the physician can provide. For the academic practice, however, the problem is more serious. Entire departments or units of the practice may rely on the revenue generated from referrals within the practice. If the practice's physicians cannot refer to the practice's radiologists, the radiology department will suffer financially. The same is true for departments of psychiatry, pathology, and physical medicine and rehabilitation which provide commonly carved out mental health, laboratory and rehabilitation services.

The practice must not assume that it can use its own laboratory, its own mental health services, or even its own pharmacy. Rather, the practice must aggressively negotiate to have those services included in the contractual relationship. In some cases, the practice can contract with the organization to allow the practice's providers an opportunity to provide services to the network, or at least other providers within the practice. This may require the organization to work around a contract that the organization has signed with another group to provide the service. If the contract is non-exclusive, the practice may be able to successfully negotiate a deal. More likely, however, the contract creating the carved-out relationship grants the group providing the service a right to provide that service exclusively.

Depending on the practice's value to the organization and its negotiating strength, the practice may be able to force the organization to accept the practice's services at the organization's expense, despite an exclusive carve out. For example, a managed care organization that has an exclusive, capitated contract with a private laboratory company has paid the company to provide laboratory services to its entire patient population. If that organization also agrees to pay a group to provide those services, the organization will be paying for the same service twice.

When the practice butts up against an exclusive, carved-out relationship, the practice's best strategy may be to attempt to develop a relationship with the carved-out entity. By negotiating directly with a national laboratory company, for example, the academic practice may be able to provide services not only to the patient population covered by the managed care organization at issue, but also to patients participating in other managed care organizations with which the national lab is affiliated. Thus, a successful contract with the national lab allows the academic practice's lab the opportunity to serve not only the practice's patients, or a particular organization's patients, but it may also allow the lab to serve patients throughout the state or larger geographic region in which the medical school is located. For example, the academic practice may be able to provide certain specialized lab work locally that a national laboratory might otherwise be required to send out of state. Or the practice's lab may be able to provide service nationally, via mail, express mail and computer, at a greater discount than can be provided by other bidding laboratories. In any event, when ancillary, diagnostic and carved-out services can be provided to a group larger than the managed care organization or the practice itself, the practice benefits both because its physicians can refer to those units and because those units will have greater opportunity in an ever shrinking market.

Make sure the practice retains the right to increase or decrease the number of providers that can participate in the plan based on employment at the medical school. The academic medical practice is an environment that requires physician mobility. Unlike the traditional private practitioner who has generating revenue as a primary objective, the academic practitioner is often driven more by academic interests and opportunities. As a result, it is not uncommon for academic providers to move from one institution to another as educational opportunities become available, programs change, or the faculty member develops new interests or collaborative endeavors.

The academic medical practice must account for the mobile nature of its provider population when it enters into managed care contracts. Specifically, the practice must attempt to ensure that all providers employed by the practice who otherwise meet the reasonable criteria established by the organization, can participate with the organization's products. Primary care physicians will generally be welcomed into most managed care organizations. It is the specialists that the practice may need to assist.

The practice can assist its specialty care providers by making sure that all who wish to participate with a particular managed care organization are able to do so (subject, of course, to appropriate credentialing). The practice then must attempt to negotiate language allowing the organization to accept new specialists who join those departments. The organization might get nervous, however, to the extent that it has adopted a closed-panel philosophy and the practice wants language in the contract allowing new specialists in new specialty fields. Despite the organization's concerns, it should be possible to negotiate language allowing the practice to add specialists, and additional physicians in general, within parameters of reasonableness.

Ensure the contract incorporates appropriate safeguards on use of the university name. One of the academic practice's greatest assets is its reputation. By virtue of its affiliation with a medical school, the academic practice can avail itself of the school's, and the larger university's, reputation and success. While the practice must use great care and specificity when authorizing an organization to use its name, the organization will legitimately need to utilize certain provider information on marketing brochures and the like. Indeed the practice should want the organization to market the practice. The practice must be careful, however, to insure that the organization is not authorized to market the practice's name or affiliation in any way that will damage the reputation of the practice or the larger university. The practice can solve this problem simply by authorizing the organization to include each provider's name, address, phone number, and specialty in brochures developed for the purpose of informing members about providers participating with the organization. Any additional marketing would require the authorization of appropriate practice or university officials on a case-by-case-basis.

Ensure term and termination provisions are appropriate for the academic group practice. Because, as noted before, the academic practice may have significant provider turnover, the term and termination provisions of the contract must be drafted accordingly. Two issues are of particular concern. First, it is not uncommon for the makeup of the practice to change significantly over time. In the event that a provider or group of providers leaves the practice on short notice, the practice must be able to terminate the contract quickly as it relates to those providers. For example, an academic practice might include two neurosurgeons. Those surgeons may have a carved-out relationship with several managed care organizations, providing those organizations with a discounted fee-for-service arrangement in return for the right to exclusively provide neurosurgical care to the organization's patient population. If those physicians were to leave the practice on short notice, the practice would need either to replace them or terminate the contract of those physicians to avoid a breach of contract. To effectuate this required termination, the practice should insist upon without-cause termination language; i.e., providing that either party may terminate the contract for any reason upon prior written notice. Between 30 and 90 days notice is typical.

A second problem common to the academic medical practice is that the practice may want to terminate the contract for certain providers but not others. In the previous example, if only one of the neurosurgeons had left the practice and the remaining surgeon could cover the workload, the practice might want to terminate the relationship only as it applied to the departing surgeon. Thus, the practice would want to include termination language that is provider specific as well as language that is practice-wide. The contract might provide that it can be terminated as to individual providers under certain circumstances (i.e., failure to maintain a license or failure to be employed by the university), yet it can be terminated as to the entire group should other circumstances occur (i.e., if the organization files bankruptcy or the organization fails to maintain a required license).

Ensure provider performance incentives are appropriate. Managed care may be defined, at a theoretical level, as a means by which providers are given incentives to make patients healthier at less cost. If one accepts that definition, provider performance incentives become a necessary element of the managed care contract. Therefore, the academic medical practice, or any practice, that participates in products offered by a managed care organization may be required to agree that the groupís providers will meet certain criteria and that some portion of their earnings may be retained as an ìincentiveî to encourage the providers to meet those goals. With that understanding, the academic medical practice must ensure that the incentives proposed by the organization are fair and appropriate given the unique characteristics and structure of the academic medical practice.

Any incentive must account for the academic provider's practice style. The academic provider, by virtue of his or her academic interests, is a part-time practitioner. As a result, any incentive plan must test the provider so as to not discriminate against the part-time practitioner. For example, an incentive plan that requires a provider to maintain a certain panel size, or requires the provider to compete on any basis relative to panel size, must be weighted appropriately. This can be accomplished in some instances by simply multiplying the quantity criteria by the percentage of FTE that the academic provider practices.

Other incentive measures may also be problematic for the academic practice. Patient satisfaction surveys, for instance, may discriminate against the part-time practitioner. A question asking whether a patient can get in to see his or her provider as needed is not a fair question to ask of the patient of a provider on sabbatical. (Of course, the patient who cannot get an appointment with any provider during that time has a legitimate complaint.) Another problematic question might ask the patient whether he or she can get in to see his or her primary care physician for urgent care on the same day. Because the academic physician also teaches and conducts research, the physician may not always be able to see patients on a same-day basis. Nevertheless, patients are aware, at least in theory, that decreased availability is a price one pays to see an academic physician, and patients do so with that understanding. Finally, because academic providers have priorities in addition to patient care, they tend to see fewer patients and are more likely to close their practices to new patients. Therefore, any incentive or requirement for a practice to remain open must be carefully considered. In sum, the academic practice must carefully review any provider performance incentive to ensure that it does not unduly penalize the academic provider merely by virtue of his or her status as an academic provider.

Ensure monitoring of compliance with the contract. Once the contract has been signed, the academic medical practice must carefully monitor contract compliance. As with everything in the academic medical practice, this process is made more difficult by the diverse and fragmented structure inherent in most academic practices. One means of solving this problem is to encourage centralization of the contracting and subsequent monitoring of managed care contracts. Several fundamental processes can simplify this process such as:

- Requiring centralized review of all contracts to promote uniformity and to ensure that the full power of the practice is behind all contracting initiatives;

- Creating a tickler file of all anticipated payments under the contract which the compliance officer can regularly review to ensure that all payments are received on time and in the correct amount; and

- Creating a tickler file of all contract termination dates to ensure that contract renewal negotiations are undertaken well in advance of the termination date.

In short, instituting only a few fundamental processes will allow the academic medical practice to monitor contract compliance with some success.

The future of managed care contracting for the academic medical practice

In large measure, the future of academic managed care contracting will be determined by the future of academic medical practices and academic medical centers. To the extent that practices and medical centers continue to consolidate, striving to develop Integrated Delivery Systems (IDSs) in varying forms, or at least more cohesive and "business-oriented" practices and medical centers, the academic contract administrator must respond accordingly. The contractor's efforts will likely be focused on developing the IDS, or other organizational structures focusing on practice integration, by creating relationships between the various university players and community physicians who may become participants in the integrated structure.

This trend toward integration does not appear to be waning. For at least the past ten years, academic medical management studies have emphasized that the success of academic medicine hinges on the ability of academic medical centers and practices to pursue integration and coordination both inside and outside of the academic institution.[11] Credible publications continue to reach similar conclusions today.[12] The academic contractor's mission must be to proactively anticipate and create opportunities for the practice and to take advantage of those opportunities when they arise. Through the turn of the century, many of those opportunities are likely to involve increased integration and coordination. This integration and coordination may be internal to the university; it may include the creation of an IDS-type organization with significant involvement from community providers; or it may be some combination of the two.

Regardless of the form of the change, it is, while trite, wise to recognize that the only constant well into the next century will be a continually changing health care industry. The contractor's role in this process is both exciting and challenging. The skilled academic contract administrator, in this time of turmoil, will face new challenges with every contractual relationship and will be well served to remember the words of Reinhold Niebuhr: "God, grant me the serenity to accept the things I cannot change, the courage to change the things I can, and the wisdom to know the difference."

References

1 The purpose of this chapter is to provide to the reader additional insight into contracting issues as they relate to the academic medical practice. This chapter does not constitute legal advice. The reader is urged to seek legal advice from his or her legal counsel.

2 F. Scott Fitzgerald, *The Crack-Up*, (New York: James Laughlin, 1956), p. 69.

3 Abraham Flexner, *Medical Education in the United States and Canada*, (New York: The Carnegie Foundation for the Advancement of Teaching, 1910).

4 Ibid., pp. 28-51.

5 The increased interest in the financing of medical care is exemplified by the proliferation of publications addressing managed care and other financing mechanisms, a small sample of those publications constitute the majority of this chapter's bibliography.

6 John D. Blair, Ph.D.; Myron D. Fottler, Ph.D.; Andrea R. Paolino, M.A.; Timothy M. Rotarius, M.B.A.; William M. Dwyer, M.B.A., (eds.); *Medical Group Practices Face The Uncertain Future: Challenges, Opportunities and Strategies*, p. 9, Center for Research in Ambulatory Health Care Administration, Englewood, CO 1995.

7 An addendum in the form of a glossary is provided to clarify how acronyms common to the health care industry are defined for the purposes of this chapter.

8 The term "provider" is intended to encompass the myriad of health care professionals who may, as faculty, provide patient care. These individuals may include, but are not limited to, physicians, physician assistants, nurse practitioners, nurses, physical and occupational therapists, psychologists, and technicians.

9 Robert W. McAdams, Jr., J.D.; Mary L. Gallagher, J.D.; Charles D. Weller, J.D. (eds.), *Managed Care Contracts Manual,* Aspen Publishers, Gaithersburg, Maryland, 1996; and Peter R. Kongstvedt, (ed.), *The Managed Health Care Handbook* Second Edition, Aspen Publishers, Gaithersburg, Maryland, 1993.

10 See, for example, Vargo v Sauer, 215 Mich App 389; 547 NW2d 40 (1996).

11 Albert P. Williams, Grace M. Carter, Glenn T. Hammons, Dennis Pointer; (eds.), Managing for Survival, p. 62; RAND Publications; Santa Monica, CA, October 1987.

12 John D. Blair, Ph.D., Myron D. Fottler, Ph.D., Andrea R. Paolino, M.A., Timothy M. Rotarius, M.B.A., William M. Dwyer, M.B.A. (eds.), *Medical Group Practices Face The Uncertain Future: Challenges, Opportunities and Strategies*, pp. 31-41; Center for Research in Ambulatory Health Care Administration, Englewood, CO 1995.

Managed care glossary

Capitation****
Under capitation, providers – hospitals and/or physicians – agree to accept a set advance payment in exchange for providing health care services for a group of people, usually for a year. Hospitals and/or physicians receive payments per member per month for a comprehensive set of services, or for a more specialized service, such as cardiac care. Whether a member uses the health service once or a dozen times, a provider who is capitated receives the same payment.

Fee For Service****
The traditional method for financing health services pays physicians and hospitals for each service they provide. Fee-for-service is the system of payment used by conventional indemnity health plans.

Health Maintenance Organization ("HMO")****
HMO members receive comprehensive preventative and hospital and medical care from specific medical providers who receive a pre-paid fee. Members select a primary care physician or medical group from the HMO's list of affiliated doctors. In turn, primary care doctors coordinate the patient's total care, which is free from hassles involving deductibles or claim forms. When using medical services, members pay a small co-payment, usually between $5 and $15.

HMO – Group Practice Model****
A physician group - usually one with a large number of primary care and specialist physicians - contracts with an HMO to provide services for a fixed advance payment. Rather than paying physicians individually, the negotiated payment goes to the group. The group bears the accountability to compensate physicians and to ensure the health of the members for which they are responsible.

HMO – IPA Model****
Physicians in private practice contract with an HMO to provide medical services through an Individual Practice Association for a set fee, paid in advance. The same physicians typically provide care for members of a variety of health plans.

HMO – Staff Model****
Physicians act as employees of the health plan and provide care exclusively to plan members. Often, a broad array of services are found in one location in staff model HMOs.

Independent Practice Association ("IPA")/Independent Practice Organization ("IPO")*

An IPA or IPO (generally, used synonymously) is a legal entity, often a corporation, that contracts on behalf of physician members and often provides administrative services to those members.

Managed Care***

A system of health care financing and delivery which is designated to effect the cost, volume and manner of service delivery through organized relationships with health care providers.

Managed Care Organization ("MCO") ****

A managed care organization may be a physician group, health plan, hospital or health system - i.e., any organization that is accountable for the health of an enrolled group of people. In contrast to organizations that provide services at a discount but do not attempt to coordinate care, managed care organizations actually have responsibility for the health of enrollees and, as a consequence, seek improvements in both the results and cost-effectiveness of the services provided. Most managed care organizations still care for those with traditional indemnity insurance in addition to patients insured under managed care health insurance products.

Physician-Hospital Organization ("PHO")****

A PHO is an entity governed equally be a hospital and a group of physicians; the purpose of which is to jointly participate in managed care products.

Point of Service Plan ("POS")****

Point-of-Service networks provide subscribers free choice of physicians and hospitals for many services, but require a higher co-payment and often a substantial deductible if the provider is not part of the HMO or designated provider network

Preferred Provider Organization ("PPO")***

Preferred Provider Organizations offer the option for beneficiaries to receive services from providers who are not part of the "preferred," or contracted, panel. Members pay a much higher portion of costs in exchange for this freedom of choice. Typically, annual deductibles must be met before members take advantage of some benefits.

*Robert W. McAdams, Jr., J.D.; Mary L. Gallagher, J.D.; Charles D. Weller, J.D. (eds.). *Managed Care Contracts Manual*, p. 6:57; Aspen Publishers, Gaithersburg, Maryland, 1996.

**Bruce A. Johnson, J.D., M.P.A., Consultant (ed.); *Managed Care Contract Performance and Review*, p. 4; Medical Group Management Association, Englewood, Colorado, 1995.

***Peter R. Kongstvedt, (ed.)., *The Managed Health Care Handbook*, Second Edition, p. 14; Aspen Publishers, Gaithersburg, Maryland, 1993.

****Integrated Healthcare Association, “Managed Healthcare – A Brief Glossary.” Cited November 1, 1996. Available from http:// www. ihe. org/gloss.htm/;INTERNET.

Chapter 13

Clinical information systems in the academic medical practice

by Howard Tepper, MBA, FACMPE

If knowledge is power, then data is the raw material needed for knowledge. As with most raw materials, without processing, it is of little use. Physicians have always been the gatherers and keepers of important clinical data. Traditionally, its organization and analysis have been, at best, time consuming. Because the costs associated with collection and organization are so high, the economic factor has outweighed the benefits. Physicians traditionally have kept their own information for inpatients on index cards and relied on hospital records. For outpatients, they have used their own medical records, both systems relying on paper systems.

Problems of paper charts

The complex nature of the data collected and large numbers of elements have made the search for specific data on a patient difficult. Searching and analyzing data elements over a number of patients or over a period of time is nearly impossible. Paper charts physically can only be in one place at one time, allowing for viewing by only one party at a particular time. It comes as no surprise to anyone involved in health care that paper charts also can be difficult to locate. Even more difficult is ensuring that all elements of a chart such as test results, ancillary reports, etc., find their way to the correct chart. This becomes more evident as the amount of paperwork increases. The amount of paperwork generated yearly in the health care industry grew 35 percent between 1987 and 1993 to 950 billion pages.[1]

Written in fulfillment of the requirements for advancement to Fellowship Status in the American College of Medical Practice Executives, 104 Inverness Terrace East, Englewood, CO 80112-5306; 303-397-7869

In recent years, paper-based approaches have increasingly been replaced by computer-based systems. In turn, the number of patients seen has increased. The Galen Medical Group reports that, since the implementation of an electronic medical record, four internists have gone from seeing 16 to 18 patients per day, to seeing 20 to 24 patients, including six comprehensive visits.[2]

The transition from paper to electronic records is accelerating. Some reasons include: the cost of computer hardware has decreased; telecommunications and networking are less costly and more reliable; a consensus exists in reducing the administrative costs of health care; and electronic standards are emerging to exchange data between organizations and applications.[3]

The introduction of computer technology into physician practice has made the collection and analysis of data simpler and of more value. However, while there is little disagreement that computers can be useful, it has been difficult to gain consensus on their role. After various attempts at development of clinical systems, the one that has emerged for use in the physician's office is an electronic medical record. A recent listing of software companies selling electronic medical records systems listed over 50 companies.[4] An industry analysis by Robertson, Stephens & Co. shows the market for electronic medical records is growing by 70 percent annually.[5] These electronic medical records cover a broad range of systems. The simplest collects a patient name and a diagnosis. The more complex involves artificial intelligence and decision-making and takes the place of a paper record.

The need for an electronic medical record

The need for an electronic medical record has become more important as physician practices need to operate more efficiently in the age of managed care. More than ever, there needs to be an increase in the throughput of physician offices. The financial calculation for a fee-for-service patient is simple. The more patients seen means more billable services. For capitated patients, an increase in capacity means increasing the number of capitated lives.

An electronic medical record can increase the efficiency of a practice in a number of ways. Staff time saved just for the pulling of charts can be substantial. The time saved in looking for charts and in manually completing information is additional savings. Having lab tests, vital signs and past history immediately available increases practitioner efficiency. Studies indicate that physicians devote 35 percent of their time and nurses 48 percent of their time charting and doing paperwork.[6]

A review of dozens of studies on paper records conducted by Arthur Little, Inc., found 20 percent of paper records had items from another patient's chart. Additionally, paper charts were missing for between 6 to 18 percent of patient visits, and information clinicians required was missing 18 to 20 percent of the time. This required repeated testing or consults for 32 to 54 percent of patients.[6]

While the move to managed care may be the largest trend in health care, underlying issues have involved defining and measuring quality in health care. While quality in health care has always been an issue, the development of measurable and definable quality elements has begun.

One way to measure and define quality is to measure outcomes. The basis in measuring patient outcomes is to measure a patient baseline and show improvement. The clinical record contains this data. Measurement of the data elements only occurs by organizing data for analysis. An electronic medical record offers the data in an analyzable format.

Traditionally, managed care companies' cost-control efforts had to reduce provider rates and utilization. In the future the focus will be not just on reducing costs but managing them. To manage these costs there must be accurate real-time data.[7] The electronic medical record will provide the backbone for managing this data. Creation of the Health Plan Employer Data Information Set (HEDIS) was a joint effort between health plans and employers to standardize the collection and reporting of health plan data. The National Committee for Quality Assurance (NCQA) assumed responsibility for continued development of HEDIS. Health plans that wish to receive accreditation by NCQA submit data to HEDIS on a regular basis. Health plans use the data from specific providers to profile providers by companies and to rate them within plans. The data used comes from patient data usually supplied by providers. Few practitioners track their own HEDIS elements or validate the data used. Electronic records can ease analysis of the data elements and can provide real-time information to highlight areas that need improvement.

When most health care reimbursement systems used cost reimbursement, payment was the cost of a procedure or service. There was little financial risk in high-cost items because these items simply increased reimbursement. With capitation and negotiated rates, the actual cost elements of a procedure or service play a crucial role in the financial profitability of services. Introduction of cost-accounting systems that record elements and their cost is necessary to determine the cost of services. Computerized records allow for the capture of all services performed and analysis of data collected. This will assist practitioners in choosing not only the service with the best clinical outcome, but within the best clinical choices, the one with the best financial profitability.

According to a survey conducted by Andersen Consulting, 81 percent of hospitals have protocols and 19 percent have some type of automated decision support. Electronic medical records are providing the data necessary to create the system to implement guidelines that physicians can use when making treatment decisions.[8]

To be a successful practice, the patient must be the focal point. Successful clinical information must also revolve around the patient. Since the medical record contains all the patient medical information, it is the center of the information system.

Gaining acceptance of the system

While the need for an electronic medical record has become recognized in the health care industry, gaining acceptance for usage is the major challenge. As with any technology or new product, there are those who are quick to adopt new ideas. Geoffrey Moore has written extensively on the subject of marketing and selling high-tech products. A successful implementation requires the treating of physicians as customers of high-tech products. He defines the various types of groups in the acceptance of technology. These groups translate well into the acceptance and implementation curve of electronic medical records in physician practices.

The first group are the innovators. In medical practice these are the physicians participating in clinical trials and the first to use and purchase new medical technology. They have an interest in technology and enjoy not only what the technology brings to a given application, but also the pleasure of using new technology. Next are the early adopters. These are physicians who can understand and appreciate the potential benefits of the new technology. They see the new technology as a way to make them more efficient and implement it fairly soon after it is introduced.

The third group are the early majority. They too understand and appreciate technology but are pragmatists. They are willing to hear the sales pitch and can relate to the need for the new technology, but they have seen "many come and go." They will wait and see if the innovators and early adopters have successfully implemented the technology. The fourth group is the late majority. They not only want to see a successful implementation of others before they try it, but their biggest concern is discomfort with new technology. They will wait until there is a clear standard and then only use the standard if there is a lot of support.

The last group are the laggards. They simply do not want anything to do with any new technology. These are the physicians who fondly remember the good old days before e-mail, voice-mail and when regular mail came twice a day.

Understanding these groups is important to successfully implementing a clinical record. Just as important as understanding the groups is understanding the "chasm" between the groups in the timeline.[9] What makes a success with one group creates a total failure with another. Furthermore, being successful with the innovators who are the smallest subgroup does not guarantee success with the whole group.

Patient attitudes toward electronic medical records concern some physicians. However, studies of patients exposed to the use of electronic medical records indicate positive attitudes toward them. Patients felt the electronic medical record facilitated the visit and that physicians cared enough about them to obtain state-of-the-art technology. Although confidentiality concerns some patients, others felt that an electronic medical record was more secure than a paper record.[10]

Regardless of the group, the most important point to get across in gaining acceptance is that the system adds value. Understanding the group will be of assistance in understanding how each defines value. Some functions available with the records provide added value to all groups. These are: availability of records; access to lab data; and prescription writing. Physicians need to view the system as something that gives to them, such as automated lab results, not something that just takes *from* them, such as data entry time.

Most important, because physicians are in the business of caring for patients, it needs to be made clear that the use of an electronic medical record will benefit patients in terms of accessibility, completeness and analysis.[11]

Implementing an electronic medical record system

The success of computerized patient record implementation depends on the implementation team. All parties need representation, but the size of teams needs to be workable. There should be a project team that acts as an executive steering team. Members should include the chair of the implementing department, the practice medical director, the practice manager, the departmental administrator and the lead information system person. This group is a policy-setting committee and indicates to the organization that successful system implementation has a high-level organizational importance.

Reporting to this committee should be three functional committees. One is the physician committee. Representation in the group should include the various medical specialties using the system. The group should deal with clinical issues and be chaired by the medical director. By involving clinicians in planning they will understand what the system will do when installed and will be more supportive. Most implementations that fail are directed by administrators or nurses who may not fully understand the physician's needs.[11]

The next is the operational committee. The practice administrator chairs the group and membership includes members of practice staff. The major charge of this committee will involve workflow issues and implementation of the new system. Before new system implementation, and even before the decision made to purchase a specific system occurs, this committee needs to fully understand and chart the current workflow process. This analysis needs to begin from the patient's entry into the clinic, through the medical visit, and up until they exit. It also needs to look at other non-face-to-face contacts, such as phone and mail interactions. By fully understanding the pre-electronic record system, the committee will ensure the new system meets all the needs of the practice. Prior to implementation, documentation of new system workflow should occur. This should clearly document any new processes, and which processes will no longer be necessary after the electronic medical record's implementation.

The third committee is the information systems committee. Their charge is all computer-related issues. This committee will deal with issues of hardware, software and integration with other systems. Integration with other systems includes development of interfaces with lab systems, financial systems and other systems used in the practice. If the practice is part of a larger organization of a hospital or medical school, there should be representation of information system staff from these entities. The issue of training falls under this committee. The committee must develop a process to train staff and physicians not only in the new system but also in the use of computers. Computer training should begin long before system installation. All staff should have a basic knowledge of computers and the chosen operating system(s) (DOS, Windows, Windows 95, etc.). Organized communication between all the committees must occur for the implementation to be successful.

Many a well-chosen and installed system has failed because of inadequate training. Development of a training plan for all those using the system is crucial. An electronic medical records system has two main user groups, physicians and office staff. Each uses the system differently and, therefore, has significantly different training needs.

Training of both groups in the general use of computers can begin right after making the decision to use an electronic system. The training programs need to match the different formal education levels of the groups. The initial training should start with the basics for turning on a computer, mouse and keyboard control and the printing functions. Once the groups have mastered computer basics, specific system training can begin. Each group needs to understand all the functions available in the system but only needs detailed training in the functions they will be using. Physicians need to know the system schedules patients, but if scheduling is to be handled by the front office, they do not need to know the details of scheduling.

Training cannot be a close-ended process. There needs to be ongoing training for existing staff as well as a process to train new staff and physicians. Ongoing support for the system should include review training of existing functions and training of any new enhancements that come with upgrades. Handling of support issues can be by clinic staff or the software company. Training for senior members of the clinic staff directly by the company as "super users" is advisable. This staff can act as a local support group and should be able to handle most system questions. This staff should also act as liaison between the users and software company. Channeling of all questions through this group will properly organize issues forwarded to the software company.

Choosing a system

After making the decision to implement and selecting committee membership, the process of choosing a system begins. There are many systems labeled as electronic medical records systems covering a large range of features. The first step is outlining the features required by the practice. If the clinic is multispecialty, the system needs to allow for customization by specialty. The segregation of data by location, practice and department is important, if the practice represents many departments in different locations and practices. Design of some system is for physician offices and not for academic practices. They cannot roll data up into practice specialties, divisions and departments. While not necessary for some physician practices, it is important data in the academic setting.

To be successful, the system needs to give individuals the ability to customize viewing of data while maintaining standards. Customizable summary screens can accomplish this. The screen will display patient data in customized formats according to provider preference. The ability to customize to the provider level is crucial in obtaining buy-in from providers who may be hesitant to try a new system. Viewing new data and data that was never before available in a format of their choosing, will likely make physicians regular users of the system.

Another measure of the success of a system is its use as a real-time system, by entering patient information at the time of a visit. A system should have the ability to accept entry of progress notes during a patient visit.

A successful method to decrease the amount of data entry required is the use of preformatted visit templates. Studies of physician dictation practices show that about 80 percent of the dictation does not change patient to patient.[12] Patient type and disease are the basis for template creation. This is also very valuable in complying with evaluation and management code requirements, managed care requirements and clinical guidelines. Meeting these requirements occurs by preformatting data element requirements by type of visit, patient and disease. Many physicians carry cards listing the evaluation and management documentation requirements by CPT code.

If a system can accommodate preformatted visits, then by choosing a new patient and the visit level, all the documentation requirements will be on the screen. Example: If the visit is for a diabetic patient, the questions to be asked, labs to be taken and systems to be examined, are shown on the screen. This will greatly reduce the amount of data entry and ensure reviewing of all medically required systems. The system should also have the ability to accept free-form notes that give the practitioner the option of modifying to include all patient elements being observed or examined. If payer auditors cannot find or read the chart, the auditor may deem that a service did not occur and the submission of a bill was fraud.

The system should provide the practitioner the ability to prescribe medication from formulary lists. Some systems allow for choosing from multiple formularies based on the patient's health plan. The system should also check for drug interactions and allow for the transmission of prescriptions electronically. Additionally, it should print instructions such as the purpose of the medication, potential side effects and other special instructions. The drug information portion of the system was the most frequently used part of a records system for a group of internists using an electronic medical record.[13] Boston's Brigham and Women's Hospital, estimates it saves $10 million annually by physicians alerted to medication-related problems such as duplicate prescriptions or allergies.[14]

As important as preformatted visits are, a similar and important function is the ability for the system to use protocols. In a paper system it is difficult for a physician to check when a patient has last received the recommended diagnostic tests based upon sex, age and past medical history. A system should offer the ability to enter protocols based on the outpatients' sex, age, past medical and family history. Upon entry of patient information against the protocols, the system would determine what, if any, tests are due or overdue.

As an example, a protocol for women over the age of 40 might contain an annual mammogram and pap smear. When the patient comes for an annual exam or for a specific medical complaint, the system will alert the physician if the patient is due for the annual mammogram and pap smear. Not only does this assist the physician in providing good medical care, it is a useful tool for providing managed care companies with testing rates and compliance requirements. The system should be able to merge this data with letters to patients reminding them which tests are necessary and if they are overdue. This is especially useful in the case of suspicious test results that a physician wants redone. Prior to these types of systems, it was cumbersome and labor intensive to track follow-up tests.

One of the biggest benefits to physicians in using an electronic medical record is that it will make the lab result paper chase, during patient visits, nonexistent. Integration of lab results into the record needs to occur. This integration is more than having the result on the screen. The results must become part of the record so physicians have the ability to review lab results with vital signs and other patient information. In some systems the physician can graph the lab results with other information and build a patient timeline indicating disease progression. All these functions add value for a physician.

As managed care moves toward health maintenance and disease prevention, the system should track not only disease- and complaint-oriented visits, but also health maintenance visits, tests and information. This information can be valuable in marketing physician groups to managed care companies. It provides a measurable level of health maintenance activities provided to patients. Using data from the record outcomes of patients who have had health maintenance visits can be compared with those who have not.

Any system should allow the user to search data. For the search to be successful, the system must contain a user-friendly search engine. More important, it must keep data as data elements. For data to be searchable, the system must recognize information from progress notes and the patient chart as data linked to a specific patient. To better understand this, compare a word processor to a database program. Word processors store words electronically. Their storage method limits the ability to search for data. The ability to link data is almost nonexistent. Database programs keep each word as a searchable and linkable data element. These differences should be within the program and be transparent to the user entering the data. It is also crucial to define the data elements before a system is chosen to ensure the system is capable of storing the type of data necessary in the future.

With the increase in graphical interfaces and the use of graphics in computer systems, the system should have the ability to graph data. As scanning technology becomes better and less expensive, systems should have the ability to scan and store graphic-based results such as EKG and x-rays. Systems that offer the options of storing patient photographs have been useful in assisting staff to identify and remember patients when providing phone assistance.

The system should have the ability to use common computer standards that allow for the easy import and export of data. If other systems use the data from the electronic medical record, make sure data can be output in formats readable by other systems. Similarly, if other systems need to upload data to the records, make sure the formats are compatible.

The system should allow for multi-level, restricted access based on passwords. If there is inactivity after a short predetermined time, logging off users should be automatic. This will prevent unauthorized access when users leave a terminal and do not return. Logging of information accessed by person, location, information received, time and date is crucial. An additional level of security such as a call back feature is necessary if the system has telephone access. The call-back feature requires the system to call-back a predetermined phone number based on the users' login.

The system should be able to store problems or chief complaints, as well as diagnosis as data elements. After an examination and interview with the patient, the physician makes a determination of a diagnosis. Patients initiate an encounter because of a "problem." The system should record the primary patient problem and secondary problems as well. Traditionally, clinical systems and billing systems only record diagnostic information. To properly record the entire encounter, the system needs to record problems as well. Similarly it should record as data elements "history of" and "rule out" since ruling out of a diagnosis is not a diagnosis itself.

To make the system easier to use and keep data standardized, it should contain the full ICD-9 list and/or Systematized Nomenclature of Medicine (SNOMED). Although SNOMED provides more detail, it is not as accepted as ICD-9.[15] Support of the current coding system and ability to upgrade to new coding systems is important.

Remote access is a requirement for clinics even if they only have one location. One important benefit of the record is its availability to all users at the same time, and at anytime. The system network should provide the ability to access the system by modem. Physicians with more than one office are especially prevalent in the academic setting. Faculty may have an academic office and not have their own office in the practice. With the use of electronic medical records, physicians can access the record from any location. Probably the most important remote access need is for off-hour emergencies. Currently physicians do not have access to the record when called by a patient in off-hours. Using an electronic medical record, physicians can call and view the record and return the patient's call. This is even more critical when physicians cover for other physicians for patients they may have never seen or examined.

To keep pace with requirements for participation in managed care plans, the system should have the ability to use specific formularies as required by the plans. It should also have the ability to receive lab data from various lab companies as may be required by the managed care companies.

Data - the raw material

The outcome of data analysis is important but how the data gets into the system is as important as the data itself. The first electronic medical record systems were simply an electronic repository for storage of the paper record. Most of the technology used was optical disk storage and stored pictures of the paper record. This may have solved some of the storage issues of paper record, but it did little to make the data more valuable since there was no simple way to analyze stored records. The next generation offered free-form entry of data into specific forms. This allowed better data control since elements were on specific forms. Both these systems still did not return usable data to practitioners, and acceptance of the systems was not widespread.

The next generation of systems began using structured data. Information was stored as discrete data elements instead of free-form. By entering a patient's vital signs, and other information, they became usable discreet elements. It was now possible to review a patient's blood pressure over a period of time, or compare that patient's blood pressure to other patients' data. For the first time, systems were able to give back to users data in a usable format and they began to see benefits in using the systems.

Having data in a structured format improved analysis but did not address entry of information into a system. The simplest method of entry is manual entry from the keyboard. Using preformatted forms makes data entry simpler. The key to gaining buy-in and use of the system is to make data entry as easy as possible. Many data element choices during patient visits can be listed from a group of choices. The simplest example is patient gender. Rather than entering male or female for each patient, there is a simple check-off box. When the user gets to a data element, the program can provide a pull-down menu with choices. Similarly, all patients in the system should be available for choosing from a pull down menu. The more information available in this manner, the more likely are users to use the system and the level of correct data increased. Another method of data entry is precoded answers on a bar code sheet. Users can choose the correct choice by dragging a wand across the proper codes associated with the correct choice. By making data entry simple for physicians and eliminating the need for transcription, a large health maintenance organization estimated its first-year transcription savings were as high as 80 percent.[2]

The easiest method for data entry to the system is voice recognition. Unfortunately, voice recognition technology is still evolving and has not yet become perfected for an electronic medical records application. Many systems offer the ability to accept transcribed dictation. Some data entry still occurs at the time of visit, but this option allows for transcription of hospital discharge notes and other dictation into the system. The dictation must follow predetermined formats and be transcribed in a format uploadable by the system.

Patient records need to be available for multiple users at the same time. To operate properly, the system requires installation of a computer network. The shared data resides on the network host. The data, therefore, does not reside at each user terminal, but resides in a central location. Electronic medical records systems that support remote clinics and multiple networks need determination of data residency location by the steering committee. When sharing with other entities such as hospitals, there may be issues of the records residing in a hospital repository. These issues are more political than data processing in nature and require resolution prior to the installation.

Many times the subject of converting old records comes up during the introduction of electronic medical records. The first systems that relied on optical disk technology scanned the current as well as old records. Storage of these records was as images and not data. The current system stores information as data. Scanning of old records does not add data to records, therefore, there is little benefit in scanning old records. At the first patient visit using an electronic record, the paper record will still need to be present. At the second visit with an electronic record, some old paper charts will be necessary. Paper records are usually not required by the third visit. Reentry of old data is always an option, but provides low benefit for high cost.

Consultation on the viewing of data with practitioners is important. Just as with paper records where pages are in a specific order, the system needs to offer the ability to tile (view) electronic pages. Users should have the ability to change the order to their liking. The first screen should be a customizable summary screen containing user definable data elements.

Workflow

To be successful, the electronic medical record needs integration into the workflow process. Prior to the implementation, the operational committee needs to understand the workflow process. Elimination of processes that are duplicative or unnecessary should occur before electronic medical record implementation. The chance of a successful implementation increases greatly if implementation occurs into a well-organized and operating practice. Addressing of workflow issue should occur prior to the implementation of the electronic medical record. The implementation of electronic medical records is complex enough without trying to implement unrelated workflow changes at the same time.

Once the workflow process is working well, then development of the new process begins. Division of clinic staff is by work function. These groups should understand how the records will change their functions and what new functions will be necessary. While the electronic medical record automates labor-intensive processes, it alone does not automatically decrease the number of employees required to operate a clinic, but an improved workflow process may. Implementation may do away with the need for certain positions, but it may add others. If employees were pulling charts, that duty will not be necessary, but new functions relating to the computer system may be.

An Arizona clinic that implemented an electronic medical record found a reduction in chart pull requests by 60 to 70 percent.[2] An increase in efficiency also occurs from reduced filing. A medical group in Tennessee found that filing was reduced by 50 percent. The group expects an additional 20 percent reduction by the sharing of consultant reports on a wide area network or through e-mail.[2] Probably the greatest time saving comes from the front-office staff not having to return calls requiring information retrieval from patient charts. Retrieval of patient information is on-line and immediate, without having to return patient calls.[2]

Security, confidentiality and legal issues

Medical records security has become such an important issue that the government has proposed the Medical Records Confidentiality Act of 1996. Some of its major proposals include: giving individuals the right to see their records regardless of who holds them; putting limits on how much information doctors, employers, insurers and others could disclose; requiring law enforcement agencies to produce warrants or subpoenas to gain access to records; establishing penalties for unauthorized disclosure of medical information; forbidding researchers to use health data without patient permission, even when anonymous without patient permission; and forbidding health information services from storing information without patient permission.[16]

The use of computers for any application brings security issues to the forefront. Confidentiality is not the only reason to provide security. Protection of the integrity of the data as well as access to the data is important. In an application such as medical records where security and confidentiality are so important, the issue of security is that much more important. The computerization of a patient's records can actually afford more security to the records than a paper record. Those who believe in not using electronic medical records because of security and confidentiality issues need to understand the current paper record is not anymore secure or confidential. Almost any physician or clinic employee has access to paper records. Copies of records are regularly made and records find their way out of the practice. A computer record allows for controlled multilevel access to records. Front-office staff who may need demographic information no longer need access to the entire record containing clinical information just to see the demographic sheet. Job function limits chart area access.

Many clinics use a paper sign-in/out sheet for records. While this system maintains a record, it is only good if it is used. Not completing the sheet does not stop access to a record. An electronic medical records system logs all access or attempts at access by user. This easily answers the question of who has a record and who has seen a record. Another security method is data encryption. Data encryption uses mathematical formulas to scramble information, making it indecipherable to unauthorized users.[17] An electronic medical record properly implemented on a properly secure network provides more security and confidentiality than a paper record.

The concern for security and confidentiality has led to an increase in state and federal regulation of records. Until recently, most laws that apply to medical records have been state laws.[18] Certain laws pertain to all records regardless of format while others pertain only to paper or to electronic medical records. It is important to make sure the software complies with pertinent laws that cover the locations of practice. Regardless of required compliance with laws, all entities should develop a confidentiality policy, explained to employees upon hire and reviewed annually. The U.S. Food and Drug Administration (FDA) concerns include medical software. In particular, electronic medical record systems that previously were mostly recordkeeping systems, but now include decision support, concerns the FDA's Center for Device and Radiological Health (CDRH). These systems bear directly on patient care by providing treatment options or recommending treatments sometimes from information collected automatically from devices. The CDRH is considering regulating electronic medical record systems.[19]

Links to other systems

The computerization of records not only offers savings in terms of storage and efficiency, but also brings the opportunity to enhance revenue by automating charge capture. Achievement of automation occurs by linking the clinical records to financial systems.

Published estimates of dollars lost because of inaccurate coding or lost charges range between 3 to 5 percent. A case review of 18 medical practices indicated lost revenue of between $10,000 to $100,000 per practice per year.[20] With an electronic medical record linked to financial systems, physicians no longer need to complete "superbills" or charge tickets. Enhancement of revenue occurs since there is no losing of data, thus billing of all services clinically documented occurs. The system needs the ability for practitioners to hold bills, and the system must generate a listing of services not billed. Verification of this information and approval by the practitioner can take place. The system will give the practice a measurable amount of unbilled services. Currently, practices estimate their service unbilled but cannot quantify the exact number of charges unbilled.

A full-featured electronic medical records system will offer the ability to upload and download data to other systems. Health Level Seven (HL-7) is a common language approved by many organizations as the standard for electronic transfer of clinical patient information.[21]

Systems should be able to read and output data in the HL-7 format. That ability is especially important in receiving lab results electronically from lab companies. Almost all national medical laboratories have the ability to transfer lab results in that format. Which other systems need to share clinical information needs careful thought. Many hospitals and integrated systems are moving to data repositories. In these repositories many specific-purpose systems deposit data that can than be shared. Rather than having each system communicate, each deposits data elements to a repository in common formats that are readable by other systems.

Return on investment

Most industries spend between 5 and 10 percent of their operating budgets on information systems. Health care typically spends 1 percent. The difference between 1 and 10 percent is spent on paying very expensive, well educated and qualified personnel to do clerical work.[22] Many of the benefits of an electronic medical record are intangible. They are intangible because some benefits of computer technology are intangible, especially in health care where the mission is more than bottom line. Health care quality is difficult to measure and so are the contributions made by electronic medical record systems.

There are, however, some clearly measurable benefits, and it is easier to estimate the costs of a system than its benefits. Costs for which there are published prices such as hardware, software training and support are the easiest. Harder to estimate are other costs such as the needing of temporary help, and temporary productivity loses. The benefits may be even harder to measure since many are qualitative.

These benefits can be divided into five areas: direct reduction of expenses; increased productivity leading to increased revenue; improved quality of patient care; improved patient satisfaction; and improved quality of work life for physicians and staff.[5] M.D. Anderson Cancer Center projected a 2.4 return on the investment of an electronic medical record. The return included a reduction of costs of 2.7 percent from improved data capture and access, a 4-percent reduction from improved decision support and a 2.2 reduction from improved business management.[23]

An early study of increased efficiency in the use of electronic medical records showed nurses were able to save one minute in pre-exam interviews. Physicians reduced total time per visit by 13 percent while spending the same time with patients. These reductions were due to faster pre-encounter chart reviews, and post-encounter data documentation. [23] These savings occurred even though the system used was significantly slower and less user-friendly than today's systems. A 1990 study found the cost of care to patients whose care provider used an electronic medical record was $596 less than those using a paper chart. Credit for reducing costs went to better preventive care and health.[24]

Malpractice insurers are realizing that electronic medical records improve documentation and quality of patient care. Insurers reward participation in risk-management activities, attending risk-management seminars, undergoing risk audits or providing patient education materials. Electronic medical record systems are the first technology insurers have considered a method to reduce risk.[25] In recognition, many offer premium credits of about 5 percent.[2] Many claims occur because of overlooking of tests or problems. To be eligible for these reductions, using approved systems that offer the ability to track tests ordered and provide reminders is required. In addition to preventing mistakes, the systems help document care, preventing the lack of data which makes malpractice suits difficult to defend.[26]

While electronic medical records do not completely do away with the need for paper storage and filing, there is an estimated $3 per patient saving in filing reduction.[27] Recapture of space used for record storage occurs with the use of an electronic medical record. Some estimates are as high as 99 percent of space recaptured. For practices that are using offsite storage, the cost saving can be even higher.[28] The University of Wisconsin Hospitals and clinics estimate a reduction of its storage by 95 percent with an electronic medical record. Sloan Kettering estimates a 2,000 square foot saving because of implementing an electronic medical record.[2]

Workstation placement

Throughout the implementation process, it is important to bear in mind that the measurement of a successful implementation of an electronic medical record is if the provider uses the record. Even the best record system will fail if the physician does not find it easy to use. Placement of the workstation terminal must be in an easily accessible and comfortable-to-use location. Location of the terminals should be in any area where a physician would normally write notes. This includes all exam rooms, consult rooms and any area physicians would use to update charts.

The most crucial placement is in the exam room. System location should afford the physician the ability to view the screen and patient at the same time. Even those concerned with the loss of the personal touch believe that if a physician uses verbal skills and maintains eye contact, this is not a problem.[29] This can be accomplished by setting up the computer, desk, sink and counter in an L shaped configuration (Figure 13.1 at end of chapter). Location of the CPU can be inside a cabinet with only the screen, keyboard and mouse showing. During the interview process when the patient sits in the chair, the physician can speak to the patient and see the screen at the same time. When the patient is on the exam table, the physician can remain seated and face the patient at the same time. Placement in the consult rooms can utilize the traditional office setup with the screen located on the desk but off to the side (Figure 13.2 at end of chapter).

Recent advances and price drops in laptop and notebook computers make them a possible choice for location in patient exam rooms. Traditionally, connection to networks is through hardwiring. Recent developments in wireless networks provide network capability without hardwiring. These represent possible solutions, but may have line-of-sight limits and may not work properly because of interference from other equipment. As technology continues to improve, exploration of these options should occur.

Future

As computer technology continues to evolve, voice-recognition and hand-writing recognition may become workable options for data input to electronic medical records systems. If these technologies become perfected, electronic medical records will certainly make good use of the technology.

Various organizations are experimenting with the use of the Internet for medical records. This would offer the ability to provide access to records over a preexisting system and share records between institutions. As the Internet evolves and matures, this may offer a possibility. Currently it is still undergoing too many changes to provide a stable environment for an electronic record. When measuring a web-based electronic medical record system, there are eight areas to consider: 1) completeness and detail of a common information model; 2) machinable quality of the web-based electronic medical record data; 3) protection of patient confidentiality; 4) transactions supported; 5) institutional affiliation and organization; 6) inter-institutional infrastructure; 7) the degree of coupling between the web-based and "local" electronic medical record system; and 8) customizability. [30]

Development of intranets is more recent. Intranets are private computer networks that use Internet protocols and Internet-derived technologies, including World Wide Web browsers, web servers and web languages to facilitate data sharing within an enterprise.[31] They have the Internet look and feel but operate more as an in-house network because of limited access. They too are quickly evolving and may offer a home for electronic medical records systems.

Conclusion

The concept of electronic medical records has been around for some time. The time is now right to be successful in implementing systems. The costs of systems and related computer costs have decreased. The systems themselves have become increasingly user-friendly and offer the added value that physicians require to use systems. Managed care companies are requiring more clinical data and financial incentives and constraints are driving physician practices to become more efficient. The use of electronic medical records will assist practitioners in efficiently providing quality care to patients – their major goal.

Figure 13.1

Exam room workstation location

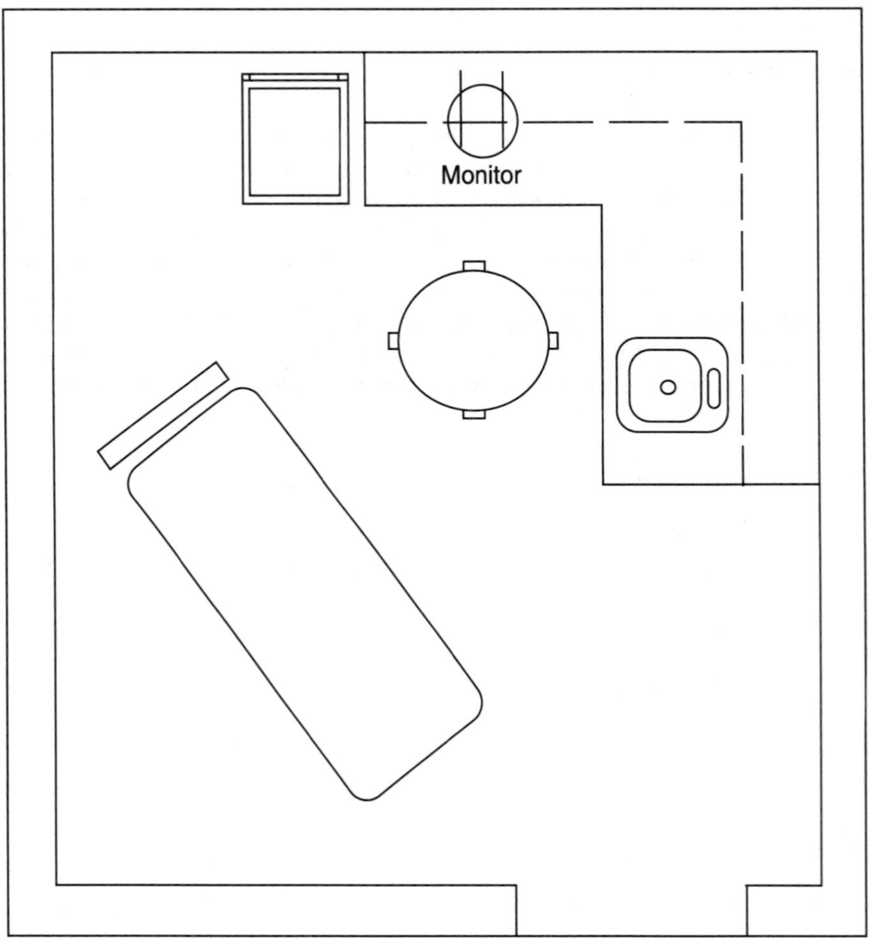

Figure 13.2

Consult room workstation location

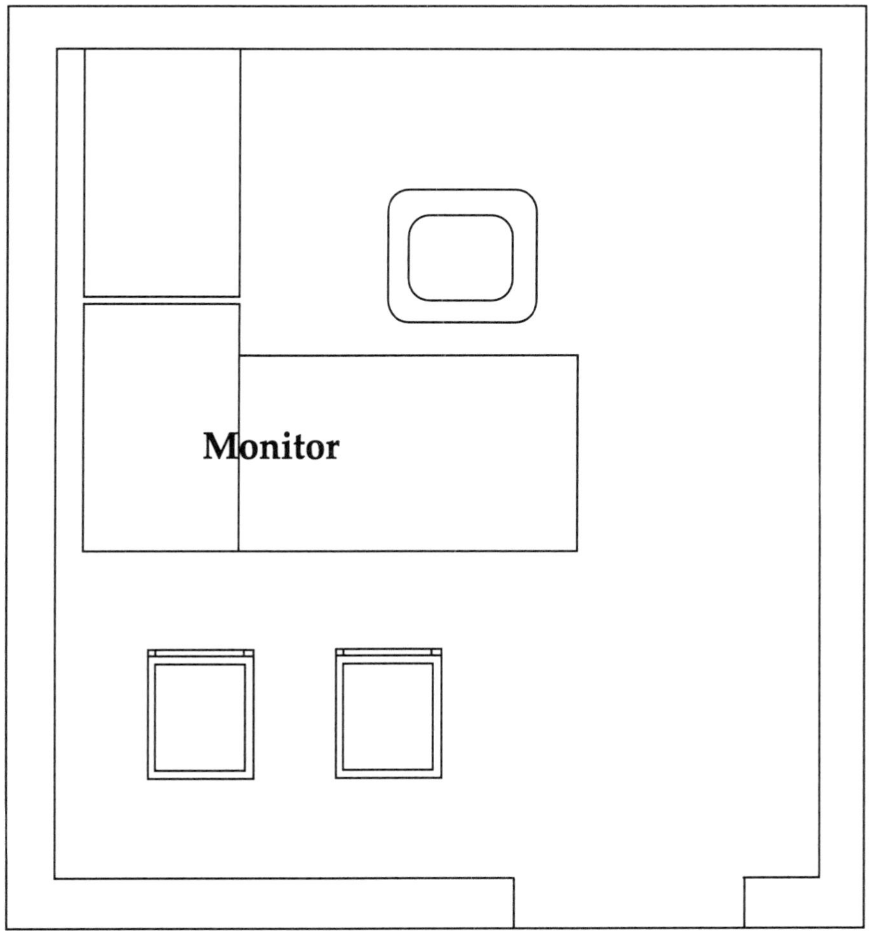

References

1. Evans JC, Hayashi AM. "Implementing On-Line Medical Records." *Document Management* 1994;12-17.
2. Renner K. Electronic Medical Records in the Outpatient Setting Part 2. *Medical Group Management Journal* 1996;43:60-64.
3. Mawhinney H, Dodge B. "The computer in the consulting room. What can it do for the physician." *Medical Group Management Journal* 1994;41:45-72.
4. Anonymous 1996"Resource Guide." Health Data Management 1995;3:
5. Op cit, Renner.
6. Drazen E., *Patient Care Information Systems: Successful Design and Implementation.* Springer-Veralag, 1995:
7. Huyser R, S., *Health Care Information Industry Review.* 1996;1-19.
8. Bunschoten B., "Automated Protocols: Will They Ever Be Commonplace." *Health Data Management* 1996;4:49-56.
9. Geoffrey MA., *Crossing the Chasm.* New York: HarperBusiness, 1991:
10. Ornstein S, Bearden A., "Patient Perspectives on Computer Based Medical Records." *Journal of Family Practice* 1994;606-610.
11. Bunschoten B., "Pushing Physicians to Give Data Entry A Spin." *The Journal of Medical Practice Management* 1996;11:82-88.
12. Howard K., "Resolved: Automate Your Medical Records System in 1994." *Professional Practice Today* 1994;5:3-5.(Abstract)
13. Safran C, Rind D, M., Sands D, Z., Davis R, B., Wald J, Slack W, V., "Development of a Knowledge Based Electronic Patient Record." *MD Computing* 1996;13:46-54.(Abstract)
14. Watson S., "Health Care's Holy Grail The Computerized Patient Record System". *Computerworld Health Care Journal* 1996;h11-h14.(Abstract)
15. Cimino JJ., "Coding Systems in Health Care." *1995 Yearbook of Medical Informatics* 1995;71-85.(Abstract)
16. Roder W., "Keeping Medical Records Cybersafe." *Inter@ctive week* 1996;(Abstract)
17. Bunschoten B., "Striking a Balance between Access and Security," *Health Data Management* 1996;4:69-72.
18. Gilbert F., "Confidentiality of Computerized Health Records," *The Journal of Medical Practice Management* 1995;11:42-46.
19. Anonymous. FDA Reveals Proposal to Regulate Clinical Software and Telemedicine, *emed News* 1996;1-2.(Abstract)
20. Damsey L., "Limit Losses With Correct Coding," *Family Practice Management* 1994;51-54.
21. Thompson T., "Easier Said Than Done," *Hospitals & Health Networks* 1996;70:29-32.
22. Korpman R, A., "Electronic Medical Records: Integration-Key for Physicians.," *The Journal of Medical Practice Management* 1994;9:282-286.

23. Kian L, A., Stewart M, W., Bagby C, Robertson J., "Justifying the Cost of a Computer-Based Patient Record," *Health Care Financial Management* 1995;
24. Hammond KW, Prather RJ, Dave VV, King CA.," A Provider Interactive Medical Record System Can Favorably Influence Costs and Quality of Medical Care," *Computers in Biology and Medicine* 1990;20:267-279.
25. Cross M., Malpractice Insurers Endorse Electronic Records as a Way to Reduce Risk," *Health Data Management* 1996;4:67-72.
26. Anonymous. "Malpractice Insurers Offer Discounts For Doctors Using Electronic Medical Records," *The Journal of Medical Practice Management* 1995;14
27. Nieburgal D., Canton D., *Cost Benefits of the Computer-Based Patient Record in Doctors' Offices.* 1993;304-308.(Abstract)
28. Henry SB, Holzemer WL., "A comparison of problem lists generated by physicians, nurses, and patients: implications for CPR systems," *Proc Annu Symp Comput Appl Med Care* 1995;382-36.
29. Ridsdale L., Hudd S., "Computers in the Consultation: The Patient's View," *British Journal of General Practice* 1994;367-369.
30. Kohane IS., "Exploring the Functions of World Wide Web-Based Electronic Medical Record Systems," *MD Computing* 1996;13:339-346.(Abstract)
31. Siwicki B., "Intranets in Health Care," *Health Data Management* 1996;4:36-47.

Chapter 14

Preserving market share and payer mix through facilities placement and operation

by Diana V. Shaw, MPH, MBA

As the environment has continued to change over the past ten years, it has become increasingly apparent that the academic medical practice must also change. Ever-growing competition, a steady gain in managed care, and decreasing federal dollars are paramount in leading practices to face this need for change. Change is never easy, and for academic medical practices change is particularly difficult due to their affiliation with academic teaching facilities. This affiliation means that they provide education and clinical research, treat high-cost, complex patients, and practice within large academic teaching facilities which are often located in the inner-city where costs are higher and a disproportionate share of free care is present.[1] These factors immediately establish the dynamics for being a high-cost, high-quality, highly specialized provider competing in a low-cost, good-quality, generalist-driven environment.

The question then becomes: How can academic practices compete effectively in this type of environment? The answer is actually imbedded in the very environment that has created the strife – the new market-driven, business-oriented environment. Health care is now being viewed as any other "product" or "service." And it is this new attitude that provides us with the opportunity to explore the tools and techniques used by other businesses to compete effectively. Let's look at two goals important in today's competitive environment – one common to any business and one particular to health care – and review how they would be dealt with by the traditional academic model versus the new business model:

1. Gaining, or at least preserving market share; and
2. Developing a favorable payer mix.

What strategies would be used to achieve these goals? How would the approach differ under the traditional academic practice model versus the new business model?

Traditional academic model -- the "ivory tower plan"

Under the traditional academic practice model, if these two goals were even contemplated, they would be approached using what I will call the "ivory tower plan": We are the medical Mecca. They will come to us. We have the best medicine, the best doctors, and the best technology and facilities. We will manage our facility in a manner that is efficient for our providers. The patients and payers will come to us, in spite of minor inconveniences, simply because we are the best.

This "plan" would result in an academic medical practice functioning within the medical center footprint. Patients, when referred from one specialty to another for their care, would meander throughout the vast facility, toting x-rays and medical records under arm, being registered time and again at each new stop. They would often have to recite their list of medications to each new provider and have their care documented in separate and distinct charts. They would also received separate and distinct bills for each service rendered.

From the medical care perspective, patients would receive the "best of the best."[2] From a process perspective, the patient would have to deal with a disorganized, confusing flow as each physician functioned as an independent practitioner. Patients, therefore, would most likely prefer to seek routine care from community physicians in an effort to avoid having to deal with the vast, cold, inconvenient academic medical practice. A common sentiment would likely be to seek care from the community physicians and community hospitals if your problem were routine and you could afford to pay for health care services. If your problem were unknown or uncommon, or if you could not afford to pay for health care services, you would then seek care from the academic medical practice. The result? The academic medical practice would develop with both complex, ill patients (i.e., high cost) and patients who had limited or no other access to the health care system due to their inability to pay for services.

In this traditional model, each physician would rent space from the hospital or medical school for patient care activities. In some cases, hotel services such as check-in and check-out services and other staff support, would be part of the rental fee. In other cases, the practice would supply its own staff. Under either scenario, the rental assessment for this space would often entail a complex calculation, interwoven with patient care, education and research costs. Other overhead expenses inherent in maintaining the large facility would also become part of the rental structure (i.e., cost of developing and maintaining a medical library suitable to support education and research activities, maintenance of the vast, aging physical plant itself, etc.). As a result, space square footage rates would likely be higher for a practice within the academic medical center than for a practice offsite paying the average external market rate.

Some improvements have been made recently in academic medicine – a sort of modified "ivory tower plan." Ambulatory-care buildings have been built (usually contiguous to the medical center buildings or at least on the campus) to consolidate all ambulatory activities under one roof in an attempt to achieve some economy of scale and to bring a small measure of convenience to the patient (in the form of "one-stop-shopping"). These facilities do provide increased convenience for patients currently within the academic medical practice system in that they no longer have to wander among the facility's different buildings to see their providers (i.e., helping the academic medical practices maintain current market share). However, these new buildings do not address issues such as cost structure, increasing market share or diversifying payer mix – thereby still not truly addressing the goals we have established as important and necessary for successful competition.

Business model

This model differs from the traditional academic model in that managers are aware of factors such as market share, cost and competition. The business of health care is no longer seen as sheltered or protected, and academic practices must compete for business with successful, non-academic, independent rivals. Now the academic practices need to apply business management strategies and tools to position their practices so that they can achieve a competitive advantage and the goals noted previously. Now goals like achieving increased market share and diversifying one's payer mix become important and a matter of strategic planning.

Environmental/industry review

Begin by reviewing the industry to determine where it resides in the product-life cycle and how we got where we are today. Health care today is most appropriately described as being a mature industry. Its characteristics include surplus capacity, declining demand, reduced customer confidence, loss of control over policymaking and conversion from a seller's market to a buyer's market.[3] At this stage in the life cycle, competition usually shifts to a focus of decreasing costs. Attempts will also be made to differentiate one's product and create a competitive advantage.

Michael Porter, a Harvard University economics and business strategy professor, suggests that, in general, the degree of competition within an industry hinges on five forces: the threat of new entrants, the bargaining power of customers and/or suppliers, the threat of substitutions, and the maneuvering among current participants.[4] In health care's mature market, a threat of new entrants is quite high – usually in the form of low-cost, for-profit health care corporations. The bargaining power of customers (i.e., the payers and patients) is also quite high due mostly to the abundance of suppliers (i.e., the providers). A threat of substitutions is created through the use of lower-cost providers (i.e., skill mix changes). In addition, there is considerable maneuvering among those currently in the industry – trying to be among the few survivors who will continue to grow and prosper in health care.

Success depends upon understanding these competitive forces, how they work in the industry and how they affect your organization in its particular situation.[5] The manager's goal is to find a position where the company can either best defend itself against these forces, or influence them in its favor.[6] Let's look at "threat of entry" as it applies to the current health care industry. Potentially six major barriers exist for entry: economies of scale, product differentiation, capital requirements, cost disadvantages independent of size, distribution channel access and government policy. But for health care, these factors do not appear to form a formidable barrier to entry currently.[7] As a result, competition will likely increase as rivals enter the arena, potentially decreasing the academic practice's market share and skimming the more desirable payers from the academic practice's plate.

Three other factors can have a limiting effect on rival entry: incumbents possessing substantial resources to fight back, incumbents' ability and willingness to cut prices to maintain market share, and slow industry growth.[8] These factors could limit competition by creating a barrier to entry, but in today's health care environment entities interested in entering this "industry" are most likely for-profit corporations. And these new competitors – being more cost-effective and efficient than academic medical practices – are actually in a better position to cut prices lower than current incumbents, and, in many cases, have far more in resources with which to fight the current incumbents. Further, even though health care as an industry is experiencing a reduced rate of growth, it is still viewed by many as being quite profitable. Therefore, even these factors would not limit entry but, rather, actually create an attractive environment for entry. Hence, competitive pressures continue to increase for the academic medical practice.

If we next look at the competitive force of powerful suppliers and buyers, we see that the "ivory tower plan" was one that developed from powerful suppliers (i.e., physicians, hospitals, medical centers, etc.). Many communities could be dominated by a single academic medical center, few alternatives existed, products (i.e., health care services) were considered to be highly unique, and medical centers could integrate forward into the buyers' (i.e., payers, insurance companies) market. Our current environment, though, shows the buyers to be the dominant force: health care is now seen as a commodity (i.e., no longer needing to rely exclusively on the academic medical practices' unique, highly differentiated, expensive services). The products being purchased represent a significant fraction of the buyers' cost. The buyers have demonstrated a willingness to integrate backward. Further, the buyers have determined that there are substitutes available for the services formerly provided by academic medical practices. These substitutions come in the form of for-profit corporate chains offering health care services, insurance-owned HMOs, independent physician practices (especially those not affiliated with academic medicine, free of the additional expense of education and research) providing good quality services at a much lower cost. While the academic practice's services are still thought of as unique, the buyers seem to feel that the extra cost does not balance against the additional value contributed by the "uniqueness" of the service.

The lack of barriers, availability of substitution, and power of the buyers results in increased rivalry between existing competitors – jockeying for position, use of price competition, product or service introduction and "advertising slugfests."[9] In this environment, while a company must learn to live with some factors, it also has the ability to improve the situation somewhat through strategic planning and choice. As such, in today's health care market, the "buyers" (i.e., the payers) appear to be mainly motivated by price, and secondarily by differentiation. So while the academic medical practices must learn to accept these factors, they must also use this knowledge to strategize and gain a competitive advantage.

Creating competitive advantage

Competitive advantage falls into two basic categories: lower cost than rivals or creating a differentiation that will justify a premium price.[10] But competitive advantage must be looked at in conjunction with competitive scope. Hence, an organization would desire to achieve a competitive advantage within a certain geographic location, product/buyer segment served, and degree of vertical integration. In an attempt to make appropriate strategic choices, Porter suggests that one should view this process as a dynamic process, using a resource-based view.[11] This view suggests that competitive advantage is based upon a firm's valuable resources or competencies. These resources or competencies are often intangible assets, such as skills, reputation, etc. Seen as relatively steadfast, these resources are viewed as strengths to be cherished and developed, and should be the basis for guiding one's choice of strategy. The benefit of this view is that it helps the corporate strategist plan for the long haul, by focusing on core competencies and resources – attributes that will enable sustaining a favorable competitive position over time. Academic medical practices should be able to capitalize on their reputation and brand names – a valuable resource and competency.

Porter further suggests that competitive advantage might be rooted in the environment in which the firm is based. This environment defines many factors with which the firm must deal, as well as the information, incentives and pressures that should guide strategic choices. The four attributes of the environment are depicted through the use of a diamond diagram.[12] These attributes (firm strategy, structure and rivalry; demand conditions; factor conditions; related and supporting industries) represent the information firms have available with which to make their strategic decisions.

The diamond represents a manageable method to determine demands, trends and incentives. For example, factor conditions for the academic medical practice represent highly specialized skills necessary to produce health care services. Demand conditions include the buyers' demands to purchase these services at low cost but with good quality. Related and supporting industries represent those entities that are part of the health care system and interface directly or indirectly with the academic medical practice (suppliers), patients (users) and payers (buyers), and are rather plentiful – even though quality is variable. And lastly, firm strategy, structure and rivalry represent the academic practices themselves–their strategy to increase market share and diversify payer mix (in our example) as well as limitations presented by their structure and inherent rivals. These tools, when applied to our example, clearly signal that for the academic medical practice to compete effectively and create a competitive advantage, they need to decrease the cost of health care services, while simultaneously capitalizing on their differentiated "products." These two actions will enable the achievement of the two goals identified earlier.

Academic medicine's response to the new model

Academic medicine has responded to the call for change with a proliferation of collaborative alliances, joint ventures and mergers – all in an attempt to gain a competitive advantage.[13] Examples include University of California, San Diego Medical Center; University of California, San Francisco Medical Center; the Washington University Medical Center and BJC, Inc., St. Louis; the University of Chicago Medical Center; the West Virginia University Health Science Center, Morgantown; Columbia Presbyterian Medical Center and Columbia University Health Sciences Center, New York City; and the Partners Health Care System, Boston (consisting of the affiliation of Massachusetts General Hospital and Brigham and Women's Hospital).[14]

These institutions, after viewing their environments and analyzing their strengths and weakness, determined that they had several options available to them. They could market their services to private purchasers (most commonly accomplished through networking by establishment of an integrated health care system capable of providing a complete range of services at, hopefully, a competitive price – i.e., vertical integration). They could reduce clinical service costs (through traditional approaches such as reducing administrative overhead, closing beds, as well as non-traditional approaches such as total quality management, reengineering of clinical care activities and development of clinical pathways). They could increase their sales to government purchasers (i.e., development of inner-city and rural primary care networks and community health centers – aimed at increasing the number of Medicaid patients, as well as reaching the privately insured inner-city patient). They could market non-clinical services such as research (often taking the form of conducting research for interested biomedical industries and selling of intellectual property) or teaching (developing educational products with potential to generate revenues). And they could reduce the costs involved with teaching and research (i.e., consolidation of activities across network partners).

Much of the networking activity is aimed at accomplishing the goals we have focused on in this chapter – increased market share and diversification of payer mix. Often the approach used to accomplish these goals is the provision of care at a variety of sites throughout the community. This approach appeals to the managed care companies covering many lives throughout a specific region,[15] as well as appealing to the patients themselves. These sites can be developed by the academic practices as part of their affiliation with the medical center or jointly with community physicians being brought on board. For the academic practices, this model presents an opportunity to enlarge their market share and also to diversify their payer mix, through facility placement and operation throughout the community.

An example of a successful facility placement and operation of integrated academic practices and community practices is the Dartmouth-Hitchcock Medical Center, Hanover, NH. Here academic medicine practices have successfully reorganized for the new environment. This system has a shared governance approach representing the average faculty member, the department level and the institutional level; an integrated practice with all practice operations shared and managed through the group practice; a faculty focus with recognition of separate but complementary roles of the clinician and researcher; and regionalization through expanded facility placement and operation of clinical sites in both primary care and specialty disciplines over a broad geographic area. Today, two out of every three ambulatory visits are seen off the main campus.[16] Operationally, these offsite practices are administered and governed the same as the campus group practice.

The Emory System of Health Care, Atlanta, provides another example of successful reorganization of academic practices. This system has as its mission the development and operation of comprehensive, geographically distributed, integrated medical and health care services.[17] Major steps included the establishment of the Emory University School of Public Health; the establishment of a Department of Family and Preventive Medicine within the School of Medicine; the creation of a "Center for Personal Physicians"; the creation of network comprised of both academic practices and community affiliations with facilities placed strategically throughout the state; aggressive pursuit of managed care contracts; and creation of interdisciplinary centers. Again, we see a pattern similar to that of Dartmouth-Hitchcock Clinic in the creation of networks with facilities that are geographically dispersed and utilize the skills of both the academic practices and the community practices.

Stanford (California) University Medical Center's experience has been similar. Its strategy is comprised of three main elements: building or buying into external medical groups to create a primary care network with the academic practices; creation of a regional outreach arm to develop a referral relationship; and formation of partnerships with other large institutions.[18] Brigham and Women's Hospital, Boston, an affiliate of the Partners HealthCare System, is geographically dispersing its facilities and clinical operations by both purchasing community practices and arranging for its academic practices to provide services at inner-city and suburban sites.

Many of the efforts noted above focus on dispersed facility placement and operation to diversify the entity's payer mix (often increasing the proportion of more lucrative payer activity) and increase its market share[19] – our two goals. Additionally, some practices will enjoy the added benefit of decreased costs by renting space in an offsite facility (denuded of the high overhead associated with the medical center and hospital inpatient facilities).

Conclusion

The environment has changed dramatically–forcing the academic medical community to change also. Whereas, academic practices in the past have benefited from their association with academic medicine, this very affiliation today is considered to be somewhat of a handicap. The buyers are insisting on lower costs, higher patient satisfaction, excellent access, and medically appropriate care.[20, 21] In the past, academic practices have been slow to change and have thus fallen short of meeting the buyers' expectations.

Academic medicine is now responding with many different models. But among the most frequently seen – and seemingly among the most successful at creating a competitive edge – is the development of networks that utilize diverse geographic facility placement and use both community physicians and academic medical practices. These networks provide geographic coverage in a manner that provides excellent accessibility to a broad range of patients, with a diversified payer mix, and can result in an increase in market share and lower costs. Additionally these practices are stressing the importance of meeting both patient satisfaction expectations (i.e., maintaining a service focus), as well as the buyers' expectations (i.e., providing cost-effective, medically appropriate care).

It is imperative that health care managers utilize traditional business tools in assessing the environment, the industry and the position of their practice. A good understanding of the nature of competition and the motivating forces is also necessary. But development of a true competitive advantage is the real key for the academic medical practice's survival. Facility placement in diverse geographic locations, bringing the unique skills of the academic practice to the patients, appears to be a good way to achieve a competitive advantage, accomplish the goals of increased market share and a diversified payer mix, and respond to the changing environment with the tools readily available through use of a business model.

Bibliography

Blumenthal, David and Meyer, Gregg S. "Academic Health Centers in Changing Environment," *Health Affairs.* Vol 15, No 2:p. 200-215.

Cohen, Richard L. "Academic Medical Centers Tooling Up for the Future," *Health Care Marketing Report.* July 1994, Vol 12, No 7:p. 1-4.

Goben, Ronald. "Stanford Restructures to Beat the Teaching Hospital Blues," *Medical Network Strategy Report.* January 1995, Vol 4, No 1:p. 4-6.

Golembesky, Henry E. "New Market Forces are Special Challenge to Academic Health Centers," Academic Medicine Centers: *Physician Executive.* October 1995, Vol 21, No 10:p. 18-22.

Haley, Michael. "Positioning Doctors for Convenience Medicine," *Hospital & Health Services Administration.* July/August 1984, Vol 28, No 4:pp. 95-110.

Jones, Wanda J. "Reality-Based Strategies for Real Times," *Health Care Strategic Management.* June 1989:p.16-19.

Kent, Christina. "America's Teaching Hospitals: Descending the Ivory Tower," *Medicine and Health* (Perspectives insert). March 14, 1994:p. 1-4.

Porter, Michael E. "How Competitive Forces Shape Strategy," *Harvard Business Review.* March-April 1979:p. 137-145.

Porter, Michael E. "Towards a Dynamic Theory of Strategy," *Strategic Management Journal.* Vol. 12, 1991:p. 95-117.

Shires, Edwin D. "Managed Care: Competitive Strategies for Academic Medical Centers," *MGMA College Review.* Spring 1995:p. 77-87.

Townsend, Roy W. "Rolling with the Changes: The Emory System of Health Care," *Academic Medical Centers: GFP Notes.* February 1993, Vol 6, No 1:p. 1-5.

Wietecha, Mark. "The Dartmouth-Hitchcock Clinic: One Model for Academic Group Practice," *Academic Medical Centers: GFP Notes.* January 1993, Vol 6, No 1:p 17-19.

Zuckerman, Alan M. "Strategic Responses of Academic Medical Centers to the Growth in Ambulatory Care," *Medical Group Management Journal.* January-February 1994:p. 62, 64, 66-7.

Chapter 15

Risk management for the academic medical practice

by Anne-Elizabeth McGeary, BSN, MHA

Academic health centers are often the location for a wide range of teaching programs and their students, from residents in highly specialized medical programs to student nurses learning to take a patient's temperature. All of these students expose their host institution and supervisors to potential legal problems. The academic group practice manager must have an effective risk management plan in place to deal with all the risks involved, whether that be an internal physician practice-based program or one that works in concert with one developed by an academic medical center.

Special risks inherent in academic medical practices

Aside from being a high-technology environment, academic health centers in general, are places where patients come who are often gravely ill, are in pain or discomfort, and are often nervous and frightened. Under these circumstances, repetitive examinations or interruptions from physicians-in-training and their supervisors could add to the discomfort or the unhappiness of the patient.

Academic health centers are often the site for experimental procedures and research protocols. Perhaps no other area of health care policy development except reproductive management, specifically abortion policy, engenders more emotional debate than human experimentation. The mix of experimentation and patient care makes academic health centers very risky places, indeed.

Legal liability in the academic environment

One of the biggest challenges for academic medical group managers is to develop risk management strategies that eliminate the potentially hazardous elements that exist in every aspect of delivering medical care. To avoid the situations that result in lawsuits and to anticipate the legal consequences of the actions of physicians and staff, an academic medical group practice manager needs to begin with an understanding of the legal theories of liability that may be alleged against a health care provider.

Theories of liability

Negligence is the most common foundation of medical malpractice liability claims. When a plaintiff brings a negligence complaint, the plaintiff has the burden of proving:

1. Duty (what the defendant should have done for the plaintiff);
2. Breach of duty (what the defendant did not do for the plaintiff or failure to carry out the duty owed);
3. Proximate cause (that the defendant's failure to carry out the duty injured the plaintiff);
4. Damages (the injury that the plaintiff suffered).

Patient care liability, or as it is more frequently known, medical malpractice liability, is based on the legal concept of tort. Tort liability is a form of civil violation that does not result from the breach of a contract or a broken agreement. The different types of torts include negligence, intentional torts and strict liability. The liability imposed on a health care provider, such as a hospital, may be either direct or vicarious liability. For example, the hospital may be directly liable for failing to care for a patient, or the hospital may be held vicariously liable for the tortious acts of its employees. The theories of liability are also different for each accountable party within the health care delivery system.

Liability and the academic medical center

Direct corporate liability

In the past, academic health centers were considered by the law to be places where physicians cared for their patients. The hospitals simply provided the facilities and supplies for the treatments that the independent physicians prescribed for their patients. While hospitals have always been liable for the actions of their own employees, if the physician's treatment was found to be negligent, the physician alone was liable to the patient. Their legal responsibilities changed in the 1960s with litigation that imposed liability on the hospital for deficiencies in the quality of medical care provided to patients by the physicians practicing in their facility, and established the concept of corporate liability in the health care environment.

Corporate liability in the medical environment refers to the duty on the part of hospitals or institutional providers to exert reasonable and due care in the recruiting, retention, and supervision of medical and health care providers and in the condition of the physical plant available and quality of supplies. Corporate liability is different from vicarious liability because it arises from the hospital-patient relationship and not from the principal-agent relationship between hospital and employee. A claim for corporate negligence must establish that the employee breached some duty of care to the patient because the corporation can only act through its agent. The hospital's liability is not derived from the actions of others, however, it arises out of the hospital's independent duty of care to its patients.

Medical center hospitals have been held liable for failing to provide adequate supplies, and for failure to properly staff or equip its facilities. In Fjerstad v. Knutson, a hospital was sued successfully for failing to have the services of an on-call physician available for emergency services.

The theories of corporate liability with respect to health care centers have been continually evolving since 1965, when the Darling v Charleston Community Memorial Hospital case established that hospitals have a duty to care for their patients that is separate and distinct from the physician. It was also determined that hospitals have a duty to exercise reasonable care in the selection, supervision, and retention of physicians and that hospital bylaws and regulations in themselves do not conclusively determine or insure the standard of care.

Since the Darling case, a number of cases have recognized hospitals' responsibility to patients for failing to exercise reasonable care in granting hospital staff privileges to independent physicians and in reviewing the credentials and competency of the physicians practicing in their facility. In Johnson v Misericordia Community Hospital, a patient successfully sued his treating physician and the hospital after the physician attempted without success to remove a pin fragment from the patient's hip. A complication of the surgery was that the patient's femoral nerve and artery were damaged and as a result, his thigh muscles were permanently paralyzed. At the trial, the expert testimony established that the surgical procedure was not conducted according to standard orthopedic practice. After hearing this testimony, the jury rendered a sizable verdict for the patient against both the physician and the hospital.

The basis of the plaintiff's claim against the hospital was that the hospital was negligent in granting orthopedic surgical privileges to the surgeon because it had a duty to know that he was not competent to perform surgery. It was disclosed at the trial that there had been no review of the surgeon's qualifications when he made application to the hospital's medical staff. It was further disclosed that the physician's application was incomplete and contained inaccuracies. Review of the application would have revealed that the orthopedic surgeon's privileges at other health care institutions had been restricted and terminated on several occasions, including a censor on his privileges at another hospital only two months before his application to the hospital in question. Not only did his physician peers in the community not consider him a competent surgeon, there were ten pending malpractice claims filed against him in the local court.

Respondeat superior

Academic health centers employ personnel to work in its treatment and laboratory areas. If a patient experiences injury or bodily harm as a result of their actions or omissions, the institution can be held responsible under the doctrine of respondeat superior. This doctrine holds the employer responsible for the harmful behavior or actions of employees within the scope of their assigned duties. As more academic health centers hire faculty physicians to provide medical services in the hospital, their potential risk of exposure to malpractice claims under the doctrine of respondeat superior will increase.

Currently, residents and interns are normally hospital employees and the hospital has the right to govern and control their activities, even though their acts are professional in nature. Thus, their negligence will result in liability for the hospital. Negligent acts of house physicians and other professionals who are employed by the hospital can result in hospital liability as well.

It is also generally recognized that respondeat superior is not applicable to the relationship between health centers and independent contractors and, therefore, the health center is not usually held responsible for their actions.[6]

Ostensible agency

In recent years, however, there has been a clear trend toward imposing vicarious liability upon hospitals for the negligence of their "physicians/independent contractors."[7] Courts have begun to invoke the agency doctrine of apparent authority when the hospital causes a patient to believe that the physician is an agent or employee of the hospital.

This theory has been applied in cases involving hospital-based physicians, such as anesthesiologists, radiologists, or especially emergency-room physicians, in which the hospital has assigned or provided a physician or physician service that the patient does not really choose. This doctrine can also be applied to medical students and teaching hospitals. Past court rulings have usually differentiated between the entities and found the medical schools responsible for the actions of its students and faculty. Medical school faculty are usually also members of the hospital's medical staff and the institution could be held responsible if it failed to adequately credential or monitor the actions of the faculty or the students.[8]

Agency by estoppel

Under the theory of agency by estoppel, an academic health center may be held liable for the actions of an independent physician if the institution intentionally or inadvertently allows a patient to believe the physician is an authorized agent of the hospital. Agency by estoppel differs from ostensible agency slightly in that the patient believes the provider is an agent of the hospital and the hospital fails to notify the patient that this belief was mistaken.

Another group of doctrines that formerly protected health centers from liability was those known as the "borrowed servant" and the "captain of the ship" doctrines. The borrowed servant was traditionally an employee of the institution, but since the employee was acting at the direction of the physician, any negligence was attributed to the physician.

The "captain of the ship" doctrine was specifically related to circumstances involving the operating room. The surgeon, as the captain of the ship, supervised the members of the operating room team based on the needs of the patient as determined by his or her condition in the operating room. Now that hospitals have contracted with hospital-based anesthesiologists and employ operating room nurses who are highly trained and specialized, the notion that the surgeon controls all the actions related to patient care is outmoded.

Liability and the academic health care provider

Medical school physician faculty members have the same professional responsibilities as independent physicians in private practice. Although they are acting as teachers and supervisors, medical school faculty members are still licensed medical practitioners and the courts can still impose the same legal duties and responsibilities upon them. Most of those duties arise from the concept known as the physician-patient relationship.

Physician-patient relationship

The physician-patient relationship is a consensual agreement usually created when a patient seeks and obtains treatment from a physician. The decision to enter into the relationship is the choice of the physician after the patient has given consent. Once initiated, however, the relationship can be legally concluded only if: (1) it is ended by the parties' mutual consent; (2) it is revoked by the patient; (3) the physician's services are no longer needed, or the physician withdraws from the case after reasonable notice to the patient. Limitations can be put on the relationship if they are stated at the outset. While little empirical data exists to prove that a good physician-patient relationship prevents dissatisfaction and subsequent litigation, it often seems that physicians who routinely have more difficult outcomes and have good physician-patient relationships are sued less often than physicians who do not communicate effectively.

Once this relationship exists, the physician has contractual obligations implied in the relationship. Some of these obligations include the maintenance of confidentiality and the duty to treat. A survey of malpractice defense attorneys, stated that 70 percent of suits were attributed to failures in the doctor-patient relationship and communication.[10]

Informed consent, adequacy of disclosure

The doctrine of informed consent requires physicians to inform patients of the risks of a proposed treatment and of any alternatives. Liability for failure to obtain informed consent may arise under a negligence theory in some jurisdictions and a battery theory in others. Over the past 30 years, the law has developed far beyond a patient simply giving consent to a procedure. The law now requires that the patient be informed of the risks, as well as the probable outcomes or benefits, of the proposed procedure and that any consent given by the patient be derived from a complete understanding of those risks and outcomes. Regardless of the actual outcome of a procedure, a physician may still be found negligent if the patient was not adequately informed about the procedure and its risks and any possible alternatives.[11]

In such cases, the plaintiff has to prove that:

- the physician failed to disclose the existence of a material risk to the patient;
- the disclosure of the risk would have led a reasonable patient in his or her position to reject the medical procedure or choose an alternate therapy; and
- there exists the possibility of an injury.[12]

Obviously, the most effective way to prevent malpractice claims associated with informed consent is to prepare the patient with a good understanding of any proposed procedures or therapy and any associated risks. In addition, a detailed, specialized consent form should be used.

Physician liability and managed care

A new area in which a third-party has attempted to enter the physician-patient relationship, although economically, is through managed care contracting. Managed care programs are protected by an exemption in the ERISA legislation from malpractice liability, but this exemption does not protect physicians who are treating their patients. Physicians should be very careful in reviewing managed care contracts, since most managed care-related malpractice claims are based on a provider improperly denying treatment based on the language of the provider agreement.

To date, there has been little litigation involving managed care due to the relative youth of the managed care industry. However, this can be expected to increase because changes in the utilization review practices used by managed care organizations and the increasing credibility of managed care resulting in the national health care reform debate. Both have empowered these plans to become more aggressive in enforcing their treatment policies. Physicians have two choices when faced with a difference in a managed care treatment plan. They can ignore the utilization recommendations and continue to treat the patient according to their best judgment and risk economic loss, or discontinue seeing the patient and refer the case to another physician. Also, to further protect from exposure to managed care related claims, physicians must consider managed care contracts carefully. They must understand the requirements for sharing confidential patient information, and understand how their professional liability insurance carrier will consider and defend potential managed care cases.

Liability in the teaching environment

There are two specific, potential areas of liability for academic medical providers:

1. the teaching and supervision of unlicensed practitioners, such as medical students and residents; and
2. the conduct of medical research.

Medical students

Since most medical students do not hold a medical license in the state where they are training, they hold the same legal status as laypeople. Yet, they are often given the authority to make medical decisions and participate in treatments and procedures. Sometimes, residents are held to the same standard as licensed practitioners. Other states view residents as physicians in transition.[15]

Medical students are supervised by a licensed physician, which is permitted under most medical practice acts. This does not absolve the licensed practitioner or the medical student from liability from negligence; it only avoids prosecution from the unauthorized conduct of medicine. The teaching faculty as well as the medical student are still subject to professional negligence claims and for claims relating to improper supervision or for fraud.

Fraud

Fraud in many forms is a risk whenever medical students and residents are involved, in two major ways. The first is when the patient is led to believe, intentionally or unintentionally, that a medical student or resident is a fully qualified physician or graduate of a specialized training program. The second circumstance is when the services of a medical student or resident in training are billed to a patient, when the medical faculty are not in attendance.

One potential type of fraud action unique to the academic practice involves the disclosure to patients that they may be treated by medical students. Care should be taken to disclose to the patient and obtain their consent to treatment specifically by students.[16] If the hospital consent form informs the patient that it is a teaching hospital with student involvement, the supervising physician is not required to advise the patient of the individual qualifications of each resident who assists in the patient's treatment.[17] The Court of

Appeals of North Carolina approved the following language of a hospital consent form in light of an informed consent and constructive fraud claim against both the University and the supervising physician of the medical student:

TEACHING INSTITUTION

> I understand that Duke University Medical Center is a teaching institution, and I agree that students training to be physicians, nurses, and allied health personnel may assist in providing my care and that my medical records may be used for purposes of research, education, and patient care.[18]

In Bowlin, the court found that it was standard practice to use medical students to assist in procedures at teaching hospitals, thus the consent form and standard of using medical students defeated the informed consent claim. Similarly, while the court recognized the fiduciary relationship of the attending physician to the patient, the court refused to impose an affirmative duty on the physician to advise the patient of the particular students' abilities or qualifications and rejected the constructive fraud claim.

Medicare, fraud and abuse

"Teaching Physician" Documentation. In December 1995, in response to a federal review, physicians from the University of Pennsylvania agreed to pay $30 million to settle federal charges that the physicians billed the Medicare program for charges they had coded inaccurately or for services they had not actually provided. The senior officials at the University of Pennsylvania apologized for the billing errors but admitted no wrong doing. The wide-ranging investigation focused on the time period from 1989 to 1994 and alleged that the physicians lacked the billing records and the medical documentation to prove they performed the services for which they had billed Medicare.

One source reported that an anonymous caller contacted Pennsylvania Blue Shield officials about a year before the investigation and the same source contacted federal officials. As result of the federal investigation, Pennsylvania Blue Shield auditors began a review of Penn's bills from its traditional fee-for-service product and its local HMO, Keystone Health Plan East.

One Revolution: Managing the Academic Medical Practice in an Era of Rapid Change

In the December 8, 1995, the Health Care Financing Administration (HCFA) published a final rule with comment period on Medicare payment for services and revisions with respect to payment policies and adjustments to the relative value units. The rule clarified the existing payment policies related to the implementation of the IL-372 Guidelines. The three areas initially targeted by the guidelines were supervision of residents, transfers versus discharges and home health services. Although there continue to be very limited exceptions, the physical presence of the teaching physician remains required to bill a Part B fee for a service that involves medical residents. The provisions in the law, which affect physicians practicing in all teaching settings in approved graduate medical education (GME) programs, relate to documentation that went into effect on July 1, 1996.[20]

According to the Medical Group Management Association, by August 1996, at least 15 academic centers received letters from the government informing them of their intent to audit their Medicare billing programs. In a statement released to the press, the faculty practice of Thomas Jefferson University, the Jefferson Faculty Foundation negotiated a settlement agreement with the government in which they agreed to pay $6 million in overpayments and $6 million in fines. The Department of Health and Human Services (DHHS) audited the billing records of the Jefferson Faculty Foundation and identified billing errors which resulted in this settlement.

Thomas Jefferson University was the first institution to take part in PATH or "Physicians at Teaching Hospitals," a voluntary disclosure program that was developed by DHHS in which an external accounting firm audits a random sample of Medicare admission records to identify inaccurate billing practices. As a result of an agreement between HHS and the Jefferson Faculty Foundation, 100 Medicare charts were audited which found that billings by faculty physicians were not supported by adequate medical documentation.

The settlement for the Jefferson Faculty Foundation is estimated to be double the amount of damages estimated by the audit for the years from 1990 to 1994. However, the Federal False Claims Act provides for up to triple damages and penalties in cases found to be false claims. The settlement amount was also determined with respect to the nature of Jefferson Faculty Foundationís full and open cooperation with the audit. In addition to the settlement, the faculty must continue implementation of a Corporate Compliance Plan, that includes mandatory education for all physicians and billing personnel, internal and external, independent audits of the billing practices, establishment of hotlines to report any billing improprieties and regular, formal reporting to HHS on compliance on all aspects of their compliance program.

Improper supervision

Liability of supervising faculty physicians occurs outside the traditional physician-patient relationship. In fact, a supervising physician may never even treat a patient and still be held liable for negligent supervision.[21] Such liability is based in negligence for the specific responsibility to supervise. Liability is not based upon derivative forms of responsibility such as respondeat superior,[22] or, the doctrine of borrowed servants. [23]

To establish the liability of a physician for negligent supervision, expert testimony should be required. The expert must prove that the nature and extent of supervision did not meet the standard of care of a supervising physician under similar circumstances.[24] Courts will also consider factors in determining the supervising physician's negligence such as: (1) the complexity of the procedure performed by the resident; (2) the level of knowledge and skill of the resident; and (3) applicable hospital rules and regulations.[25] In this regard, availability for telephone consultations has been held by a court to not necessarily constitute negligence per se, without consideration of the surrounding facts.[26] Similarly, a supervising physician cannot be held responsible for actions of residents or students occurring before the physician was contacted by the residents.[27]

The remaining elements of a patient's negligence action as discussed before still apply; i.e., the negligence of the supervising physician must still be the legal or proximate cause of the harm to the patient.[28] Another court found that a medical school professor would not be liable for the negligence of the student unless the professor could have prevented the harm to the patient[29] Thus, while most reported cases focus on the duty owed by a supervising physician, the element of causation also provides a line of defense to improper supervision claims.

In summary, claims of improper supervision arise when injuries to a patient result from improper delegation of authority by the medical faculty or from unauthorized acts rendered at the initiative of the student.[30] These functions of the faculty must also be planned with consideration of the standards of accepted medical education, the specific facts of the procedures and students involved, and full consent of the patient in order to minimize the risk of legal claims for improper supervision.

Liability related to the conduct of research

A lesser known but growing area of potential liability applicable only to federally funded academic medical practices conducting research are known as qui tam actions. These actions are also known by the federal act amended in 1986 known as the False Claims Act.[31]

The term "qui tam" is taken from a Latin phrase[32] meaning "who brings the action for the king as well as for himself." As a United States statute, the qui tam action dates back to the civil war when President Lincoln urged Congress to pass a statute that provided for criminal and civil penalties against defense contractors who defrauded the government.[33]

Qui tam cases often arise in the context of Medicare funding,[34] but can also arise from National Institutes of Health funded research. Potentially any federally funded activity can create the basis for a disgruntled employee or researcher. Most, if not all, of the claims against an academic medical practice will come from within, or from former employees, because the Act requires the relator to be an "original source" of the information with personal knowledge.[35] As the relator, the plaintiff receives a percentage of any award received by the government. Although the percentage may vary, the relator recovers a percentage whether the U.S. Justice Department decides to intervene or not.[36]

The most effective way of monitoring the risk of a qui tam lawsuit may be to carefully follow the NIH and Medicare requirements for funding. However, some consideration should be given to what extent the data and research become the property of the academic medical practice in the event that a researcher or other practice member is terminated. In such situations where the academic practice has a claim to ownership, retention of the study data or other documentation may help to thwart a potential claim.

Charitable immunity and governmental immunity

Immunity from suit, while an intriguing defense strategy/risk management tool at first blush, is of limited value in practical application. This is due to the trend of the courts in most states in eliminating both defenses.

Charitable immunity has essentially vanished. The defense is not valid in most states and only appears in a few instances under very limited circumstances in those states which still recognize the validity of this doctrine.[38] Most notably, the courts of Georgia still apply the doctrine of charitable immunity in select factual scenarios.[39]

The Court of Appeals of Georgia recently considered the charitable immunity of a hospital and private physicians.[40] The court upheld the defense as to the hospital on the basis that the plaintiff had received charitable care and did not provide sufficient evidence that she was a paying patient.[41] The court refused, however, to extend the immunity protection to the private physicians involved in the patient's care.[42]

The doctrine of governmental or sovereign immunity also has enjoyed only limited application by the courts to protect health care providers in recent years. Application may vary state to state based upon each state's governmental or sovereign immunity statute. For example, a Federal District Court has considered the state employee status of resident physicians at a state university medical center under the Tennessee Code.[43] The court held that the resident physicians should be dismissed from the case because they were state employees acting within the scope of their employment for the University of Tennessee. Important factors in the court's decision included the fact that the residents were paid by the state, the hospital did not completely control their work, and the language of the Tennessee statute.[44]

The decision under Tennessee law can be contrasted with decisions of other courts refusing to find governmental immunity. Specifically, the Ohio courts have found that the provision of medical care by a professor is outside the scope of the professor's state employment.[45, 46] In doing so, the Ohio courts looked to the nature of the conduct in determining whether the shield of governmental immunity would apply. Thus where a physician acted "more like a physician in private practice than like a teacher"[47] and where the "physicians' actions were not related to their university duties of performing research and teaching,"[48] the defense of governmental immunity was held not to apply.

Despite these highlighted cases analyzing the immunity defenses, it is important to note that most states do not bar recovery on immunity grounds.[49] Similarly, the potential immunity defense for federally employed health care providers has been eliminated by statute.[50]

Risk management for the academic medical practice

The greatest dilemma for health care providers for the 1990s and beyond is to reduce the cost of health care while preserving and enhancing the quality of health care services. An important part of solving the problem of diminishing resources is the preservation of capital, achieved in part by avoiding financial losses from malpractice litigation. Financial losses related to malpractice claims are paid in many ways, such as legal fees and payment of insurance premiums, as well as excessive medical tests ordered in the practice of "defensive medicine." All these losses have effectively reduced the resources for medical advances as well as necessary patient care services. To prevent these losses, the academic practice group practice manager must operate a risk management program as part of an overall quality program.

The ideal solution to quality control would be to prevent risks by avoiding all errors and mistakes when providing medical care. Unfortunately, the delivery of medical care is unavoidably accompanied by the occurrence of some injury.

The term "risk management" was coined by the insurance industry in 1963 and related primarily to the funding and control of predictable losses in a business activity.[51] Risk management has been traditionally defined as the process of planning, organizing, directing and controlling the resources and activities of an organization and its functions to minimize the adverse affects of accidental losses to that organization at the least possible cost.[52] In the health care industry, the focus of risk control programs is patient safety and quality of care.

During the 1970s, in response to an insurance crisis which caused many insurance companies to leave the medical liability insurance field, the medical and health professions were faced with a wave of consumerism which placed their services and hospital operations under public scrutiny. "Patients' Rights" laws were enacted in many states and the rapidly escalating cost of health care became an issue of national concern. Also at this time the Joint Commission on Accreditation of Hospitals placed new emphasis on quality assurance in hospitals, requiring that quality assurance activities be more problem focused and results oriented.[53]

The response to these forces caused many hospitals and medical institutions to develop their own internal, formal risk management program. The goals: to improve quality control efforts and patient satisfaction, both of which ideally would lead to reduced financial losses.

Although the development of the risk management process in the medical setting is still a relatively new phenomenon, there are nonetheless unique applications that make medical risk management a specialty within its own right. The traditional definition of risk management may have little application in the medical sciences. Thus, a working definition for hospitals and physician groups might be:

Risk management for the academic medical practice

> The process of applying sound management technique to identification, assessment and resolution of problems to prevent medical mishaps, and minimize the adverse effects of injury and loss to patients, employees, visitors, and the hospital corporation.[54]

While risk management and quality improvement were treated as separate and distinct programs in the past, it is now accepted that they are two different approaches to the goal of ensuring quality of care and patient safety.[55]

According to the Joint Commission on Accreditation of Hospitals, the essential components of a sound quality assurance program in the aggregate include:[56]

1. Identification of important or potential problems or related concerns in the care of patients;
2. Objective assessment of the cause and scope of problems and concerns, including the determination of priorities for both investigating and resolving problems;
3. Implementation of decisions or actions that are designed to eliminate identified problems;
4. Monitoring activities designed to assure that the desired result is achieved and sustained; and
5. Documentation that reasonably substantiates the effect of the overall program.

Risk management programs utilize a similar model for directing essential activities, through incident reporting, protection of documentation and relevant evidence, evaluation of potential claims, modifying potentially hazardous situations, and ongoing monitoring to prevent further untoward occurrences. In January 1989, the Joint Commission on Accreditation of Health care Organizations updated the formal risk management activities it requires for accreditation.[57] It now requires increased participation by physicians in risk identification, analysis and risk reduction/loss prevention. While the Joint Commission does not specify exact methods for data collection and analysis, the guidelines require health care organizations to have ongoing, objective review of clinical services and request that they identify potential high risk areas for patient injury.[48]

Risk management checklist

The following checklist,[49] when part of a coordinated team approach by all health care providers in the academic practice, can assist in prevention of claims. Of course, each practice has unique factual scenarios and opportunities to avoid claims, but these serve as a set of suggested areas to monitor:

1. Audit medical records. Establish a procedure for auditing medical records to determine whether documentation is appropriate for quality of care and payment issues. The audit should consider whether the record is accurate, objective, legible, timely, comprehensive and secure. Monitor the procedure's operation;
2. Audit billing records. Flag billing records in cases with questionable outcomes, or, review medical records in cases with unusually delinquent payment histories. Take care not to create a patient's reason to sue by pressing for collection on a procedure or treatment with a questionable or less than optimal outcome;
3. Inspect practice sites. Practice sites should be inspected to determine that they are in compliance with state public health laws, accreditation requirements and other relevant standards;
4. Confidential reporting of incidents. Establish and maintain a confidential program for reporting incidents to a peer review committee.;
5. Teach physicians how to handle an adverse outcome. Procedures for adverse outcomes should be reviewed with physicians before incidents occur. These include: immediate consultation for the patient if indicated, and any equipment involved in the incident should be tagged and stored in a secure location. Any medical records, x-rays, fetal monitoring strips and other documentation should also be secured. The physician and support staff should be reminded of patient confidentiality and instructed not to speak to the media. It is important for the physician to have prompt factual contact with the patient including potential consequences of the adverse outcome without a direct admission of guilt as appropriate;[60]
6. Review insurance coverage. Analyze the scope of coverage, exclusions, limits and costs;
7. Examine premiums. Determine whether the costs of premiums are appropriate based on the cost of insurance available in the market;

8. Review claims-management services. Review the operation and costs of claims-management services, fees for insurance brokers, retention of legal counsel and legal fees;
9. Loss-control programs. Determine the need for and implement educational programs about loss-control for faculty and staff of the practice; and
10. Monitor risk-management activities. Establish a calendar to monitor expiration dates of insurance policies, regular audits and other risk-management activities.

Alternative approaches to reducing the cost of professional liability

The present malpractice crisis has caused widespread frustration and dissatisfaction with the current legal system and has influenced the relationships between physicians and their patients. The impact of malpractice suits on the physician and medical community has been described by the Reverend Edward Reading as the "Malpractice Stress Syndrome." In the same way that other diseases and "stressing" situations have a deleterious effect on the human body which, in turn, have an impact on the patient's family or social constellation, the malpractice stress syndrome can cause emotional insecurity and instability and even physician impairment and organizational stress. Clearly the losses from medical malpractice present not only potential financial loss but also loss in the areas of human suffering and the integrity of the medical profession. Many medical societies and hospitals have developed new proposals for reducing malpractice claims, which go beyond formal institutional risk management programs.

Clinical standards for professional liability

In 1983, a group of anesthesiologists from the Harvard University-affiliated hospitals developed the first set of written patient-monitoring standards developed not just to improve patient care but also to reduce malpractice claims. At first the standards were considered by most clinicians to be little more than a written recitation of current treatments. But after national publication of the standards, they were thought to be of more use to the legal profession than physicians. Many consumer groups and the media appreciated the efforts by the physicians and since adoption of the standards, the Harvard institutions' malpractice losses have been decreasing.[61]

Informed consent guidelines: the experience of the Harvard medical institutions

In 1983, the Risk Management Foundation (RMF) of the Harvard Medical Institutions began developing and documenting informed consent guidelines for institutions insured by the Controlled Risk Insurance Company, LTD (CRICO). In July 1989, the Foundation undertook a comprehensive study to evaluate (overall and by institution) compliance with those guidelines and their effectiveness.[62]

The review examined all CRICO claims or suits from the time period of April 1976 to June 1990 that involved failure to obtain consent as an allegation. In nearly 232 claims, an alleged poor or unexpected outcome of treatment had occurred, which had resulted in a malpractice action for failure to obtain consent. The sole complaint in 21 percent of those cases was failure to obtain consent. As a result of this review, several Harvard institutions have developed programs to address problems associated with informed consent.

The Harvard institutions endorsed the use of procedure-or-risk specific consent forms which include specific complications for the planned procedure and a space for additional comments. It was determined that since the risks for anesthesia and the transfusion of blood or blood components are separate from the risks associated with surgery, several of the Harvard institutions now use separate consents for those treatments. On the Children's Hospital Consent for Medical and Surgical Procedure form, there is (in addition to the signature line for the parent) a space for the signature for the patient over 12 years of age or older to be used at the discretion of the physician. Clearly what can easily be drawn from their experience is that the more individualized the consent form, the more powerfully it can be used as a loss control prevention practice tool.

The Michigan malpractice arbitration program

The Michigan malpractice arbitration program was a legislative response developed to decrease the cost of resolving a wide range of disputes. Although not without its critics, it preserves the legal tradition of using an adversarial system, while eliminating the more costly aspects of court-based litigation. Currently, 10 states, including Illinois, have enacted laws that offer arbitration as an option before a claim arises. Of these states, only Michigan has advanced its law and implemented a program which:

- informs patients of the option of arbitration;
- maintains an agency to process the cases; and
- provides the funding needed to make arbitration a viable statewide alternative.[63]

Medical malpractice tribunal

Another alternative to the current legal-based system that has been proposed by Abramson and David, is the creation of a medical malpractice tribunal. The medical malpractice tribunal would be composed of a general physician, a physician who is known as an expert in the specialty area that the claim is based on, an attorney, and a layperson. The tribunal would be responsible for investigating the facts of the claim, gathering evidence and listening to testimony from the relevant parties. The tribunal could then employ statistical information about treatment-related injuries and then make findings as to physician liability and patient compensation. Such a system, they propose, would reduce legal costs and through predictability, increase malpractice prevention and mitigate the practice of defensive medicine. The authors also recommend giving the tribunal the power to recommend sanctions against substandard providers and requiring those found guilty of malpractice to contribute subsidies to a compensation fund.[64]

Peer review and credentialing

The process of peer review is a system of ongoing monitoring and evaluation of another's performance, with the understanding that physicians who engage in this process have a duty to restrict the activity of colleagues who endanger patient safety or quality of care. In the past, peer review was largely shielded from supervision or intervention from those outside the medical profession. In the past two decades, increasing scrutiny has been directed toward physician peer review. As part of the consumer movement, the general public has requested access to information regarding physician credentials and clinical expertise. Expanded application to the medical profession of federal antitrust law by the U.S. Supreme Court has encouraged litigation in connection with peer review actions considered to have been conducted in bad faith. Court decisions that have permitted plaintiffs to recover damages from hospitals as well as physicians have put ever-increasing pressure on hospitals for enhanced credentialing.[65]

Peer review also can be a valuable risk management tool to aid in the defense of medical malpractice actions. Many states have enacted peer review statutes protecting information from discovery that is part of the peer review process.[66] The legislative rationale for the protections from discovery is to allow a complete and open review and critique of procedures and specific incidents in the hope that the quality of care may be improved and similar future incidents avoided.[67]

Therefore, it is important for the medical practice group manager to implement policies and procedures based upon a careful review of the local state statutes applicable to the practice. One should take care to cloak investigations and information created by the peer review organization with the protection of the local peer review statute by having regular review meetings with members of the medical practice. By way of example, the Pennsylvania Peer Review Protection Act provides in part:

> "The proceedings and records of a review committee shall be held in confidence and shall not be subject to discovery or introduction into evidence in any civil action against a professional health care provider arising out of the matters that are the subject of evaluation and review by such committee...."[68]

However, the statutes in some states allow for voluntary disclosure by peer review participants in certain instances and information readily obtainable or discoverable from independent sources is not protected by the peer review process.[70] Nonetheless, the focus of investigations should be a "peer review investigation" at either the health care provider level, or the faculty level, rather than an incident report.[71] States differ as to the extent academic faculty review, in the absence of health care peer review, may be confidential or privileged information. Similarly, review should be undertaken on behalf of physicians initially, not necessarily with legal counsel.

By comparison, if the only meaningful review occurs in response to a threatened suit or in anticipation of litigation, the confidentiality of gathered information and reports could be compromised. The medical practice manager should take care to establish a legitimate and meaningful program of peer review to protect the information gathered, not merely a procedural "sham" to withhold otherwise discoverable facts and critiques of medical care. To set up a valid peer review program, the medical practice plan manager would be wise to seek assistance from legal counsel who will actually be defending malpractice claims for the academic medical practice.

Insurance for the academic medical practice

The "malpractice crisis"

Although some authorities may question its severity,[72] it is generally accepted that there exists a "malpractice crisis" in the medical profession. According to studies by the American Medical Association, the number of claims filed against physicians increased from an average annual rate of 3.0 per 100 (3/100) physicians before 1980 to 10.2 per 100 (10.2/100) in 1985, although the rate has dropped to 6.4 per 100 (6.4/100) in recent years.[73, 74] The cost associated with this litigation ranges in the billions of dollars nationwide.[75]

The traditional way of protecting against these losses is to purchase professional liability insurance in the commercial market. Since the 1970s, the cost of these premiums has continued to soar, which gave rise to alternative forms of protection of assets, most notably the creation of self-insurance companies. Among the first medical professional liability self-insurance programs created were those associated with academic medical institutions.

When the academic group practice considers whether or not to purchase insurance in the commercial market or self-insure, several factors should be carefully reviewed. Some of these factors include the size of the potential insured, the claims history of the risk pool including analysis of the subspecialties involved, and the administrative costs associated with creating and maintaining such a complex program. The most common allegations by specialty are shown in Figure 15.1 at the end of the chapter. Self-insurance can be highly regulated by state insurance departments. While regulations vary on a state-by-state basis, it can be difficult to qualify a self-insurance program. In fact, some states require a successful claims history and lead time before they will authorize the self-insurance company. This can be true whether it is a domestic insurance program or an off-shore insurer seeking to do business in the state. The practice plan manager should consult legal counsel and carefully weigh the costs of a self-insurance program versus the availability and cost of commercial insurance before making any decision or recommendation.

State insurance funds

In response to the perceived malpractice crisis, several states have formed state patient compensation funds.[78] Depending on the state, these funds serve as either primary or secondary sources of indemnification to health care professionals. Thus, they may integrate with commercial insurance or self-insurance. Most of the state funds, however, charge mandatory premiums. The effectiveness and cost savings associated with these state-operated funds is open to debate, but it does increase the availability of insurance coverage.

Settlement costs unique to academic medical institutions

As discussed in the previous section, academic medical institutions face the unique challenge of training and insuring medical students and residents. Residents often do not have substantial assets or access to the insurance markets. Similarly, they are often employees of the hospital where they receive their training. Therefore, the responsibility for insuring these individuals often falls upon the academic medical centers. Whether the insurance is purchased commercially, through the state fund or from self-insurance, the burden and expense of the premiums fall upon the licensed physicians and medical centers. In situations where the premium-paying institution is state-funded, or, the insurance to be purchased is obtained from a state fund, the taxpayer also shares in this burden.

Conclusion

The process of risk management requires a significant commitment of time, resources, and support from medical leadership to be truly effective. When administered properly, it can be a powerful method for avoiding patient injuries and financial loss.

Figure 15.1

Most Common Allegations by Specialty

General Surgery
1. Negligent trauma management
2. Negligent treatment of fracture
3. Damaged structures during surgery
4. Failure to diagnose and/or treat appendicitis
5. Nerve damage during surgery
6. Post-operative wound infection

Orthopedic Surgery
1. Negligent treatment of fracture
2. Failure to diagnose fracture
3. Post-operative complications due to negligent surgery
4. Post-operative nerve damage
5. Negligent total hip replacement
6. Surgery, wrong side/limb
7. Post-operative wound infection

Obstetrics/Gynecology
1. Negligent performance of elective sterilization procedure
2. Complications during vaginal delivery (involving mother)
3. Injury to infant at birth
4. Retained sponge, surgical instrument, etc.
5. Complications after total abdominal hysterectomy
6. Negligent pre-natal care

General/Family Practice
1. Negligent drug therapy
2. Failure to diagnose carcinoma
3. Negligent treatment of cardiac condition
4. Failure to diagnose fracture
5. Negligent management of diabetes
6. Negligent obstetrical care

Internal Medicine
1. Negligent drug therapy
2. Damaged structure during treatment
3. Negligent management of cardiac condition
4. Negligent administration of chemotherapy

Figure 15.1 (continued)

Neurosurgery
1. Negligent treatment of head trauma
2. Negligent management of disc problems
3. Negligent treatment of back pain/injury
4. Post-operative emboli
5. Bovie burns during surgery
6. Post-operative wound infection

Radiology
1. Failure to diagnose fracture
2. Negligent administration and management of contrast media
3. Failure to diagnose carcinoma
4. Perforation of bowel during barium enema

Emergency Medicine
1. Negligent treatment of laceration
2. Failure to diagnose fracture
3. Negligent treatment of trauma
4. Failure to remove foreign body

Anesthesiology
1. Tooth damage
2. Damaged structures due to negligent anesthesia management
3. Cardiac arrest during surgery
4. Post-operative brain damage
5. Esophageal intubation

FROM: Pennsylvania Medical Society Liability Insurance Company's Risk Management Documentation. As reproduced in: Grand Rounds on Medical Malpractice, pg. 62.

References

1. Tottenham, Terry O. and Joy, Louise, M., "Liability for Patient Care, HEALTH LAW PRACTICE GUIDE," Vol. 1, *National Health Lawyers Association*, Page 9-9.
2. As above, Page 9-4.
3. Fjerstad v. Knutson, 271 N.W. 2d 8 (S.D. 1978).
4. Darling v. Charleston Community Memorial Hospital, 221 N.E. 2d at 253 (Ill. 1965), cert. denied, 383 U.S. 946 (1966).
5. T Tottenham, Terry O. and Joy, Louise, M., "Liability for Patient Care," HEALTH LAW PRACTICE GUIDE, Vol. 1, *National Health Lawyers Association*, Page 9-30.
6. Monagle, John F., Risk Management - A Guide for Health Care Professionals, Aspen Systems Corporation, pg 4, 1985.
7. T Tottenham, Terry O. and Joy, Louise, M., Liability for Patient Care, HEALTH LAW PRACTICE GUIDE, Vol. 1, National Health Lawyers Association, Page 9-30.
8. Id.
9. Campion, F.X., M.D., Grand Rounds on Medical Malpractice, Risk Management Foundation of the Harvard Medical Institutions, Inc., 1990, pg. 15.
10. Avery, J.K., Lawyers Tell What Turns Some Patients Litigious. Medical Malpractice Prevention July/August 1986, pp. 35-37. Quoted in "Maintaining Effective Patient Relations," A Risk Management Series, St. Paul: The St. Paul Fire and Marine Insurance Company, 1989:2.
11. Devlin, Mary, J.D., The Doctrine of Informed Consent, The Journal of Medical Practice Management, Volume 11, Number 5, March/April 1996, pp. 244-245.
12. Devlin, Mary, J.D., Informed Consent—Part One Recent Cases, The Journal of Medical Practice Management, Volume 7, Number Two, pg. 141.
13. Richards, Edward P., Rathbun, Katharine C., Medical Risk Management, Aspen Systems Corporation, pg. 205, 1983.
14. Centman v. Cobb, 581 N.E.2d 1286 (In. 1991).
15. Reuter, Professional Liability in Postgraduate Medical Education, 15 Journal of Legal Medicine 485 (1994).
16. Bowlin v. Duke University, 108 N.C.App. 145, 423 S.E.2d 320 (1992).
17. Bowlin, 423 S.E.2d 320, 323.
18. Bolin v. Duke University, 108 N.C.App. 145, 423 S.E.2d 320, 323 (1992).
19. Bowlin, 423 S.E.2d at 424.
20. The Philadelphia Inquirer, Blue Shield to Investigate Fees by Penn,
21. Gilbert M. Gaul, December 22, 1995.
    Mozingo v. Pitt County Memorial Hospital, 101 N.C. App.578, 400 S.E.2d 747 (1991).
22. Otnott v. Morgan, 636 So.2d 957 (La. 1994).
23. Rouse v. Pitt County Memorial Hospital, 343 N.C. 186, 470 S.E.2d44 (1996).

24. Dine v. Williams, 830 S.W.2d 453 (Mo. 1992).
25. Jackson v. Oklahoma Memorial Hospital, 909 P.2d 765 (Ok. 1996).
26. Mozingo v. Pitt County Memorial Hospital, 331 N.C. 182, 415 S.E.2d 341 (1992).
27. Rivera v. Prince George's County Health Department, 102 Md.App. 456, 649 A.2d 1212 (1994).
28. Brooks v. Goldhammer, 608 So.2d 394 (Ala. 1992).
29. Otnott v.Morgan, 636 So.2d 957 (La. 1994).
30. Reuter, Professional Liability in Postgraduate Medical Education, 15 Journal of Legal Medicine 485 (1994).
31. 31 U.S.C. Sec. 3729 et. seq.
32. qui tam pro domino rege quam pro se ipso in hac sequitur.
33. Robertson, The False Claims Act, 26 Arizona State Law Journal 889 (1994).
34. Callahan, Do Good and Get Rich: Financial incentives For Whistleblowing And The False Claims Act 37 Villanova Law Review 273, 309 (1992).
35. Robertson, The False Claims Act, 26 Ariz. St. L. Jo. 889 (1994).
36. Robertson, supra.
37. Matthew Bender, Treatise on Health Care Law, Vol 2. Sec. 12.01[2][a] and Cumulative Supplement (1995).
38. Id.
39. Id., citing, Harrell v. Louis Smith Memorial Hospital, 197 Ga. App. 189, 397 S.E.2d 746 (1990).
40. Bagley v. Fulton-DeKalb Hospital Authority, 216 Ga. App. 537, 455 S.E.2d 325 (1995).
41. Id.
42. Id. 455 S.E.2d at 328.
43. Thompson v. Regional Medical Center At Memphis, 748 F.Supp. 575 (W.D. TN 1990).
44. Id.
45. Newton v. School of Osteopathic Medicine, 91 Ohio App.3d 703, 633 N.E.2d 593 (1993)
46. Klingel v. Ohio State University Hospitals, 72 Ohio Misc.2d 25, 655 N.E.2d 457 (1993).
47. Newton v. School of Osteopathic Medicine, 91 Ohio App.3d 703, 633 N.E.2d 593 (1993).
48. Klingel v. Ohio State University Hospitals, 72 Ohio Misc.2d 25, 655 N.E.2d 457 (1993).
49. Matthew Bender, Treatise On Health Care Law, Vol. 2, Sec. 12.01[2][b] and Cumulative Supplement (1995).
50. Id.
51. Orlikoff J.E., Fifer W.R., Greeley H.P: Malpractice Prevention and Liability Control for Hospitals. Chicago: American Hospital Association, 1981, pp. 28-29.
52. Head G.L. The Risk Management Process. New York : Risk and Insurance Management Society, 1978, pp. 8-16.

53. Campion, Francis, Grand Rounds on Medical Malpractice, Risk Management Foundation of the Harvard Medical Institutions, Inc., 1990, pp. 196- 200.
54. Campion Supra.
55. Richards, E.P., Rathbun K.C., Medical Risk Management, Aspen Systems Corporation, 1983, pp 11-48.
56. Joint Commission on Accreditation of Hospitals: Accreditation Manual on Hospitals, 1981. Chicago: Joint Commission on Accreditation of Hospitals, 1981, pp. 151-154.
57. 1989 Accreditation Manual For Hospitals. Chicago, IL: The Joint Commission on the Accreditation of Health care Organizations; 1988.
58. Draft Scoring Guidelines For Hospital Risk Management Functions, 1989. Chicago, IL: The Joint Commission on the Accreditation of Health care Organizations; 1988.
59. The checklist was taken substantially from Managing the Academic Medical Practice: The Two Headed Eagle, First Edition, pps. 65-66 (1992).
60. Campion, Francis, X., M.D., Grand Rounds On Medical Malpractice, Risk Management Foundation of the Harvard Medical Institutions, Inc., 1990, pp. 163-164.
61. Campion, F.X., M.D., Grand Rounds on Medical Malpractice, pp. 82-93.
62. Finan, I. The Impact of Informed Consent Guidelines At the Harvard Medical Institutions. Forum: Risk Managment Foundation of the Harvard Medical Institutions Inc. 1990; 11:3-7.
63. Schut, David, J.D., The Michigan Malpractice Arbitration Program, The Journal of Medical Practice Management, Fall 1992, Volume 8, Number 2, pp. 140-144.
64. Abramson, E.M., David, D.S., Medical Malpractice: a Non-Adversarial Suggestion, American Journal of Medicine. 92(2):197-201, 1992 Feb.
65. Campion, Francis, X. M.D., Grand Rounds on Medical Malpractice. pp. 301-311.
66. See e.g. The Pennsylvania Peer Review Protection Act, 63 Pa.C.S.A. Sec. 425.1 et. seq.
67. See e.g. 63 Pa. C.S.A. Sec. 425.2 and the definition of a "Review Organization" contained therein.
68. 63 Pa.C.S.A. Sec. 425.4.
69. Zitter, J. Right of Voluntary Disclosure of Privileged Proceedings of Hospital Medical Review or Doctor Evaluation Process, 60 A.L.R. 4th 1273.
70. E.g. 63 Pa. C.S.A. Sec. 425.4.
71. McMahon, M., Academic Peer Review Privilege In Federal Court, 85 A.L.R. 4th 691.
72. Weiler, P., et. al., A Measure Of Malpractice, 15 Journal of Legal Medicine 479 (1994).
73. Socioeconomic Characteristics of Medical Malpractice 1989. Chicago, IL: American Medical Association Center for Health Policy Research, 1989: 18-20.

74. Reynolds, R.A., Rizzo, J.A., Gonzalez, M. L., The Cost of Medical Professional Liability. Journal of the American Medical Association. 1987; 257: 2776-2781.
75. Medical Malpractice: Insurance Costs Increased but Varied Among Physicians and Hospitals. Washington, D.C.: 1986; U.S. General Accounting Office Document (GAO) HRD-86-112.
76. Richards, Edward P. , Rathbun, Katharine C., Medical Risk Management, Aspen Systems Corporation, pp. 38-48, 1983.
77. Matthew Bender, Treatise on Health Care Law, Vol. 2. Sec. 14.01 et. seq. and Cumulative Supplement (1995).
78. Grand Rounds on Medical Malpractice, Appendix, pg. 347. Footnote 44 Corpus Juris Secondum Sec. 59(d).

Chapter 16

The future of the academic medical practice

by David J. Bachrach, MBA, FACMPE/FACHE

I had second thoughts when I was asked to prepare the summary chapter of this book on *The Future of Academic Medical Practice.* After all, who can predict the future with the level of accuracy that we can detail the past? The fact is, as I look back on a similar chapter penned by Russell Coile in the 1992 book, *Managing the Academic Medical Practice: The Two-Headed Eagle,* I find he did a pretty good job of predicting the challenges that would face academic health centers and faculty practice plans during the middle five years of the 1990s.

In the following pages I will highlight the prognostications and recommendations of the plenary speakers at the April 1997 meeting of the Academic Practice Assembly; I will relate Bill Nicholas' findings from his Spring 1997 survey of faculty practice plan and clinical department administrators; and, I will offer my own observations of what may come to pass as we move through the millennium and into the next century. As one of the purposes of this book is to provoke dialogue as well as change, you may choose not to agree with me. That's perfectly "OK." Let us plan to meet at the 26th annual APA meeting in the Spring of 2002 and look back together on what has occurred. I am sure that then, as now, our hindsight will be closer to 20-20 than our foresight.*

---

*Readers may wish to comment on this chapter and other parts of the book. Please feel free to drop me an e-mail at dbach@notes.mdacc.tmc.edu (you may wish to confirm my current e-mail address by checking the MGMA On-Line Directory at http://www.mgma.com/iwd/mem)......DJB

One Revolution: Managing the Academic Medical Practice in an Era of Rapid Change

Proceedings from the 21st meeting of the Academic Practice Assembly

The membership of the Academic Practice Assembly has convened annually for more than 20 years to share information and exchange ideas. A key feature of each conference has been comments from experts about the trends and directions which may drive these practices in the future. In April 1997, the APA met for the 21st time. Two speakers spoke directly to this topic and their most poignant comments follow. These comments are taken from articles prepared by Dennis Barnhardt, MGMA's Communications Director, as reported in the June 1997 *Medical Group Management Update*.

Jeff Goldsmith, PhD, president of Health Futures of Charlottesville, VA, opened the conference with these key points:

1. Academic practices must be converted to risk-sharing enterprises; "cross-subsidization" patterns must be dealt with. This occurs when cost and price lines are blurred between the primary missions of teaching, research and clinical care. The total costs of teaching and research, for example, often have been subsidized by other revenue streams. "The road to hell is paved with cross-subsidies...in a competitive environment individual lines of activity will increasingly have to stand on their own economic foundations. Persistent economic loss in any major activity in an institution is a symptom which must be cured. The individual missions of the institutions are going to have to be self-supporting. You will not be able to subsidize research - it will have to be scaled back to break even. Managed care is not going to pay for teaching";

2. To survive, academic institutions, which heretofore have shielded faculty from economic risk, must undergo fundamental transformation of clinical and political cultures inside academic faculties. Such change is necessary for academic institutions to function effectively in training physicians to practice in a resource-limited environment;

3. Economic risk is being shifted to providers of care, principally physicians, and in most cases bypassing hospitals. The ability of physicians to organize collectively to bear and manage risk will eventually determine if they survive. This shift has lead to a significant reduction in the rate of inflation of health care costs to

an annualized rate of 6 percent; even now we are in a disinflationary environment;

4. The idea of bearing and managing economic risk, which has produced problems for everyone, is totally foreign to academic culture. Academic cultures were constructed to protect faculty against external forces, and that makes it difficult for faculty to think about what society needs;

5. Despite these challenges, Goldsmith noted that academic medical centers have proven themselves extraordinarily resilient. One great opportunity lies in their ability to develop and report their outcomes research, which demonstrates empirically the benefits of certain course of care. He noted that the emergence of evidence-based medicine fits the academic culture. Further, he noted that many of the academic medical centers are already vertically integrated, having achieved what many in the private sector are only now trying to achieve.

Dr. Thomas C. Royer, MD, chairman of the board of governors of the Henry Ford Health System, closed the general session with the following imperatives, as reported by Barnhardt:

1. Academic medical centers will survive if we can return to our roots; to a time when people entrusted their lives and the lives of their children to us. We can and must move from the fragmented, disease-oriented, acute and cost-management systems to one which provides a continuum of care, managing preventive and primary care over populations and leading to managed care as a style of practice. He said that, "We absolutely, as academic medical centers, can be successful in creating integrated delivery systems where patient care is the driver of research and education, and where we can maintain clinical delivery and service delivery at the highest level. But we can no longer focus on a system that is based on merely treating individual disease; rather we must focus on maintenance of the health of the population";

2. Royer's guiding principles for development of an integrated health network are:
   - Focus on the customer;
   - Conserve and appropriately manage community resources;
   - Protect and enhance the valuable "name brand" of the academic practice;

- Empower employees, physicians and clinical personnel; and
- Create an infrastructure to serve employees, physicians and clinical personnel, "one that works together and talks together.".

3. Royer noted that academic medical centers have a unique card to play in marketing their services. While they generally provide access to essential and typically high-cost services, and managed care contracts provide an avenue for obtaining those services under more favorable economic terms, teaching hospitals offer prestige and significant name value. These are critical features as managed care plans compete for enrollment. He went on to say that academic medical centers possess the leading, state-of-the-art technological equipment and treatment methods which, in many cases, can improve outcomes and reduce the long-term cost of care. Further, academic centers are generally regarded as the provider of superior quality care;

4. But Dr. Royer noted some negatives as well. These included:

   - A diffuse decision-making structure at academic centers often makes managed care contracting agreements slow to be approved and even difficult to reach;
   - Due to high overhead costs associated with large physical plants, high-tech services and more complex case mixes, academic medical centers tend to be more expensive than their community-based competitors;
   - With easy access to sophisticated equipment and the propensity to use it for teaching purposes, academic hospitals have a greater potential for the inefficient utilization of high-tech and costly resources;
   - The facilities have typically provided poor patient access to care since academic institutions frequently were not physically designed with patient convenience and service as a priority;
   - Since most academic physicians also maintain responsibility for teaching and research, their schedules do not provide patients the flexibility and convenience found in a community-based setting; and
   - There tends to be a focus on "special cause" diseases rather than "common cause" diseases with a broader focus on prevention, chronic care and the continuity of care.

5. Dr. Royer spoke to the need for academic medical centers to recognize and emphasize their core competencies if they are to be successful. These include:

   - Creating and sustaining a system culture;
   - Managing relationships with and among customers, patients, community, payers, physicians, other providers and employees;
   - Maintaining and demonstrating quality and cost performance;
   - Maintaining the health of a defined population;
   - Developing leading-edge information technology; and
   - Implementing the strategic plan.

6. Lastly, Dr. Royer noted these major challenges facing, and opportunities available to academic medical centers:

   - Developing a commitment to the "tricycle model," where the front wheel is patient care and the back two wheels are research and education;
   - Developing relationships and defining a comprehensive patient care system including provider, purchaser and insurance relationships; focusing on value - not on quality or cost;
   - Focusing on cost-effective and quality outcome measures;
   - Identifying and pursuing an appropriate primary care strategy incorporating both educational and patient care delivery;
   - Restructuring internally to allow the hospital, faculty and community physicians to work effectively together by improving the integration of academic departments;
   - Maintaining the importance of the "core event" in health care delivery;
   - Assuring the stability and integration of the tripartite missions of patient care, education and research; and
   - Moving away from the hospital paradigm and removing excess capacity.

Trends in academic medical management related to centralization

During the Spring of 1997, William Nicholas, PhD, conducted a survey of faculty practice plans throughout the country. His findings were presented at the 21st annual APA meeting and highlights follow. Nearly 400 questionnaires were sent to the 133 American medical schools (MD and DO) that report having faculty practice plans. Inquiry was made of the senior faculty practice plan administrator along with the administrators of the departments of surgery and internal medicine. The response rate (i.e., usable questionnaire responses) was 46 percent; considered representative and statistically significant.

For purposes of the survey, these definitions were used in describing the different types of faculty practice plans:

Multispecialty model: A high degree of common governance; one overall governing board; a central administrative and management structure; income is pooled;

Integrated model: A transitional model between the multispecialty and the federated plans; income is not pooled;

Federated model: Has some measure of common governance; a central advisory committee to address issues of common management systems; income is credited to the unit that generates the revenue; and

Departmental model: Departments are autonomous; there is no common governance and little or no common management systems; income is not pooled.

The findings were summarized as follows:

- Faculty practice plans are currently organized as:

  43 percent Integrated
  21 percent Federated
  18 percent Multispecialty
  18 percent Departmental

- A large number of FPPs are now undergoing reorganization. Not all respondents agreed on the direction to go but the composite response was that, following this period of reorganization, the mix of plans will have the following profile:

  53 percent Multispecialty
  26 percent Federated
  21 percent Integrated

That is, there would be virtually no departmental practice plans in place five years from now. Of significance, the surgery and internal medicine department administrators saw their jobs changing dramatically during this period and many saw themselves making job changes; if for no other reason then with the loss of FPP responsibility would likely come a reduction in compensation.

- The forces motivating these changes are several, but there was general agreement that five major forces were driving this change. Equal weight was given to the first three:

  - Economics: The need to adapt or stabilize the organization's financial base;
  - Managed care: The need to adapt academic behavior to a different way of doing business; and
  - Competition for patients: A response to private sector movement to dominate traditional academic markets.

  Of slightly lesser weight, but also viewed as important were:

  - Government pressures: A response to legislation and regulation; and
  - University pressure: A concern that adverse financial risks associated with the medical practice could seriously harm the university.

- Faculty practice plans were considering several responses to these pressures. In descending order, preferred organization models were:

  - Independent practice corporation;
  - Merger or joint venture with not-for-profit;
  - Foundation under the university; or
  - Merger or joint venture with for-profit.

- The respondents were asked to look forward and comment on what skills would be most needed by them in the years ahead, and what would happen to their current positions. Here's what they said:

  <u>The strategic moves that would get the most play in the next three years were</u>:

  -- The development of electronic interfaces and the pooling of data among the strategic partners to develop and disseminate information concerning patient care outcomes; and

-- Changing the risk-sharing methods to integrate financing and delivery of care (e.g., capitation and sub-capitation).

The management expertise required to maintain a competitive advantage includes:

Most Important:
- Knowing how to work collaboratively with medical groups, hospitals and health plans; and
- Managing diverse network interests through skills in creating a common vision and purpose.

Moderately Important:
- Managing diverse network interests through skills in negotiation and conflict management.

Least Important:
- Building referral sources through long-standing, but informal networks.

Nearly 20 percent of the respondents felt that a major share of their responsibilities would be shifted elsewhere. The largest group were the department administrators in surgery who seemed to feel that a major share of their responsibilities would migrate to the practice plan administrator or the dean's office. While the internal medicine administrator seemed to feel similarly concerning a shift to the practice plan administrator, they also saw some of their duties moving to the university; possibly reflecting their responsibilities for grants management functions. Interestingly, about 11 percent of the plan managers saw their duties shifting; two-thirds to the dean's office and one-third to the outside.

- On the basis of his survey, Dr. Nicholas offered the following findings and conclusions:

  A. Medical practices will continue to move away from the departmental model and toward the multispecialty group practice model;

  B. Health care is a local business, so the pace of change will be different in different regions of the country;

C. While the movement toward centralization is impressive, it appears to be evolutionary rather than revolutionary;

D. Over the next three years, faculty practices will see the most operational growth in the areas of electronic interfacing, pooling and dissemination of information, and changes in financial risk-sharing;

E. Today's faculty practices lack common vision. Executives skilled in creating and nurturing group vision will be important contributors to the success of their practices;

F. Economics, managed care and competition for patients appear to be the major factors influencing academic practices to change their organizational models;

G. Four in ten departments of surgery are looking at changing the fundamental relationship between the practice and their medical school;

H. When considering practice structures separate from the university, independent practice corporations are the most popular with practice plan managers and managers of departments of medicine. Surgery administrators prefer merger or a joint venture with a not-for-profit entity;

I. A master's degree is the educational norm for academic practice executives;

J. A gender gap does not exist in senior academic practice management. It is narrowest in departments of surgery;

K. For surgery practice executives, the career cycle appears to be about eight years;

L. Confidence is higher in practice plan administration, and with internal medicine administrators, that the next phase of change will not directly affect individual employment. One in four surgery administrators see their positions being eliminated in the next five years;

M. When there is employment change, most surgery administrators see themselves moving into practice plan administration.

A forecast for the next five years

Five years ago Coile told us to prepare for a rough ride and he was surely correct on that score. The past five years have seen academic medical centers buffeted by dramatic changes in the health care marketplace, and in federal and state regulation. The following trends represent what we may see as the major issues confronting academic medical centers, and what we may expect to find in the years ahead.

Academic medical center revenues will stabilize and margins shrink

FPPs continue to be the largest single source of revenue available in support of the nation's medical schools. While the top 25 research grant-supported schools continue to garner the vast share of those dollars, little increment in such funding has flowed to the majority of the medical schools. Similarly, state allocations to public and private schools (yes, some private medical schools get state allocations; Baylor College of Medicine in Houston being one example) have remained generally flat, although we have seen some increases in the 1997 legislative sessions as state coffers have been enriched during the recent surge in the nation's economy. The fact is, the FPP continues to be the dominant, most flexible source of medical schools' support.

During the early part of this decade we continued to see FPP gross revenues (charges) grow, although the net recoverable amount continued to shrink as a percentage of charges. Many of the major metropolitan markets where we find a large number of academic medical centers saw movement into the third and fourth stages of managed care. We saw discounts from established fee schedules increase. However, we didn't raise our standard fees as aggressively as we have in the past, contributing in part to what is now an increase in the Physician Fee Index of only about 1.8 percent for the 12 months ending June 1997, compared to figures of seven to ten times that level at the beginning of the decade. We now see many more academic practices participating in risk-bearing programs; either as contract providers for full scope-of-care services for a defined population, or as a "carve-out" provider of specialty services. While some academic institutions created managed care products, like the University of Michigan's M-Care developed in the 1980s, many more have initiated or are now in the process of starting their own health plans as competition for patients heats up.

We can expect to see clinical revenues grow marginally over the next five years, although physician revenue growth will outpace the rate of growth in hospital income. As a result, there will be some realignment of support from the owned or affiliated teaching hospital for support of faculty salaries, with a greater reliance on the FPP to make up this loss in support.

We will continue to see changes in medical schools' structures and resource allocation process

The structure of medical schools has traditionally followed a format that can be readily recognized by leafing through the Association of American Medical Colleges' *Directory of American Medical Education.* All surgical and internal medicine disciplines are aligned within large departmental structures (although during the past 25 years we've often seen the surgical disciplines of orthopedics, urology, neurosurgery, plastic and reconstructive surgery and cardio-thoracic surgery move out into independent units). Similarly, the disciplines of dermatology and neurology, among others, have split from their parent departments of internal medicine. This trend was the result of several factors including individual board certification, independent residency programs beginning in the first year of graduation following the elimination of the rotating internship, as well as the prestige that comes from the independence and "equal"* stature that comes with the chair title.

Medical schools have generally parceled out core resources in a fashion that places relatively more funds in the departments that have traditionally not been involved in extramurally funded research, or whose discipline does not command high professional fees; or where we don't find much ancillary or procedure-driven revenues. That is, the "haves" get a base allocation and generate the rest of their support, and the "have nots" get a disproportionate share of the dean's discretionary funds; including those funds which the dean may recover as a part of the "tax" on faculty practice plans. In an attempt to assemble a comprehensive and well-balanced medical education and clinical delivery system, many schools tried to maintain within their ranks a full complement of basic and clinical departments. The cost of doing this has become nearly prohibitive and the decline in practice revenues and allocations from affiliated teaching hospitals may make this virtually impossible in the future.

---

*While all chairs are considered equal, some would suggest that the chairs of surgery and internal medicine are somewhat more equal than others, given the size of their faculties and their larger resource bases.

We can expect to see continued pressure to reduce program costs and align costs with revenues. There will be less cross-subsidization of activities and affiliated hospitals may be less willing to shoulder a portion of the academic costs. We will probably see the consolidation of departments (possibly the return to the single, comprehensive departments of surgery and internal medicine). Some schools may contract for teaching with physicians in private group practices (a return to the old 'volunteer' faculty model in these disciplines, but probably with some compensation thrown in rather than expecting the community physicians' time to be contributed gratis).

We may see medical and dental schools within the same university return to the shared teaching of the basic sciences.

We may see schools realign their faculty into multidisciplinary groups focused around a disease rather than by clinical specialty affiliation which has been the tradition – a tradition that will be hard to change. However, some believe strongly that specialists and subspecialists from different disciplines who work closely in the continuum of care of patients within a broad category of disease may be better aligned for purposes of management and resource allocation than the traditional groupings. The disease-oriented groupings, while having their own shortcomings, are possibly better aligned with how performance of individual faculty and groups of health care providers (including physicians in the diagnostic specialties and support staff) will be evaluated in the future.

There may be an increased dependence on philanthropic support at schools which have not traditionally made that a priority It will assuredly mean that there will be increased pressure to reduce administrative costs through optimal efficiency and effectiveness measures.

We can expect to see deans look critically at not only the size and scope of all academic and research programs, but at the very necessity of maintaining these programs at all. Not every medical school will try to be "all things to all people."

And finally, we will see fewer medical schools with smaller class sizes; possibly 110 schools, down from the current 125, by the year 2005. Some schools may merge and preserve some of their history as a means of making their closure more politically acceptable (to legislatures as well as alumni); and class sizes will be smaller.

Academic medical centers will continue to restructure and reengineer

If one places academic medical centers on a continuum which compares the relative cost per unit of service (i.e., the efficiency with which they deliver a severity adjusted equivalent patient day) with not-for-profit and for-profit integrated health care systems, one would probably put the academic medical center (AMC) at one extreme and the for-profit at the other extreme. Look at the degree of difference between the "best of class" in each category. Where your organization stands along this continuum, relative to your competition, should be of great interest to you; it is to the payers in your community. (This assumes that you have accurately calculated your cost per severity adjusted equivalent patient day and have benchmark information available to you.)

There is no single "right" way to restructure and reengineer an academic medical center. However, unless you are the benchmark institution by which others set their targets, chances are you have been, are now, or will be (should be) using some of the restructuring and reengineering tools which are available and in use by others. There are many qualified consulting firms that have now perfected these skills with other health care organizations, including other AMCs. Institutions may wish to recruit administrative talent from other AMCs that have been successfully through the process. Be sure that those recruited, whether consultant or staff, have experience in and a good understanding and appreciation of the mission and priorities of an AMC, and clearly understand your institution's mission, vision and philosophy of operation/code of ethics.

Strategic planning committees can be used to develop guidelines and expectations as institutions set goals for moving toward their objective cost level. This is a journey, not necessarily a destination. The degree of competition in your market and what is happening to the institution's market share will determine the urgency with which, and the timeframe within which, you pursue these efforts. Since the other institutions in your community are also working to reduce their costs, the target will continue to move; generally away from you.

Academic medical centers will continue to work on reducing their costs of delivering patient care. The move to place education and research costs "on their own bottom," (i.e., cover them entirely with their own sources of revenue) will allow for the isolation of patient care costs and a clean analysis. Considerable effort, and cost, will be expended in pursuit of a more competitive position. Even when severity adjusted, however, AMCs are still likely to be the higher-cost provider in most markets.

There will continue to be a reduction in the size of the support staff, and the size of the faculty, as efficiencies are improved and some programs are consolidated or cut.

The most successful AMCs will document and report their higher quality and accessibility to the latest diagnostic and therapeutic technologies, along with their better outcomes.

The most competitive AMCs will have developed a network of lower cost, accessible providers (physicians and hospitals) which can handle a segment of the continuum of care, and who will serve as a source of referral for that segment best handled by those physicians practicing at the AMC.

We will continue to see public (and government) sentiment swing away from strictly cost as the measure by which contracts will be written. The most successful institutions will gain an advantage by providing clearly stated and documented rationales for selecting the AMC as the provider of choice to those health plan executives empowered to make contract decisions. In fact, the most successful will set the standard for reporting outcomes in their region; forcing the for-profit and not-for-profit providers to report their outcomes in a similar format.

Fewer clinician faculty will enjoy the benefits of tenure

Tenure continues to be a hotly discussed topic among faculty at all universities. The generally higher salaries paid to clinicians at medical schools during a time when the future level of clinical income is uncertain, makes the issue even more intense. We are seeing more faculty hired on a non-tenure clinical track; some with three- to five-year contracts but no long-term commitments. They will have clinical teaching commitments, and some may participate in clinical research and pharmaceutical trials, but they will not be given research laboratory space. There is not likely to be the expectation about publication in refereed journals that one finds among their tenure-track colleagues. In exchange for the lesser permanence of their appointments, these faculty may find greater upside earning potential and the opportunity to work as an active clinician with the support of the energetic, bright, young physicians in residency and fellowship training.

The era of the triple-threat faculty member may largely be past. William N. Kelley, MD, chair of Internal Medicine at Michigan during

---

the 1970s and 80s, coined the terms "physician scientist" and "clinician scholar" to designate those individuals on the tenure track who would be given release time to engage in scholarly activities. Physician scientists would have a light clinical load and would likely have a research laboratory and plenty of time to engage in investigative work and writing. Their students would more often than not be doctoral candidates and post-doctoral fellows, as well as residents and clinical fellows completing their laboratory experience. Clinician scholars would maintain a relatively large clinical practice and would deliver care while engaged in teaching third- and fourth-year medical students, residents and fellows. Both groups of faculty would be judged eligible for tenure based upon their academic productivity by the traditional means.

The faculty on the non-tenure clinical track, on the other hand, would not have the protection of tenure, but likely would enjoy the opportunity to have a greater total level of compensation driven by the volume (and quality) of their clinical service. They would be engaged in the clinical teaching of residents and fellows, but would commit the vast majority of their time to the efficient practice of high quality patient care.

We can expect to see fewer faculty in the tenured ranks and more on the clinical track in the future. The pressure to reduce the ranks of tenure track faculty will come not only from a concern about the economic stability of the school as a whole, but will be the result of the pressure placed on individual faculty to commit more time to practice. Department chairs will not be able to offer as much release time to faculty to engage in independent research and writing; laboratory assignments will be more critically reviewed; reassignments will occur more rapidly if meaningful, measurable productivity is not forthcoming. There will be an expectation that clinical research studies will recover their full costs from sponsors, or from extramural sources of funds other than patient care revenues. Further, faculty will be evaluated, in part, on patient satisfaction as fed back to the affiliated hospitals and health plans which will expect physicians to be more available and involved in the direct care of the patient. One key measure will be waiting time to schedule an appointment, as well as the time kept waiting once the patient arrives for the appointment.

Base faculty salaries will decline or be frozen; increases will be in the incentive component

We are seeing, with increasing frequency, a reduction in total or base faculty salaries. While base salaries may be held steady or reduced, increases will come in the incentive component. FPPs have worked with the medical school dean on the creation of performance measures which look critically at faculty productivity in both the academic (teaching and research) and clinical areas. Faculty who wish to maintain or increase their total income have had to shoulder a greater clinical load. This means not only more patients, but also a willingness to learn the contemporary lexicon and tools of patient case management; clinical pathways and patient care guidelines. Physician outliers who consume too many resources in the care and management of their patients, when their practices cannot be justified by the severity or complexity of illness, may find themselves under critical review by their colleagues charged with responsibility for case management and guidelines.

We can expect to see an increasing percentage of clinician faculty salaries in the incentive component, and the criteria for receipt of this component will become more firmly applied. Criteria will include not just the volume of patients seen, but such factors as patient satisfaction measures tied to the timeliness of appointments and the physician's ability to communicate. Also critical will be adherence to peer-developed pathways and guidelines, and compliance with peer-established resource utilization criteria.

Hospitals will reduce their support of graduate medical education

Reduced hospital reimbursement impacts the faculty practice plans in several ways. First, almost all medical schools depend upon the hospital's support of faculty salaries for the provision of Part A services; i.e., services to the hospital in the form of supervision of clinical service programs such as radiology, anesthesiology and pathology, as well as the supervision of the hospital-based residency programs. Reduced hospital income (we used to call it "reimbursement" but the more accurate term today is "payment" since costs are rarely reimbursed, per se), coupled with the forces of competition will lead hospitals to carefully scrutinize expenses. Graduate medical education (GME) is getting special attention these days.

We are seeing increased pressure to reduce the size of GME programs. These programs grew to their present size under pressure from several fronts including: the increase in the number of specialty designations (including family medicine); an extension from three to four years for most training programs; the need for more physician personpower in indigent care, generally inner city hospitals; the reduction in the number of hours residents could be expected to work; and the fact that up until the mid-1980s, Medicare would pay for these costs, no matter how great!

Our domestic training programs not only served the graduates of American medical schools but offered training opportunities to those from foreign medical schools as well. The current federal budget reduction strategies include a major focus on Medicare costs. As a result, the reimbursement of GME costs is getting a great deal of scrutiny. The target is to have a national program that includes first-year positions equal to 110 percent of the number of graduating domestic medical students; a number that will allow a training opportunity for each of these graduates, and those U.S. citizens who are getting their medical education abroad, with a few slots left over. This move, coupled with the pressure to reduce the number of physicians in non-primary care training programs and increase the number of primary care trainees (and reduce the reimbursement for physicians in training above the first certification level), points toward a realignment in the number and distribution of physicians in this country; an exercise which has been elusive to the policy makers for the past 50 years.

It is likely that there are few readers who haven't been involved in some sort of cost-reduction or reengineering program during the past few years; not only within the FPP and the medical school, but with our affiliated teaching hospitals. In the course of that effort, we may expect that many hospitals have revisited the costs which they are supporting relative to: the size and scope of their residency training programs; the presence of international medical graduates; and the amount of off-site ambulatory training which they are paying for. If, in the course of this examination, they find that they are assuming too great a burden (i.e. they are bearing more cost than they are being paid for by third parties), they may propose a cut in these programs or a shift of all or a portion of these unrecovered expenses back to the medical school. With limited flexible resources with which to assume these costs, the dean invariably turns to the FPP to assume these costs, if not on a long-term basis, at least until the size and scope of the programs can be reduced as new classes of trainees are made smaller and previously enrolled classes move through their training years.

The size of GME programs will decline as: hospital margins shrink; the federal government reduces Medicare reimbursements; state governments reduce Medicaid payments; and managed care plans refuse to pay any education costs. The market is increasing the rewards for primary care and decreasing payments for those in the procedure-driven specialties. This may realign student demand for graduate training opportunities in these disciplines. Certainly the absence of good employment opportunities following completion of four or more years of residency will be a factor as well in reshaping our GME programs.

Changes in federal rules concerning attending physician billing for patient care services when supervising residents will significantly impact FFP revenues (IL-372)

Within five years of the introduction of Medicare and Medicaid in the late 1960s, the federal government's regulatory arm noted its concern with what it perceived as "double dipping"; payment of resident salaries through Part A of the hospital cost-reimbursement formula and the billing of physician services by the attending (faculty) physician who was supervising residents in the care that they delivered as a part of their practical learning experience. Medicare and Medicaid was developed during a period when house staff (residents) were, in most cases treating a largely indigent population of patients under relatively "loose" supervision (the knowledgeable reader clearly understands this construct), and the attending staff often saw their private (i.e., paying) patients largely independent of the teaching experience. This had not been anticipated to be a problem since attending physicians previously weren't billing this teaching patient population previously; in fact, no one was billing for these patients. It quickly became apparent to some that the previously unreimbursed patient now had a source of payment and attending physicians became more involved in their care, to varying degrees. More significant, the business structures established at medical schools began to capture fee income for all patients. The result was that the Part B costs of Medicare and Medicaid grew at well above forecast levels.

Intermediary Letter-372 was sent by the Health Care Financing Administration (HCFA) to those intermediary organizations contracted to process reimbursement for the Medicare program. It offered guidance to the intermediary in what to look for in the form of documentation of services provided by the attending to justify submitting a Part B bill for services. In general, the expectation was that for a bill to be rendered, the attending would be involved in the care of the patient and present and/or available to directly care for the patient during the essential/critical part of the illness or treatment. Further, the attending would supervise the care delivered by the resident, either directly or in a time period immediately proximal to the event of care and would document that supervision by a note in the patient's chart and/or the counter signature of the resident's note in the chart.

Compliance by the intermediaries around the country was unevenly applied and specific regulations, while drafted, were never uniformly adopted. Government interest in this area peaked and waned several times during the 1970s and 80s, but definitive regulations were not adopted and applied by the intermediaries.

Therefore, it was with some surprise that the Office of Inspector General (OIG) emerged with such vigor during the fall of 1995 with its compliance audit findings at the University of Pennsylvania Medical School. In a settlement with the OIG, Penn made a payment of $30 million, representing $10 million in erroneous billings and false claims and $20 million in treble damages and penalties. Their Philadelphia neighbor, Jefferson Medical College, settled after a similar finding with the payment of $12 million. All medical schools have been put on notice by HCFA and the OIG that they will be audited. Virtually one-third have already received notice letters as of mid-1997 and the others are reacting as if their letter will arrive shortly.

The result has been stunning. Even in the absence of clear and definitive guidelines, schools are writing their own, often "worst case" scenarios and are training attending and resident physicians alike in the proper documentation of charts and when it is, and is not appropriate to render a bill for professional services. Schools have been invited to submit to PATH I or PATH II audits of past billing practices dating back to the period 1994 and 1995. (This period was well before the latest HCFA interest was apparent and still in the absence of clear and unambiguous regulations. Such regulations could reasonably be applied prospectively, but are seemingly unfair to apply retroactively. Nevertheless, they are being applied by the OIG.)*

PATH (Physicians at Teaching Hospitals) involves either a government audit (PATH I), or an audit initiated by the medical school, at its own expense, by a government-approved auditor (PATH II). It is implied that there will be degree of leniency extended by the government with respect to the penalty portion of the fine for those schools which initiate (and fund) their own audits and make full restitution.

---

*Note: In mid-July 1997 the Secretary suspended many of these audits when she was unable to find evidence that the Intermediary had provided unambiguous guidelines.

The dollars involved are huge - hundreds of millions of dollars! These are dollars that have been pulled from institutional and departmental reserves and, in some cases, from the reserves of the university. This has caused several universities, which previously were most worried about the solvency of their teaching hospitals, to give thought to whether they can afford to maintain their medical schools when this reality is coupled with the forecast of the impact managed care will have on future income. The direct and indirect (e.g., the time of physicians going through the required training) costs of training attending and resident staff is also enormous. Maybe the greatest long-term impact is the likely reduction in billing income when the new standards for determining a billable event are applied; some schools are seeing their Medicare Part B billings drop by 20-30 percent!

Whether fair or not, this has been the event that may define practice plan activity during the 1996-98 timeframe.

Both Houses of Congress and the Executive Branch agreed in late July 1997 on a plan for a balanced federal budget before the end of the decade. The Medicare and Medicaid programs are a major target for cost cutting. They are now talking about changing the eligibility criteria and premium costs for seniors who participate in the program; and seniors vote! They will do something in this area but they will come down hard on what they define as fraud and abuse in the programs. They will reduce the federal share of the Medicaid program (don't expect the states to make up the loss); and will cut hospital and professional fee payments (or at least not increase payment levels by much, especially in the procedure-driven specialties, for several years).

Let's not try to forecast how long this initiative will last or how big the paybacks the PATH audits will be. Suffice it to say that Penn's payment will probably not be the largest, and that the ultimate number will have a measurable impact on our medical schools. Most important, this "lesson" is likely to drive changes that might not otherwise have occurred in: the size and scope of our training programs; the size of our faculties (and how they spend their time); faculty compensation levels; and, possibly, the very continued existence of some medical schools.

Managed care will continue to impact academic medical centers, teaching hospitals and faculty practice plans

There was a time when FPPs measured their involvement in managed care by the number of contracts they had signed, and the number of "lives" covered by those contracts. The well-managed plan today looks at the net economic impact of those contracts, and the number of patients steered to them for care. Too often we have found that our reputation for quality and access to the latest in technology was being used by the managed care plans to market their product. However, when it came to sending us patients, they steered them to lower-cost community providers. In the future, FPPs will assume a share of the risk and will actively participate in the development of guidelines and pathways (clinical protocols for care) that may prescribe care by a lower-cost community provider in the academic medical center's network when the appropriate level of service quality can be delivered in that setting. This is part of the change in mindset. Now you can be paid more for what you don't do than for what you do do!

We can expect to see a slower rate of growth in managed care penetration in many markets as the public's sentiment concerning access to new therapies and technologies offered at academic medical centers is expressed through state and federal mandates to make such care available to covered populations. There will, however, be an increase in the number of at-risk contracts assumed by FPPs as they compete for market share with their community provider group practices.

For-profit hospital corporations may have a greater impact on faculty practice plans

One of the predecessor hospital corporations to Tenet (NME) constructed the University of Southern California's private patient hospital on their campus more than 10 years ago. There has been a flurry of activity by Columbia/HCA in their effort to acquire university-owned or affiliated hospitals as a part of its strategy to have a high profile presence in every major metropolitan market in the country. Its strategy seems to include the acquisition of these tertiary/quaternary facilities as a regional source of care for the seriously ill patient needing referral within its network of health care providers. Its majority ownership of Tulane Medical Center hospital and the Medical University of South Carolina Medical Center hospital are but two examples. Columbia/HCA was unsuccessful in its bid for other hospitals, such as the Medical College of Virginia Hospitals, and it lost the contract originally signed by Humana for the long-term management of the University of Louisville Hospital.

The impact of teaching hospital ownership by for-profits on their affiliated medical schools and their FPPs is considerable. As they try to stretch more margin from their clinical delivery systems, they will expect more performance of the medical staff. They are likely to tolerate uncompensated care less; and they may be less willing to assume the unreimbursed marginal cost for graduate and undergraduate medical education.

On the other hand, the hospital corporation-sponsored physician groups are under intense scrutiny as I write this chapter. Columbia/HCA is being taken to task in Texas and Florida for some of its physician recruitment tactics and in late July 1997 its two top officers resigned. This, coupled with the rejection it has felt in several venues where it has tried to acquire hospitals will impact its growth plans. The government raids on its offices, as part of the fraud and abuse investigations, will also hinder Columbia/HCA's ability to build a larger system.

While I would not begin to underestimate the power of these corporations, it would appear that their ability to continue to grow the value of their stock is largely dependent upon their continued acquisition of hospitals and other provider groups. There are a finite number of acquisitions out there so I would forecast that we will see a major change in the size, composition and direction of the major for-profit hospital groups in the early part of the next century (possibly sooner based on the events in late July 1997).

This is a difficult area to predict as the motives and methods which drive these for-profit hospital corporations are likely to shift with changes in leadership and ownership. We can expect that there may be more consolidation in this field. We may see a closer alignment with the physician management corporations, and we may, by necessity, find our faculty practicing in teaching hospitals run from Nashville or Santa Barbara.

We will see more faculty working in community-based practice sites

We have seen FFPs reach out into the community with ambulatory delivery sites more distant from the primary site. FPPs and their affiliated hospitals have purchased the practices of community doctors and have created clinical sites and placed a mix of more senior faculty and recent trainees at locations more convenient to their patients; principally their paying patients. Few have done this as aggressively or as successfully as the University of Pennsylvania Health System, which has acquired more than 200 physician practices stretching throughout eastern Pennsylvania as well as into southern New Jersey. Partners Healthcare System, made up of the Massachusetts General Hospital and the Brigham and Women's Hospitals, the Johns Hopkins Health System, and the University of Michigan Health System are among others similarly engaged in developing a community presence throughout their respective primary service areas.

We can expect to see a greater amount of academic medical center presence in the community, at sites remote from the principal academic medical center. This will take several forms, including the integration of physicians who were previously in community-based practices as well as the placement of academic physicians at these and other free-standing sites. Academic physicians may rotate to these sites on a periodic basis, or may maintain office hours for a portion of the work week. They may have hospital privileges at the local community hospital, which will likely be a part of the academic medical center network. Services will be delivered in the lowest cost, most appropriate setting as all elements of the integrated delivery system participate in the economic risk associated with the care of the patient.

Community practitioners will aggregate into corporately owned and managed groups

We have seen a dramatic rise in the number of community physicians whose practices are owned and managed by large corporations. While five years ago we envisioned that most physicians would be practicing in groups rather than as solo practitioners, few would have envisioned the degree and speed with which these independent corporations have developed. The stunning increase in size of some of these well-run primary care and multispecialty groups, such as MedPartners and Phycor, is a trend we can expect to see continue through this decade.

As I prepare this chapter I am aware of several departmentally-based faculty practice plans which have been approached by one or more of these for-profit companies interested in developing management/ownership contracts. We may see some of these agreements signed, especially in the higher-earning specialty areas.

Faculty groups will leave the fold and go into private practice; affiliate back for teaching

We are seeing some cases where faculty groups are leaving their medical schools and setting up independent practice corporations outside the fold. These are usually the high-earning (it used to be that they earned even more, thus their motivation for leaving) specialties such as cardio-thoracic surgery, orthopedics, plastic, neurosurgery and such. They often find a willing and moneyed supporter in the local for-profit (or not-for-profit) hospital which provides the latest in operating suite equipment and a supportive environment for inpatient and sometimes outpatient care. In many cases, the move is so sudden and the market so saturated that the medical school has few options when it comes to countering with a plan to rapidly replace these faculty. One alternative is to accept the fact that this group is now operating independent of the medical school and will contract with them to teach students and residents. In other cases, the future of the impacted training programs may be in doubt, given the pressure to reduce the number of trainees in these disciplines.

In fact, as I write this chapter the following appeared in our local paper:

"Surgeons Transplant Practice to Suburbs"

Houston Chronicle, July 12, 1997

"The departure of seven top heart surgeons from the Baylor College of Medicine shows how suburban hospitals are challenging the primacy of the Texas Medical Center elite institutions." So began the lead article in the business section of this paper. It continued, "The group...was formed as a response to increasing numbers of managed health care contracts that direct patients to suburban hospitals....Managed care plans want doctors to care for their patients in the most cost-effective setting.... the services of the skilled surgeons give suburban hospitals a way to compete with the renowned heart surgery programs at Baylor and the Texas Heart Institute....said ... the chief executive officer at Columbia Clear Lake Regional Medical Center (a 400 bed community hospital)...we were always struggling with enough volume."

The article went on, "Most of Houston's heart surgeons were trained by [Dr. Michael] DeBakey or Dr. Denton Cooley...[the head of the practice said that]...he and his colleagues hope to serve as volunteers on

Baylor's faculty...The heart surgeons decided to leave Baylor's faculty because they could not reconcile their vision of a citywide cardiovascular group with Baylor's vision of a multispecialty group offering a wider range of services. According to the head of Baylor's practice plan, Baylor tries to accommodate faculty members' managed care contracting needs...when faculty members leave,...the reasons are more likely to concern independence and how the money from patient care is divided among professors." The head of the new group said, "...they can maintain the standard of care set at Baylor in other hospitals...this is exportable...we are proud to take it out into the community where the patients and the insurers want us to be."

We will see shifts of high-earning specialty faculty physicians to the private sector with contracts with the medical school and teaching hospital for the supervision of residents and fellows to a greater degree in the future. However, more creative means of distributing earnings based on productivity will make it possible for medical schools to retain some of these high earners. We may see more departmental plans contract with physician practice management (PPMs) companies like MedPartners or Phycor, if they are not forced into a school-wide centralized or multispecialty plan. It is unlikely that we will see any of the school-wide plans contract for these services during this period.

Academic medical centers will develop/advance more women and people of color into leadership roles

For most of our nation's history candidates for admission to medical school (excepting the traditionally African-America medical schools) were drawn predominantly from a segment representing less than 50 percent of the available talent pool - the pool of white males. Only during the past quarter century has there been a concerted effort by most medical schools to increase the enrollment of women and people of color. The increase in representation has been dramatic, but the current position does not yet represent the public's mandate nor academe's objectives for success. The goal least well met involves the presence of people of color in our medical school classes.

However, today there are far more women who have completed their medical training and are now advancing in rank as members of the faculty of medical schools. The Association of American Medical Colleges (AAMC), in cooperation with the Allegheny University of the Health Sciences, has developed and delivered a program for the development of women as medical school leaders. The Executive

Leadership in Academic Medicine (ELAM) program is designed to take early and mid-career women and give them an intense learning experience over an 18-month period. The second class of graduates completed the program in April 1997. The program is still in its pilot period, but is likely to be continued for at least the next several years. Each class has about 25 students and a new group commences study each September. This is a small but significant attempt to give women the tools and confidence necessary to assume leadership positions in academic medicine.

During the next ten years we can expect to see many more women assume chairs and deanships in medical schools, and executive leadership positions in academic medical centers. Programs such as ELAM will make opportunities available for women of color, but no similar program yet exists for men. Increases in the number of people of color who assume leadership positions in academic medical centers will occur, but at a far lesser rate than women during this period.

We will see more physicians in leadership roles traditionally held by non-physicians

Throughout the 1970s and 80s, and to the present, we have seen the emergence of the professionally trained medical school administrator serving in various capacities and with various titles: department administrator, practice plan director, associate dean for administration, etc. Generally these positions have been filled by individuals with master's level degrees in business administration, health care or hospital administration, or public health. This is not to imply that there are not many capable, excellent individuals in these positions who are trained at the bachelor's level with years of experience and excellent track records. But the model of those who will enter the field today is more akin to the first group than the second.

Today, however, we find an increasing interest in the administration and management of medical school programs by physicians. We are not talking about those who are necessarily in the traditional development track for department chair, but rather those who have consciously decided that they want to manage departmental budgets, faculty practice plans and clinics previously the domain of the professional administrator.

Their motivations may be many, but probably include:

1. The opportunity to advance in the academic ranks may not be as great today as it was when they entered academic practice;

2. They may not enjoy the personal delivery of patient care as much now as they did, or thought they would, what with increased regulation, documentation, etc.;

3. The income potential of a top level medical school administrator may be far greater than that of an assistant or associate professor in one of the non-surgical disciplines;

4. The stature and prestige (i.e., perceived power) of the medical school administrator has risen in recent years and thus is attractive to the physician who seeks that level of recognition.

Regardless of the motivation, we are seeing a surge in interest by physicians from within academe, as well as from the private sector, in Executive MBA degree programs, and accelerated training programs leading to knowledge and skill development as well as credentialing in business.

We can expect this trend to continue. We may expect to see more MD/MBAs in roles previously filled by the non-physician; maybe even CFOs of our major medical centers. We already are seeing several physicians in hospital COO roles, not previously within their purview! This, coupled with the consolidation of institutions through mergers, acquisitions and affiliations occurring in the field, may make for fewer opportunities for the non-physician seeking senior roles in medical school and academic hospital administration.

To the extent that some of these well-prepared physicians will achieve appointments as department chairs, medical schools will certainly benefit from their stronger skill set. These dual-trained individuals will be even more effective when paired with someone to whom they can delegate day-to-day responsibility for non-clinical/non-academic administrative duties; whether the delegate be an MD/MBA or MBA.

There will still be a role for the professionally trained and experienced administrator. One role may be that of coach; the person who quietly helps the physician (those with or without business credentials) perform effectively in their administrative role. With more physicians entering the ranks of administration (often without the opportunity to develop their administrative, management and leadership capabilities by moving through the ranks, let alone their toolbox of business, finance and human resource skills), the physician's professional coach may fill an important role in improving the effectiveness of the current and next generation of medical school leaders.

Conclusion

The next five years will be one of rapid change. As we move into the next century, we as individuals will be challenged to a greater degree and in different ways than ever before.

The future will be filled with interesting times. May we all live through it, and live through it well.